Immunisation against infectious disease

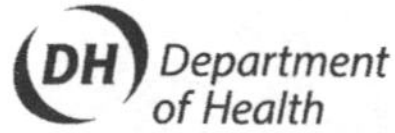

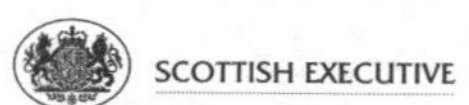

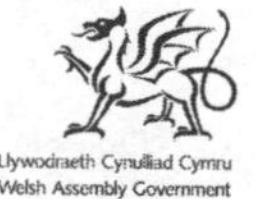

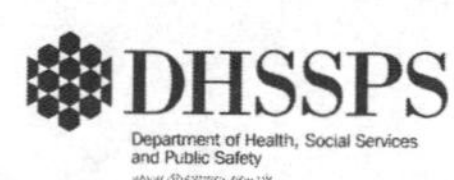

Immunisation against infectious disease

Edited by

Dr David Salisbury CB FRCP FRCPCH FFPHM

Director of Immunisation
Department of Health

Dr Mary Ramsay BSc MB BS MRCP MSc MFPHM FFPHM

Consultant Epidemiologist
Health Protection Agency

and

Dr Karen Noakes BSc PhD

Principal Scientist
Immunisation
Department of Health

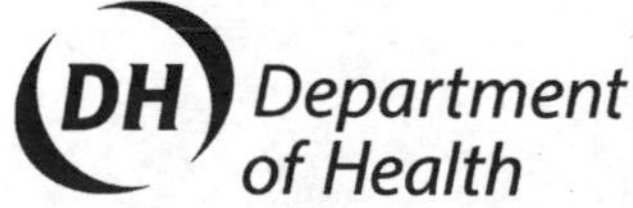

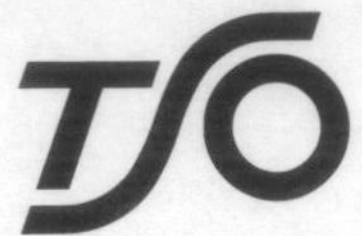

Published by TSO (The Stationery Office) and available from:

Online
www.tsoshop.co.uk

Mail, Telephone, Fax and E-mail
TSO
PO Box 29, Norwich, NR3 1GN
Telephone orders/General enquiries: 0870 600 5522
Fax orders: 0870 600 5533
E-mail: customer.services@tso.co.uk
Textphone: 0870 240 3701

TSO Shops
123 Kingsway, London, WC2B 6PQ
020 7242 6393 Fax 020 7242 6394
16 Arthur Street, Belfast BT1 4GD
028 9023 8451 Fax 028 9023 5401
71 Lothian Road, Edinburgh EH3 9AZ
0870 606 5566 Fax 0870 606 5588

TSO@Blackwell and other Accredited Agents

Published by The Stationery Office under licence from the Department of Health

Department of Health
Wellington House
133–155 Waterloo Road
London SE1 8UG

First edition 1992
Second edition 1996
Third edition 2006

ISBN-10 0-11-322528-8
ISBN-13 978-0-11-322528-6

Printed in Great Britain by The Stationery Office

N5456496 C1950 11/06

Contents

Acknowledgements

Producing a volume as complex, comprehensive and wide-ranging as this required a huge team effort from many staff at the Department of Health and the Health Protection Agency in particular. First, we would like to thank all those staff who re-drafted the chapters and the individual specialists who contributed their expertise in technical areas. Second, we must thank the members of the Joint Committee on Vaccination and Immunisation who made constructive comments on the drafts and, third, we must give special thanks to those individuals who drew the drafts together into a meaningful whole. These include Judith Moreton, Joanne Yarwood, Dr Dorian Kennedy, Dr Arlene Reynolds, and Chris Owen.

STOP PRESS

Just prior to publication, the World Health Organization published a paper entitled *Temperature sensitivity of vaccines*. See page 23 for more information.

NOTE

This edition reflects policy current at the time of going to press – November 2006
Updates are available at www.dh.gov.uk/greenbook.

Preface

The immunisation programme in the UK continues to evolve, meeting the demand to improve the control of infectious diseases through vaccination. Since the last edition of *Immunisation against infectious disease* (the Green Book), the immunisation programme has seen a number of changes, to both the vaccination schedule and to peoples' attitudes to vaccination. New vaccines have been introduced against meningococcal group C and pneumococcal infections which are the cause of serious diseases. At the same time, as the epidemiology of some diseases changes, certain vaccination schedules have been altered: the school's BCG programme has stopped and a more targeted approach to BCG vaccination has been adopted. Other changes to the immunisation schedule, such as the introduction of a Hib/MenC booster at 12 months of age and the reduction of MenC doses given as a primary course, reflect the importance of diligent surveillance and clinical trials to study the most effective way to use vaccines in the UK schedule.

The Joint Committee on Vaccination and Immunisation (JCVI) continues to play a pivotal role in advising the UK's Health Departments, providing independent scientific advice for the whole programme. JCVI meets three times a year and comprises experts from many areas of medicine and clinical practice especially related to immunisation. The members are independent of government, work to the highest international standards as recognised by the World Health Organization and publish their recommendations and advice, together with those of the various sub-committees, on the Department of Health website.

The objectives of the national immunisation programme include providing clear, evidence-based communications that meet the needs of parents and health professionals, and ensuring that those working in primary care are provided with the support required to implement vaccination programmes effectively.

Following the ill-founded MMR scare, it has become even more important for those working in the field to be able to communicate to parents the benefits of vaccination, the known side effects of vaccines and the safety and efficacy of vaccines to allay fears.

I look forward to the exciting work that lies ahead in developing an immunisation programme that offers safe and effective protection for our children and families both today and in the future.

Andrew J Hall
Chairman, Joint Committee on Vaccination and Immunisation

Part 1

Principles, practices and procedures

1

Immunity and how vaccines work

Introduction

Immunity is the ability of the human body to protect itself from infectious disease. The defence mechanisms of the body are complex and include innate (non-specific, non-adaptive) mechanisms and acquired (specific, adaptive) systems.

Innate or non-specific immunity is present from birth and includes physical barriers (e.g. intact skin and mucous membranes), chemical barriers (e.g. gastric acid, digestive enzymes and bacteriostatic fatty acids of the skin), phagocytic cells and the complement system.

Acquired immunity is generally specific to a single organism or to a group of closely related organisms. There are two basic mechanisms for acquiring immunity – active and passive.

Active immunity

Active immunity is protection that is produced by an individual's own immune system and is usually long-lasting. Such immunity generally involves cellular responses, serum antibodies or a combination acting against one or more antigens on the infecting organism. Active immunity can be acquired by natural disease or by vaccination. Vaccines generally provide immunity similar to that provided by the natural infection, but without the risk from the disease or its complications. Active immunity can be divided into antibody-mediated and cell-mediated components.

Antibody-mediated immunity

Antibody-mediated responses are produced by B lymphocytes (or B cells), and their direct descendants, known as plasma cells. When a B cell encounters an antigen that it recognises, the B cell is stimulated to proliferate and produce large numbers of lymphocytes secreting an antibody to this antigen. Replication and differentiation of B cells into plasma cells is regulated by contact with the antigen and by interactions with T cells (a type of lymphocyte), macrophages and complement. The antibody provides immunity against infection in a variety of ways. These ways include neutralising toxins, blocking adhesion and cell entry by organisms, neutralising and preventing viral replication or complement-mediated killing.

Cell-mediated immunity

Cell-mediated immunity is controlled by a subset of lymphocytes called T lymphocytes or T cells. T cells mediate three principal functions: help, suppression and cytotoxicity. T-helper cells stimulate the immune response of other cells (i.e. T cells stimulate B cells to produce antibodies). T-suppressor cells play an inhibitory role and control the level and quality of the immune response. Cytotoxic T cells recognise and destroy infected cells and activate phagocytes to destroy pathogens they have taken up.

These two components of specific immunity are closely related to each other, and T cells interact with B cells in the production of antibodies against most antigens. Specific antibodies and cell-mediated responses are induced for all infections, but the magnitude and quality of these two components vary in different infections.

Passive immunity

Passive immunity is protection provided from the transfer of antibodies from immune individuals, most commonly across the placenta or less often from the transfusion of blood or blood products including immunoglobulin. Protection provided by the cross-placental transfer of antibodies from mother to child is more effective against some infections (e.g. tetanus and measles) than for others (e.g. polio and whooping cough). This protection is temporary – commonly for only a few weeks or months.

How vaccines work

Vaccines produce their protective effect by inducing active immunity and providing immunological memory. Immunological memory enables the immune system to recognise and respond rapidly to exposure to natural infection at a later date and thus to prevent or modify the disease. Antibodies can be detected in blood or serum, but, even in the absence of detectable antibodies, immunological memory may still be present. Cell-mediated responses to some vaccines (e.g. BCG, see Chapter 32) may be detectable by skin testing but do not necessarily indicate protection.

Vaccines can be made from inactivated (killed) or attenuated live organisms, secreted products, recombinant components or the constituents of cell walls.

Vaccines such as pertussis and inactivated poliomyelitis virus (IPV) contain inactivated bacteria or viruses. Other vaccines contain only the antigens that are important for protection. For example, tetanus and diphtheria vaccines contain inactivated toxins (toxoids), influenza vaccine contains a surface protein called haemagglutinin, and pneumococcal vaccine contains the polysaccharide from the capsule. Live attenuated vaccines include yellow fever; measles, mumps and rubella (MMR); and BCG.

From birth and in early infancy and childhood, humans are exposed to countless numbers of foreign antigens and infectious agents in the everyday environment. Responding to these stimuli helps the immune system to develop and mature. Compared with exposure in the natural environment, vaccines provide specific stimulation to a small number of antigens. Responding to these specific antigens uses only a tiny proportion of the capacity of an infant's immune system (Offit *et al.*, 2002). If an infant's immune system could be exhausted by multiple vaccines, one would expect vaccinated children to be at a higher risk of serious infections. Studies to investigate whether vaccines increase susceptibility to serious infections have shown no evidence of such an effect, with infection rates generally being lower in vaccinated children (Hviid *et al.*, 2005, Miller *et al.*, 2003).

Inactivated vaccines

A first injection of an inactivated vaccine or toxoid in an individual without prior exposure to the antigen produces a primary antibody response. This response is dominated by IgM antibody initially, followed by IgG antibody. Two or more injections may be needed to elicit such a response in young infants. This is usually called the primary course. Depending on the potency of the product and the time interval, further injections will lead to an accelerated response dominated by IgG – the secondary response. Following a primary course of vaccination, antibodies may persist for months or years. Even if the level of detectable antibody subsequently falls, the immune system has been primed and an individual may be protected. Further reinforcing doses of vaccine are used to boost immunity and to provide longer-term protection. Inactivated vaccines cannot cause the disease that they are designed to prevent.

Plain polysaccharide antigens do not stimulate the immune system as broadly as protein antigens such as tetanus, diphtheria or influenza. Therefore, protection from such vaccines is not long-lasting and response in infants and young children is poor. Some polysaccharide vaccines have been enhanced by conjugation – where the polysaccharide antigen is attached to a protein carrier (e.g. Hib and MenC vaccines). This enables the immune system to respond more broadly to the antigen to provide immunological memory, even in young children. Some inactivated vaccines contain adjuvants, substances that enhance the antibody response. Most combination vaccines contain adjuvants such as aluminium phosphate or aluminium hydroxide.

Live vaccines

Live attenuated virus vaccines, such as MMR, usually promote a full, long-lasting antibody response after one or two doses. To produce an immune response, the live organism must replicate (grow) in the vaccinated individual over a period of time (days or weeks). The immune system responds in the same way as it does to natural infection. It usually does this without causing the disease itself (because the vaccine virus is weakened or 'attenuated') but, for some vaccines, a mild form of the disease may rarely occur (e.g. a rash following measles-containing vaccines).

Vaccine failure

No vaccine offers 100% protection and a small proportion of individuals get infected despite vaccination. Vaccines can fail in two main ways – known as primary or secondary vaccine failures. Primary failure occurs when an individual fails to make an initial immunological response to the vaccine. Infection can therefore occur at any point after vaccination. A good example of primary vaccine failure is the 5–10% of children who do not respond to the measles component of the first dose of MMR. The risk of measles in such children is reduced by offering an additional dose of vaccine, usually before school entry.

Secondary failure occurs when an individual responds initially but then protection wanes over time. The incidence of secondary vaccine failure therefore increases with time. Individuals who acquire infection despite vaccination may have a modified, milder form of disease and are less likely to suffer serious complications than those who have never been vaccinated. An example of secondary vaccine failure is pertussis vaccine, when protection against whooping cough after three doses is initially high but declines as a child gets older. A fourth (booster) dose is given to improve protection during the school years.

Population immunity

The primary aim of vaccination is to protect the individual who receives the vaccine. Vaccinated individuals are also less likely to be a source of infection to others. This reduces the risk of unvaccinated individuals being exposed to infection. This means that individuals who cannot be vaccinated will still benefit from the routine vaccination programme. This concept is called population (or 'herd') immunity. For example, babies below the age of two months, who are too young to be immunised, are at greatest risk of dying if they catch whooping cough. Such babies are protected from whooping cough because older siblings and other children have been routinely immunised as part of the childhood programme.

When vaccine coverage is high enough to induce high levels of population immunity, infections may even be eliminated from the country, e.g. diphtheria. But if high vaccination coverage were not maintained, it would be possible for the disease to return. Vaccination against smallpox enabled the infection to be declared eradicated from the world in 1980. The World Health Organization (WHO) is currently working towards the global eradication of poliomyelitis.

Immunoglobulins

Passive immunity can be provided by the injection of human immunoglobulin which contains antibodies to the target infection and temporarily increases an individual's antibody level to that specific infection. Protection is afforded within a few days but may last only a few weeks.

Human normal immunoglobulin (HNIG) is derived from the pooled plasma of donors and contains antibodies to infectious agents that are currently prevalent in the general population. HNIG is used for the protection of immunocompromised children exposed to measles and of individuals after exposure to hepatitis A.

Specific immunoglobulins are available for tetanus, hepatitis B, rabies and varicella zoster. Each specific immunoglobulin contains antibodies against the target infection at a higher titre than that present in normal immunoglobulin. Specific immunoglobulins are obtained from the pooled blood of donors who:

- are convalescing from the target infectious disease, or
- have been recently immunised with the relevant vaccine, or
- are found on screening to have sufficiently high antibody titres.

Recommendations for the use of normal and specific immunoglobulins are given in the relevant chapters.

References

Hviid A, Wohlfahrt J, Stellfeld M and Melbye M (2005) Childhood vaccination and non-targeted infectious disease hospitalization. *JAMA* **294**(6): 699–705.

Miller E, Andrews N, Waight P and Taylor B (2003) Bacterial infections, immune overload, and MMR vaccine. Measles, mumps, and rubella. *Arch Dis Child* **88**(3): 222–3.

Offit PA, Quarlest J, Gerber MA *et al.* (2002) Addressing parents' concerns: Do multiple vaccines overwhelm or weaken the infant's immune system? *Pediatr* **109**(1): 124–9.

WHO (1993) *General immunology.* Module 1: The immunological basis for immunization series. www.who.int/vaccines-documents/DocsPDF-IBI-e/mod1-e.pdf.

2

Consent

Introduction

Consent must be obtained before starting any treatment or physical investigation or before providing personal care for a patient. This includes the administration of all vaccines. The guidance in this chapter is based both on the current legal position and the standards expected of health professionals by their regulatory bodies. Further legal developments may occur after this guidance has been issued and health professionals should remember their duty to keep themselves informed of any such developments that may have a bearing on their area of practice.

There is no legal requirement for consent to immunisation to be in writing and a signature on a consent form is not conclusive proof that consent has been given, but serves to record the decision and the discussions that have taken place with the patient or the person giving consent on a child's behalf.

The giving and obtaining of consent is viewed as a process, not a one-off event. Consent obtained before the occasion upon which a child is brought for immunisation is only an agreement for the child to be included in the immunisation programme and does not mean that consent is in place for each future immunisation. Consent should still be sought on the occasion of each immunisation visit.

Consent must be given voluntarily and freely. The individual must be informed about the process, benefits and risks of immunisation and be able to communicate their decision. Information given should be relevant to the individual patient, properly explained and questions should be answered fully.

Consent remains valid unless the individual who gave it withdraws it. If there is new information between the time consent was given and when the immunisation is offered, it may be necessary to inform the patient and for them to re-confirm their consent. This includes new evidence of risk, new immunisations (e.g. pneumococcal vaccine) becoming available or where there is a significant change in the individual's condition, such as treatment for cancer.

Advice on consent which is specific to Wales, Scotland and Northern Ireland is available or in preparation. Please refer to the end of this chapter for further details.

What information should be provided?

Individuals, or those giving consent on their behalf, must be given enough information to enable them to make a decision before they can give consent. This should include information about the process, benefits and risks of the immunisation(s).

The four UK countries provide a wide range of information, including leaflets, posters, videos, information packs, factsheets, and websites to support all aspects of the immunisation programme. This information is based on the current scientific evidence and clinical advice and will have been tested on relevant population groups.

Written or verbal information should be available in a form that can be easily understood by the individual who will be giving the consent. Where English is not the first language, translations and properly recognised interpreters should be used.

Consent is valid if the individual, or person providing consent, is offered as much information as they reasonably need to make their decision, and in a form that they can understand. Case law on this area is evolving – more detail can be found at www.dh.gov.uk/consent

Health professionals should ensure that the individual (or those giving consent on their behalf) fully understands which immunisation(s) are to be administered; the disease(s) against which they will protect; the risks of not proceeding; the side effects that may occur and how these should be dealt with; and any follow-up action required.

In line with current data protection and Caldicott guidance, individuals should also be informed about how data on immunisation will be stored, who will be able to access that information and how that data may be used. It is important to emphasise that such information is used to monitor the safety and efficacy of the current vaccination programmes.

How should consent be sought?

The health professional providing the immunisation should ensure that consent is in place.

It is good practice to check that the person still consents to your providing each immunisation before it is given.

The Nursing and Midwifery Council's Code of Professional Conduct: standards for conduct, performance and ethics paragraph 1.3 (NMC, 2004: www.nmc-uk.org/aFrameDisplay.aspx?DocumentID=201 states that 'You are personally accountable for your practice. This means that you are answerable for your actions and omissions, regardless of advice or directions from another professional.' Giving an immunisation without consent could leave the health professional vulnerable to legal action and action by their regulatory body.

Who can give consent?

Adults

Adults are those aged 18 or over. An adult must consent to their own treatment. Under English law, no one is able to give consent on behalf of an adult unable to give consent for examination or treatment him or herself. The Mental Capacity Act 2005 is due to come into force in 2007 and sets out how treatment decisions should be made for people of 16 years of age or older who do not have the capacity to make such decisions (more information will be available at www.dh.gov.uk/consent).

If an adult has refused immunisation before losing the capacity to make a decision, this decision will be legally binding, provided that it remains valid and applicable to the circumstances. If an adult has not clearly refused the treatment before losing the capacity to make such a decision, you will be able to treat an adult who is unable to consent if the treatment would be in their best interests, e.g. in a nursing home situation where the risk of influenza could compromise the individual's health. This decision would be made by the patient's doctor in discussion with those close to the patient.

Immunisation of younger children

For young children not competent to give or withhold consent, such consent can be given by a person with parental responsibility, provided that person is capable of consenting to the immunisation in question and is able to communicate their decision. Where this person brings the child in response to an invitation for immunisation and, following an appropriate consultation, presents the child for that immunisation, these actions may be considered evidence of consent.

Who has parental responsibility?

The Children Act 1989 sets out who has parental responsibility for a child. Mothers automatically have parental responsibility for their children. A father also has parental responsibility if he was married to the mother when the child was born, or if he subsequently married her. An unmarried father may also acquire parental responsibility by:

- Parental Responsibility Order granted by the court
- Residence Order granted by the court. This will give the person with the residence order parental responsibility as well as those of the child's parents which have parental responsibility. More than one person can have parental responsibility in more than just this case. For example, two parents or the local authority and a parent where there is a care order.
- Parental Responsibility Agreement. This must be signed by both parents, their signatures witnessed by an Officer of the Court who is authorised to administer oaths, or a Magistrate or justices' clerk, or assistant to a justices' clerk, and the form sent to the Principal Registry of the Family Division (High Court) for registration after which it becomes effective.

Since 1 December 2003, an unmarried father who is the natural father of the child can also acquire parental responsibility if he is named as the father on the child's birth certificate. Unmarried fathers who are already on the child's birth certificate before 1 December 2003 will not automatically acquire parental responsibility, and would only acquire it by either later marrying the child's mother or signing a Parental Responsibility Agreement with the mother or getting a court order.

A step parent may acquire parental responsibility of a child where s/he is married to, or a civil partner of, the child's parent who has parental responsibility and either (i) there is a parental responsibility agreement to this effect or (ii) the court grants a parental responsibility order (see Section 4A of the Children Act 1989).

Routine immunisation in schools

Where immunisations are routinely offered in the school setting,* the situation differs depending on the age and competence of the individual child or young person. Information leaflets should be available for the child's own use and to share with their parents prior to the date that the immunisation is scheduled.

Young people aged 16 and 17 are presumed, in law, to be able to consent to their own medical treatment. Younger children who understand fully what is involved in the proposed procedure (referred to as 'Gillick competent') can also give consent, although ideally their parents will be involved.

If a person aged 16 or 17 or a Gillick-competent child consents to treatment, a parent cannot override that consent.

If the health professional giving the immunisation felt a child was not Gillick competent then the consent of someone with parental responsibility would be sought.

If a person aged 16 or 17 or a Gillick-competent child refuses treatment that refusal should be accepted. It is unlikely that a person with parental responsibility could overrule such a refusal. It is possible that the court might overrule a young person's refusal if an application to court is made under section 8 of the Children Act 1989 or the inherent jurisdiction of the High Court.

There is no requirement for consent to be in writing.

---

* Where a mass immunisation campaign is to be carried out in schools such as the MenC campaign 1999/2000, different guidance regarding information and consent would apply

Other issues

Although the consent of one person with parental responsibility for a child is usually sufficient (see Section 2(7) of the Children Act 1989), if one parent agrees to immunisation but the other disagrees, the immunisation should not be carried out unless both parents can agree to immunisation or there is a specific court approval that the immunisation is in the best interests of the child.

The person with parental responsibility does not necessarily need to be present at the time the immunisation is given. Although a person may not abdicate or transfer parental responsibility, they may arrange for some or all of it to be met by one or more persons acting on their behalf (Section 2(9) of the Children Act 1989).

There is no requirement for such arrangements to be made in writing. Children may be brought for immunisation by a person without parental responsibility, for example, a grandparent or childminder. Where a child is brought for immunisation by some one who does not have parental responsibility the health professional would need to be satisfied that:

- the person with parental responsibility has consented in advance to the immunisation (i.e. they received all the relevant information in advance and arranged for the other person to bring the child to the appointment) or
- the person with parental responsibility has arranged for this other person to provide the necessary consent (i.e. they asked the other person to take the child to the appointment, to consider any further information given by the health professional, and then to agree to immunisation if appropriate).

If there is any evidence that the person with parental responsibility:

- may not have agreed to the immunisation (e.g. the notes indicate that the parent(s) may have negative views on immunisation), or
- may not have agreed that the person bringing the child could give the necessary consent (e.g. suggestion of disagreements between the parents on medical matters) then the person with parental responsibility should be contacted for their consent. If there is disagreement between the people with parental responsibility for the child, then immunisation should not be carried out until their dispute is resolved.

A person giving consent on behalf of a child may change his or her mind and withdraw consent at any time. Where consent is either refused or withdrawn, this decision should be documented.

It is the duty of each healthcare professional to communicate effectively and share such knowledge and information with other members of the primary healthcare team.

Recording consent

Those who are capable of giving consent may do so in writing, orally or by co-operation. Completion of a consent form is not a legal requirement. A signature on a consent form does not itself prove that the consent is valid but it does serve to record the decision that was reached, and the discussions that have taken place. The Bristol Royal Infirmary Inquiry Final Report (2001) (www.bristol-inquiry.org.uk/final%5Freport/report/sec2chap23%5F15.htm) reported that 'too great a regard is paid to the symbolic act of signing a piece of paper rather than to the real task ...which involves explaining what is to take place.'

It is important to ensure that the healthcare record for each child – Personal Child Health Record (PCHR) and GP record (either paper or computer) is an accurate account of care planning and delivery. It is good practice for proper records of any discussions to be recorded in the PCHR and completed with the involvement of the parent or guardian.

Professional liability

Doctors and other health professionals involved in the administration of immunisation are usually not negligent if acting within their competencies and within practice that conforms to that of a responsible body of medical opinion held by practitioners skilled in the field in question (see, for example, Sidaway v Board of Governors Bethlem Royal Hospital (1985) AC 871; Bolam v Friern Hospital Management Committee (1957) 2 All ER 118). However, the courts are willing to be critical of a 'responsible body' of medical opinion and will be the final arbiters of what constitutes responsible practice.

This summary cannot cover all situations. For more detail, consult www.dh.gov.uk/consent

Scotland

There are some important differences between England and Scotland, particularly when dealing with mental health, children or adults with incapacity. The Adults with Incapacity (Scotland) Act 2000 was introduced in stages, with Part 5, Medical Treatment and Research, coming into effect in July 2002. The Mental Health (Care and Treatment) (Scotland) Act 2003 came into effect in stages from March 2004 and is now largely in force, replacing the Mental Health (Scotland) Act 1984. Both Acts provide for delivering healthcare to people who lack the ability to make treatment decisions for themselves. Full details should be provided by the health professionals involved; however, further information is available from local health councils. The Age of Legal Capacity (Scotland) Act 1991 outlines that someone has the capacity to make decisions around consent from the age of 16. However, even under the age of 16, a young person can have the legal capacity to make a consent decision on a healthcare intervention, provided that they are capable of understanding its nature and possible consequences; this is a matter of clinical judgement.

Wales

The Welsh Assembly Government is working jointly with the Department of Health in developing updated guidance on patient consent to examination and treatment. It is expected that the new guidance will be published in both England and Wales around April 2007, to coincide with the Coming Into Force date of the Mental Capacity Act. Health professionals providing immunisation and vaccination services in Wales should refer to the guidance once published. In Wales, further information can be obtained at: www.wales.nhs.uk/sites3/page.cfm?orgid=465&pid=11930

Northern Ireland

Information regarding consent for immunisation can be found at:
www.dhsspsni.gov.uk/publichealth-immuno-guidance.pdf

Guidance on consent

Guidance for patients

The following information is available from the NHS Response Line (08701 555 455) and at: www.dh.gov.uk/consent

Consent: what you have a right to expect: a guide for adults
Consent: what you have a right to expect: a guide for children and young people
Consent: what you have a right to expect: a guide for people with learning disabilities
Consent: what you have a right to expect: a guide for parents
Consent: what you have a right to expect: a guide for relatives and carers
Reference guide to consent for examination or treatment

Guidance for clinicians

HSC 2001/023: Good practice in consent: achieving the NHS Plan commitment to patient-centred consent practice.

References

Department of Health (2001) *Seeking consent: working with children*. London: Department of Health. www.dh.gov.uk/assetRoot/04/06/72/04/04067204.pdf

Scottish Executive (2006) *A good practice guide on consent for health professionals in the NHS Scotland*. www.show.scot.nhs.uk/publicationsindex.htm

3

Storage, distribution and disposal of vaccines

Introduction

Vaccines are biological substances that may lose their effectiveness quickly if they become too hot or too cold at any time, especially during transport and storage. Vaccines naturally biodegrade over time, and storage outside of the recommended temperature range – including during transport and storage – may speed up loss of potency, which cannot be reversed. This may result in the failure of the vaccine to protect, as well as resulting in vaccine wastage.

It is essential that all those handling vaccines follow policies to ensure cold chain compliance. The guidance in this chapter should be used to define local policies, including Patient Group Directions (PGDs) (see Chapter 5), and should be read in conjunction with the individual Summaries of Product Characteristics (SPCs) that are supplied by the manufacturers of the vaccines.

The terms of marketing authorisations (product licences) cover storage requirements. Unless specific advice states otherwise, including manufacturer's stability data, vaccines that have not been properly distributed or stored are therefore no longer within the terms of the marketing authorisation and should not be used.

Policies and procedures in primary care and immunisation clinics

Primary care organisations in England and equivalent bodies in Wales, Scotland and Northern Ireland should ensure that local practice is in accordance with national policy, as outlined in this chapter, for the ordering, storage, stock control, distribution, transport and disposal of vaccines. Details of local contacts for professional advice should be provided.

Each practice, clinic or pharmacy should have one trained individual, with at least one trained deputy, responsible for the receipt and storage of vaccines and the recording of refrigerator temperatures. Regular audit (at least annually) should be undertaken. Any other staff who may be involved with vaccines must be trained appropriately.

The importance of the cold chain

The cold chain is standard practice for vaccines throughout the pharmaceutical industry (see Figure 3.1).

Maintaining the cold chain ensures that vaccines are transported and stored according to the manufacturer's recommended temperature range of +2°C to +8°C until the point of administration .

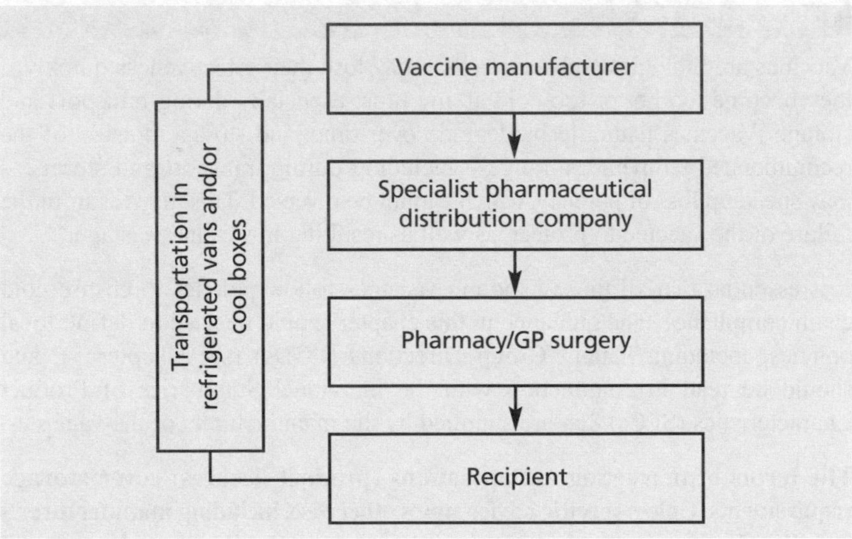

Figure 3.1 A typical cold chain system for vaccines

Storage

Vaccines should be stored in the original packaging at +2°C to +8°C and protected from light, as exposure to ultraviolet light will cause loss of potency. All vaccines are sensitive to some extent to heat and cold. Heat speeds up the decline in potency of most vaccines, thus reducing their shelf life. Effectiveness cannot be guaranteed for vaccines unless they have been stored at the correct temperature. Freezing may cause increased reactogenicity and loss of potency for some vaccines. It can also cause hairline cracks in the container, leading to contamination of the contents.

Ordering and monitoring of stock

Care must be taken in ordering vaccines, especially as certain vaccines are packaged in multiple quantities. Incorrect ordering can result in wastage and unnecessary costs to surgeries and the NHS.

Vaccine stocks should be monitored by the designated person(s) to avoid over-ordering or stockpiling.

Vaccines for the national childhood immunisation programme are ordered from a specialist pharmaceutical distribution company either through a dedicated website, by phone or by fax (in Scotland this is via vaccine holding centres in the health boards). Other childhood, adult and travel vaccines are ordered direct from the manufacturer or from the Health Protection Agency. Details of suppliers are shown throughout this book, at the end of each chapter.

Surgeries should have no more than two to four weeks' supply of vaccines at any time. This will be sufficient for routine provision. Best practice is to order small quantities on a regular, scheduled basis.

Excess stock may:

- increase the risk of vaccination with out-of-date vaccines
- increase wastage and the cost of disposal by incineration
- increase the dangers of over-packed refrigerators, leading to poor air flow, potential freezing and poor stock rotation
- delay the introduction of new vaccines until local supplies have been used
- increase the cost of replacement of stocks if the refrigerator fails
- increase the pressure on clinic refrigerators in periods of high demand, e.g. during the influenza vaccination season.

Vaccine stocks should be placed within the refrigerator so that those with shorter expiry dates are used first.

Any out-of-date stock should be labelled clearly, removed from the refrigerator and destroyed as soon as possible according to the local procedure.

Vaccines must never be used when past their expiry date.

Receipt of vaccines

On receipt of vaccines, staff must check them against the order for discrepancies and leakage or damage before signing for them. Pharmaceutical distributors and manufacturers will not accept any vaccine for return once it has left their control.

Vaccines must be refrigerated immediately on receipt and must not be left at room temperature.

Vaccine types, brands, quantities, batch numbers and expiry dates should be recorded with the date and time at which the vaccines were received.

The vaccine refrigerator

Specialised refrigerators are available for the storage of pharmaceutical products, and must be used for vaccines and diluents. Ordinary domestic refrigerators must not be used. Food, drink and clinical specimens must never be stored in the same refrigerator as vaccines. Opening of the refrigerator door should be kept to a minimum in order to maintain a constant temperature.

All vaccines are Prescription Only Medicines (POMs) and must be stored under locked conditions. Refrigerators must either be lockable or within a room that is locked when not occupied by a member of staff. Vaccines should never be left unattended at outlying clinics.

The accidental interruption of the electricity supply can be prevented by using a switchless socket or by placing cautionary notices on plugs and sockets.

Refrigerators should not be situated near a radiator or any other heat source that could affect their working, and should be appropriately ventilated.

Ice should not be allowed to build up within the refrigerator, as this reduces effectiveness. Records of regular servicing, defrosting and cleaning should be kept.

An approved cool box (with appropriate temperature monitoring – see p 21) or alternative refrigerator should be used to store vaccines during defrosting of the main refrigerator. Vaccines should only be replaced once the refrigerator has returned to the correct temperature after defrosting.

Refrigerator thermometers

The temperature within the vaccine refrigerator must be continually monitored with a maximum–minimum thermometer. This will identify when the temperature may have been outside the recommended range. Digital thermometers are the most reliable. More sophisticated temperature-recording devices are now available, including alarmed digital maximum–minimum thermometers.

Thermometers should be reset and replaced according to the manufacturer's guidance.

Temperatures in the refrigerator must be monitored and recorded at least once each working day, and documented on a chart for recording temperatures. An example can be found on p 24. The calibration of thermometers should be checked annually to ensure that they are working correctly. The records should be readily accessible for easy reference and retained until the next audit.

Refrigerator failure or disruption of the cold chain

Arrangements should be in place for back-up facilities to be available in the event of the refrigerator failing or breaking down.

Storage of vaccines

Vaccines must be kept in their original packaging when stored, so that they retain information on batch numbers and expiry dates. The packaging is also part of the protection against light and changes in temperature.

Vaccines must not be stored in the door, in the bottom drawers or adjacent to the freezer plate of the refrigerator. If there are temperature variations outside of the recommended +2°C to +8°C range, they usually occur in these parts of the refrigerator. Sufficient space should be allowed in the refrigerator so that air can circulate freely.

Patients or parents should not normally be asked to store vaccines. Exceptionally, patients may be asked to transport vaccines and/or immunoglobulins and to store them for short periods of time. Should this need arise, advice on appropriate storage should be given to the patient.

Packing and transporting of vaccines to outlying clinics

Domestic cool boxes should not be used to store, distribute or transport vaccines. Validated cool boxes (with maximum – minimum thermometers) and ice packs from a recognised medical supply company should be used. Individual manufacturers' instructions should be strictly adhered to.

Vaccines must be kept in the original packaging, wrapped in bubble wrap (or similar insulation material) and placed into a cool box with cool packs as recommended by the manufacturer's instructions. This will prevent direct contact between the vaccine and the cool packs and will protect the vaccine from any damage, such as being frozen.

Spillage

Locally written procedures should be used in conjunction with manufacturers' Control of Substances Hazardous to Health (COSHH) safety data sheets.

Spillages must be cleared up quickly; gloves should be worn. The spillage should be soaked up with paper towels, taking care to avoid skin puncture from glass or needles. The area should be cleaned according to the local chemical disinfection policy or COSHH safety data sheets. Gloves, towels, etc. should be sent for incineration.

Spillages on skin should be washed with soap and water. If a vaccine is splashed in the eyes, they should be washed with sterile 0.9% sodium chloride solution and medical advice should be sought.

Disposal of vaccines

There should be locally written procedures for the disposal of vaccines by incineration at a suitably authorised facility. These procedures must be followed.

All reconstituted vaccines and opened single and multi-dose vials must be used within the period recommended by the manufacturers or should be disposed of at the end of an immunisation session by sealing in a proper, puncture-resistant 'sharps' box (UN-approved, BS 7320).

The 'sharps' container should be replaced once it is two-thirds full and should not be accessible to any unauthorised individual.

Storage of immunoglobulins

Immunoglobulins should be protected from light and stored at +2˚C to +8˚C. Although these products have a tolerance to ambient temperatures (25˚C) of up to one week, they should be refrigerated immediately on receipt. They can be distributed in sturdy packaging outside the cold chain if needed. They should not be frozen.

Suppliers of refrigeration equipment and accessories

Advice on suppliers of refrigeration equipment and accessories, such as cool boxes, is available from:

Immunisation Policy, Monitoring and Surveillance
Department of Health
Area 512
Wellington House
133–155 Waterloo Road
London SE1 8UG

Tel: 020 7972 1227

Bibliography

World Health Organization (2006) *Temperature sensitivity of vaccines*. www.who.int/vaccines-documents/DocsPDF06/847.pdf.

This paper presents the WHO's latest recommendations on the storage of vaccines and maintenance of the cold chain.

A sample refrigerator temperature record chart

Name of health centre/GP practice/pharmacy:

....

The temperature should be between +2°C and +8°C. Check daily. If the temperature is outside the recommended range, take appropriate action as indicated in the written procedure.

Month	Current temperature	Minimum temperature	Maximum temperature	Checked by (signature)	Thermometer reset (tick)
Day 1					
Day ...					

Refrigerator defrosted and cleaned by: ....

Date: ....

4

Immunisation procedures

Introduction

Recommendations on immunisation procedures are based on currently available evidence and experience of best practice. In some circumstances, this advice may differ from that in vaccine manufacturers' Summaries of Product Characteristics (SPCs). When this occurs, the recommendations in this book (which are based on current expert advice received from the Joint Committee on Vaccination and Immunisation (JCVI)) should be followed. These Green Book recommendations and/or further advice in the Chief Medical Officer's (CMO's) letters and updates (www.dh.gov.uk/AboutUs/MinistersAndDepartmentLeaders/ChiefMedicalOfficer/fs/en) and/or in the NHS Purchasing and Supply Agency's vaccine update (www.pasa.nhs.uk/pharma/vaccines.stm) should be reflected in local protocols and Patient Group Directions (PGDs).

Doctors and nurses providing immunisations are professionally accountable for this work, as defined by their professional bodies. Nurses should follow the professional standards and guidelines as set out in *The Nursing and Midwifery Council code of professional conduct: standards for conduct, performance and ethics* and *Medicines management* (Nursing and Midwifery Council).

All healthcare professionals advising on immunisation or administering vaccines must have received specific training in immunisation, including the recognition and treatment of anaphylaxis. They should maintain and update their professional knowledge and skills through appropriate training.

More information is available in the Health Protection Agency's *National minimum standards for immunisation training 2005*.

Preparation of vaccines

The recommended storage conditions are described in Chapter 3.

Each vaccine should be reconstituted and drawn up when required in order to avoid errors and maintain vaccine efficacy and stability. Vaccines should not be drawn up in advance of an immunisation session.

The vaccine must be checked to ensure that the right product and correct dose is used in the appropriate way for each individual. Vaccines must not be used after their expiry date.

Before use, the colour and composition of the vaccine must be examined to ensure that it conforms to the description as stated in its SPC.

Different vaccines must not be mixed in the same syringe unless specifically licensed and recommended for such use.

Freeze-dried (lyophilised) vaccines must be reconstituted with the correct volume of diluent, and supplied and used within the recommended period after reconstitution, as stated in the product's SPC.

Unless supplied in a pre-filled syringe, the diluent should be drawn up using an appropriately sized syringe and 21G needle (green) and added slowly to the vaccine to avoid frothing.

Changing needles

Unless the vaccine is supplied in a pre-filled syringe with an integral needle, a new needle of a size appropriate to the individual patient should be used to inject the vaccine (see 'Choice of needle' on page 29).

Vaccine administration

Individuals giving vaccinations must have received training in the management of anaphylaxis, and must have immediate access to appropriate equipment. Adrenaline (epinephrine) must always be immediately available. Details on anaphylaxis are available in Chapter 8.

Before any vaccine is given, consent must be obtained (see Chapter 2) and suitability for immunisation must be established with the individual to be vaccinated, or their parent or carer.

Prior to administration

Vaccinators should ensure that:

- there are no contraindications to the vaccine(s) being given
- the vaccinee or carer is fully informed about the vaccine(s) to be given and understands the vaccination procedure
- the vaccinee or carer is aware of possible adverse reactions (ADRs) and how to treat them.

Route and site of administration

Injection technique, choice of needle length and gauge (diameter), and injection site are all important considerations, since these factors can affect both the immunogenicity of the vaccine and the risk of local reactions at the injection site, and are discussed in more detail below (pages 27–30).

Route of injection

Most vaccines should be given by intramuscular (IM) injection. Injections given intramuscularly, rather than deep subcutaneously, are less likely to cause local reactions (Diggle and Deeks, 2000; Mark *et al.*, 1999). Vaccines should not be given intravenously.

Vaccines not given by the IM route include Bacillus Calmette-Guérin (BCG) vaccine, which is given by intradermal injection, Japanese encephalitis and varicella vaccines, which are given by deep subcutaneous (SC) injection, and cholera vaccine, which is given by mouth.

For individuals with a bleeding disorder, vaccines normally given by an IM route should be given by deep subcutaneous injection to reduce the risk of bleeding.

Suitable sites for vaccination

The site should be chosen so that the injection avoids major nerves and blood vessels. The preferred sites for IM and SC immunisation are the anterolateral aspect of the thigh or the deltoid area of the upper arm (see Figure 4.1). The anterolateral aspect of the thigh is the preferred site for infants under one year old, because it provides a large muscle mass into which vaccines can be safely injected (see Figure 4.2). For BCG, the preferred site of injection is over the insertion of the left deltoid muscle; the tip of the shoulder must be avoided because of the increased risk of keloid formation at this site (see Figure 4.3).

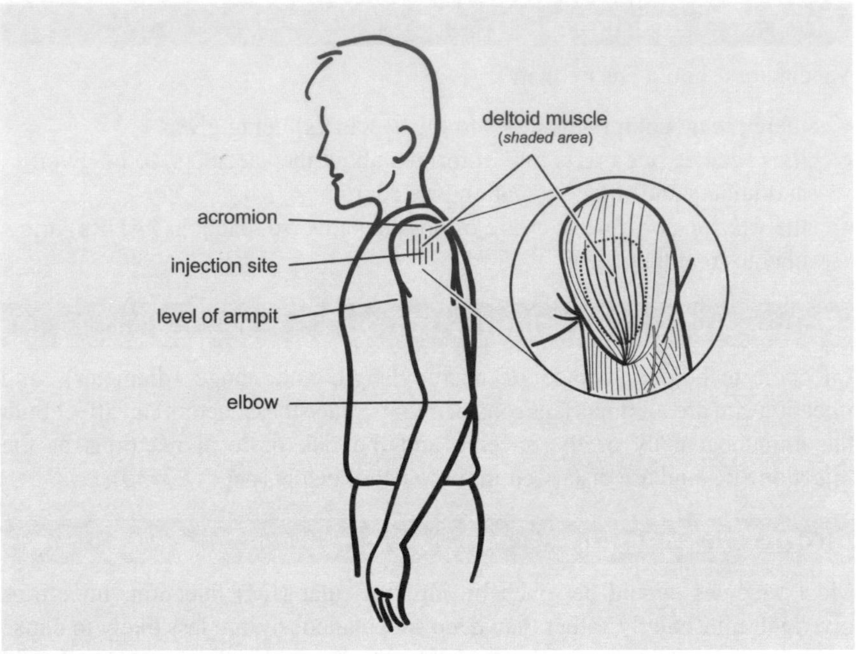

Figure 4.1 Preferred site for intramuscular and deep subcutaneous injections in older children and adults

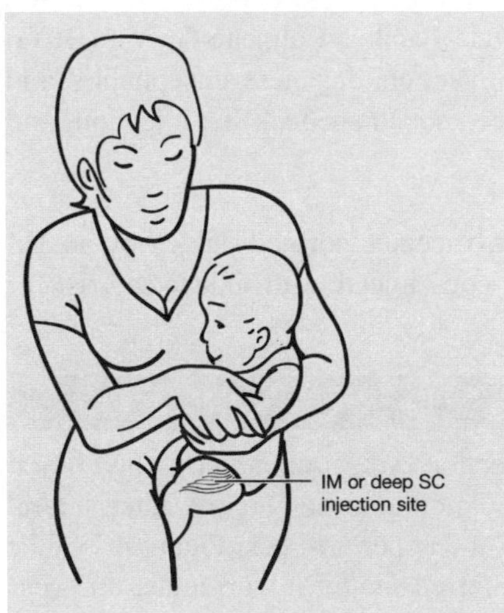

Figure 4.2 Preferred site for intramuscular and deep subcutaneous injections in infants under one year of age

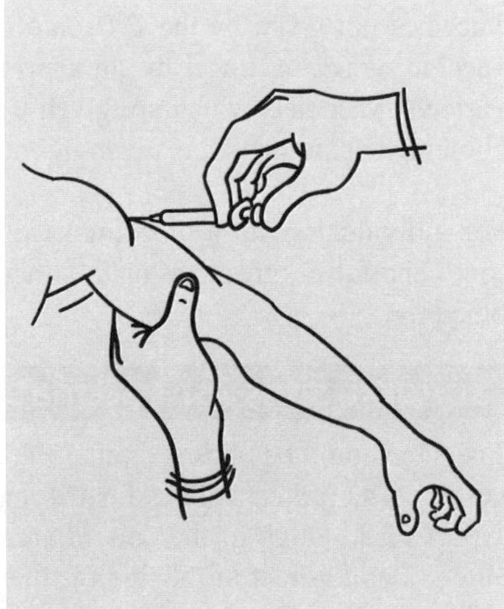

Figure 4.3 Preferred site for BCG injections in babies and adults

Where two or more injections need to be administered at the same time, they should be given at separate sites, preferably in a different limb. If more than one injection is to be given in the same limb, they should be administered at least 2.5cm apart (American Academy of Pediatrics, 2003). The site at which each injection is given should be noted in the individual's records.

Immunisations should not be given into the buttock, due to the risk of sciatic nerve damage (Villarejo and Pascaul, 1993; Pigot, 1988) and the possibility of injecting the vaccine into fat rather than muscle. Injection into fatty tissue of the buttock has been shown to reduce the immunogenicity of hepatitis B (Shaw *et al.*, 1989; Alves *et al.*, 2001) and rabies (Fishbein *et al.*, 1988) vaccines.

Suitable sites for immunoglobulin administration

When a large-volume injection is to be given, such as a preparation of immunoglobulin, this should be administered deep into a large muscle mass. If more than 3ml is to be given to young children and infants, or more than 5ml to older children and adults, the immunoglobulin should be divided into smaller amounts and given into different sites (American Academy of Pediatrics, 2003). The upper outer quadrant of the buttock can be used for immunoglobulin injection.

Rabies immunoglobulin should be infiltrated into the site of the wound (see Chapter 27).

Cleaning the skin

If the skin is clean, no further cleaning is necessary. Only visibly dirty skin needs to be washed with soap and water.

It is not necessary to disinfect the skin. Studies have shown that cleaning the skin with isopropyl alcohol reduces the bacterial count, but there is evidence that disinfecting makes no difference to the incidence of bacterial complications of injections (Del Mar *et al.*, 2001; Sutton *et al.*, 1999).

Choice of needle size

For IM and SC injections, the needle needs to be sufficiently long to ensure that the vaccine is injected into the muscle or deep into subcutaneous tissue. A 25mm needle is preferable and is suitable for all ages. Only in pre-term or very small infants is a 16mm needle suitable for IM injection. In adults, a longer length (e.g. 38mm) may be required, and anindividual assessment should be made (Zuckerman, 2000).

The width of the needle (gauge) may also need to be considered. For infants, a 23G (blue) or 25G (orange) needle should be used. For older babies, children and adults, a 23G needle is recommended. The wider bore may allow the vaccine to disperse over a larger area, thus reducing the risk of localised redness and swelling (Mayon White and Moreton, 1998).

Intradermal injections should only be administered using a 26G, 10mm (brown) needle.

Standard UK needle gauges and lengths*

Brown	26G	10mm (3/8") long
Orange	25G	16mm (5/8") long
		25mm (1") long
Blue	23G	25mm (1") long
Green	21G	38mm (1½") long

* *UK guidance on best practice in vaccine administration (2001)*

Injection technique

IM injections should be given with the needle at a 90º angle to the skin and the skin should be stretched, not bunched. Deep SC injections should be given with the needle at a 45º angle to the skin and the skin should be bunched, not stretched. It is not necessary to aspirate the syringe after the needle is introduced into the muscle (WHO, 2004; Plotkin and Orenstein, 2004).

The BCG technique is specialised and the person giving the BCG vaccine requires specific training and assessment. The skin should be stretched between the thumb and forefinger of one hand and the needle inserted with the bevel upwards for about 2mm into the superficial layers of the dermis, almost parallel with the surface. The needle should be visible beneath the surface of the skin (see Figure 4.4).

During an intradermal injection, considerable resistance is felt and a raised, blanched bleb showing the tips of the hair follicles is a sign that the injection has been correctly administered. A bleb of 7mm in diameter is approximately equivalent to 0.1ml and is a useful indication of the volume that has been injected. If no resistance is felt, the needle should be removed and reinserted before more vaccine is given.

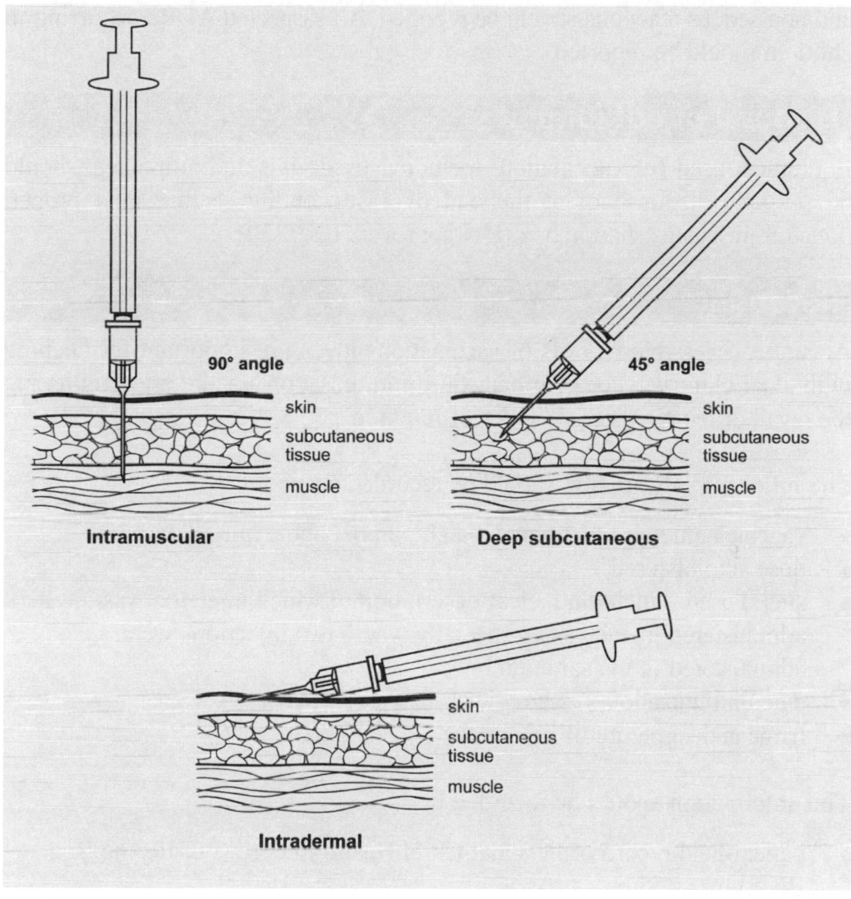

Figure 4.4 The three injection techniques

Post-vaccination

Recipients of any vaccine should be observed for immediate ADRs. There is no evidence to support the practice of keeping patients under longer observation in the surgery.

Advice on the management of ADRs can be found in Chapter 8.

Suspected ADRs to vaccines should be reported to the Commission on Human Medicines using the Yellow Card scheme (described in detail in Chapter 9). For established vaccines, only serious suspected ADRs should be reported. For newly licensed vaccines labelled with an inverted black triangle (▼), serious and non-serious reactions should be reported. All suspected ADRs occurring in children should be reported.

Disposal of equipment

Equipment used for vaccination, including used vials and ampoules, should be properly disposed of at the end of a session by sealing in a proper, puncture-resistant 'sharps' box (UN-approved, BS 7320).

Recording

Accurate, accessible records of vaccinations given are important for keeping individual clinical records, monitoring immunisation uptake and facilitating the recall of recipients of vaccines, if required.

The following information should be recorded accurately:

- vaccine name, product name, batch number and expiry date
- dose administered
- site(s) used – including, clear description of which injection was administered in each site, especially where two injections were administered in the same limb
- date immunisation(s) were given
- name and signature of vaccinator.

This information should be recorded in:

- patient-held record or Personal Child Health Record (PCHR, the Red Book) for children
- patient's GP record or other patient record, depending on location
- Child Health Information System
- practice computer system.

References

Alves AS, Nascimento CM and Granato CH *et al.* (2001) Hepatitis B vaccine in infants: a randomised controlled trial comprising gluteal versus anterolateral thigh muscle administration. *Rev Inst Med Trop Sao Paolo* **43**(3): 139–43.

American Academy of Pediatrics (2003) Active immunisation. In: Pickering LK (ed.) *Red Book: 2003 Report of the Committee on Infectious Diseases,* 26th edition. Elk Grove Village, IL: American Academy of Pediatrics, p 33.

Del Mar CB, Glasziou PP, Spinks AB and Sanders SL (2001) Is isopropyl alcohol swabbing before injection really necessary? *Med J Aust* **74**: 306.

Diggle L and Deeks J (2000) Effect of needle length on incidence of local reactions to routine immunisation in infants aged four months: randomised controlled trial. *BMJ* **321**: 931–3.

Fishbein DB, Sawyer LA, Reid-Sanden FL and Weir EH (1988) Administration of the human diploid-cell rabies vaccine in the gluteal area. *NEJM* **318**(2): 124–5.

Mark A, Carlsson RM and Granstrom M (1999) Subcutaneous versus intramuscular injection for booster DT vaccination of adolescents. *Vaccine* **17**(15–16): 2067–72.

Mayon White R and Moreton J (1998) *Immunizing children: a practical guide.* 2nd edition. Oxford: Radcliffe Medical Press.

Nursing and Midwifery Council *NMC code of professional conduct: standards for conduct, performance and ethics.* www.nmc-uk.org

Nursing and Midwifery Council. *Medicines management.* www.nmc-uk.org

Pigot J (1988) Needling doubts about where to vaccinate. *BMJ* **297**: 1130.

Plotkin SA and Orenstein WA (eds) (2004) *Vaccines,* 4th edition. Philadelphia: WB Saunders Company.

Shaw FE, Guess HA, Roets JM *et al.* (1989) Effect of anatomic injection site, age and smoking on the immune response to hepatitis B vaccination. *Vaccine* **7**: 425–30.

Sutton CD, White SA, Edwards R and Lewis MH (1999) A prospective controlled trial of the efficacy of isopropyl alcohol wipes before venesection in surgical patients. *Ann R Coll Surg Engl* **81**(3): 183–6.

The Vaccine Administration Taskforce. *UK guidance on best practice in vaccine administration (2001)* London: Shire Hall Communications.

Villarejo FJ and Pascaul AM (1993) Injection injury of the sciatic nerve (370 cases). *Child's Nervous System* **9**: 229–32.

World Health Organization (2004) *Immunization in practice: a guide for health workers.* WHO.

Zuckerman JN (2000) The importance of injecting vaccine into muscle. *BMJ* **321**: 1237–8.

5

Immunisation by nurses and other healthcare professionals

Introduction

The preferred way for patients to receive medicines is for trained healthcare professionals to prescribe for individual patients on a one-to-one basis. However, in some circumstances, it may be more appropriate for a patient to receive a medicine, including a vaccine (i.e. have it supplied and/or administered) directly from another healthcare professional. Unless covered by exemptions to the Medicines Act 1968, there are two ways of achieving this: either by Patient Specific Direction (PSD) or Patient Group Direction (PGD).

This chapter describes what PSDs and PGDs are and their use in immunisation.

Patient Specific Directions

A PSD is a written instruction from an independent prescriber (doctor, dentist or independent nurse prescriber) to another healthcare professional, to supply and/or administer a medicine directly to a named patient, or to several named patients.

Patient Group Directions

PGDs are defined as written instructions for the supply or administration of medicines to groups of patients who may not be individually identified before presentation for treatment (SI 2000/1917).

PGDs are not a form of prescribing but provide a legal framework for the supply and/or administration of medicines by a range of qualified healthcare professionals (nurses, midwives, pharmacists, optometrists, podiatrists/chiropodists, radiographers, orthoptists, physiotherapists, ambulance paramedics, dietitians, occupational therapists, prosthetists/orthotists and speech and language therapists). Employing organisations must ensure that all users of PGDs are fully competent and trained in their use.

When is a PSD appropriate?

PSDs are used once a patient has been assessed by a prescriber and that prescriber (doctor, dentist or independent nurse prescriber) instructs another healthcare professional in writing to supply or administer a medicine directly to that named patient or to several named patients. As a PSD is individually tailored to the needs of a single patient, it should be used in preference to a PGD wherever appropriate.

The usual method for the supply and administration of vaccines in the routine childhood immunisation programme is via a PSD. The authorisation for this is usually the responsibility of the GP or an independent nurse prescriber at the six to eight-week check and is recorded as an instruction in the Personal Child Health Record (PCHR or Red Book). This agreement allows immunisations to be given in GP surgeries or clinics. Where a PSD exists, there is no need for a PGD.

When is a PGD appropriate?

PGDs should be reserved for those limited situations where this offers advantage for patient care without compromising patient safety. With regard to immunisation, these situations may include nurse-led travel clinics, nurse-led immunisation sessions in schools and prisons, and nurses working with disadvantaged groups such as refugees, asylum seekers, looked-after children and drug users. In future, and with the development of new roles and new ways of working, such services will also involve a wider range of healthcare professionals working to deliver an immunisation programme.

Use of black triangle (▼) vaccines

Black triangle (▼) vaccines used in immunisation programmes may be included in PGDs, providing they are used in accordance with the recommendations of the Joint Committee on Vaccination and Immunisation (JCVI) (Health Service Circular, 2000/026). The PGD should state that a black triangle medicine is being included.

Use of unlicensed vaccines

In some circumstances, it may be necessary for the Department of Health to recommend vaccines that do not have a marketing authorisation (previously called a product licence) in the UK. For example, imported vaccines that are otherwise identical to the normal UK product but with overseas labelling may be required to maintain supplies. Such products cannot be administered using a PGD but require a PSD (see above). For convenience, where several individuals require vaccination, a list of these named individuals can be printed and authorisation signed by the prescriber.

Writing a PGD

The legislation governing PGDs specifies those professionals who should be involved in their development. These are:

- a senior doctor (see below)
- a senior pharmacist (see below)
- a senior person in each profession required to operate within the direction (see below)
- the clinical governance lead or their equivalent (see below) as organisational authority.

Good practice recommends that local drugs and therapeutics committees, area prescribing committees and similar advisory bodies should also be involved in drawing up the directions.

The legislation further specifies that each PGD must contain the following information:

- the name of the business to which the direction applies (i.e. primary care organisations (PCOs) in England, administrative regions in Wales and health boards in Scotland)
- the date the direction comes into force and the date it expires*
- a description of the medicine(s) to which the direction applies
- the class of healthcare professional who may supply or administer the medicine
- signatures of a doctor and a pharmacist
- a signature of a representative from an appropriate health organisation
- the clinical condition or situation to which the direction applies
- a description of those patients excluded from treatment under the direction
- a description of the circumstances in which further advice should be sought from a doctor and arrangements for referral
- details of the appropriate dose and maximum total dosage, quantity, pharmaceutical form and strength, route and frequency of administration and minimum or maximum period over which the medicine should be administered

* The legislation requires that the direction should be reviewed every two years, but in the case of immunisations this may need to be more frequently.

- relevant warnings, including potential adverse reactions
- details of any necessary follow-up action and the circumstances
- a statement of the records to be kept for audit purposes.

All PGDs must be signed by a senior doctor and a senior pharmacist, both of whom should have been involved in developing the PGD. For each profession required to operate within the direction, a senior person must sign as being responsible for the competencies, qualifications and training of the relevant authorised professionals. In addition, the clinical governance lead or their equivalent (who must not be the author of the PGD) must sign on behalf of the authorising NHS organisation, such as a primary care trust (PCT) or health board.

All professionals must be individually named and have signed the PGD. They must act within their appropriate code of professional conduct. PGDs should conform with the advice given in the latest relevant chapters of the Green Book.

Healthcare professionals are reminded that in some circumstances the recommendations regarding vaccines given in the Green Book chapters may differ from those in the Summary of Product Characteristics (SPC) for a particular vaccine. When this occurs, the recommendations in the Green Book are based on current expert advice received from the JCVI and should be followed. These Green Book recommendations and/or further advice from the Department of Health should be reflected in PGDs.

The PGD should also be in line with information in the Chief Medical Officer (CMO) letters and updates (www.dh.gov.uk/AboutUs/MinistersAndDepartmentLeaders/ChiefMedicalOfficer/fs/en) and/or in the NHS Purchasing and Supply Agency's *Vaccine Update* (www.pasa.nhs.uk/pharma/vaccines.stm).

Further information

The National Prescribing Centre has produced a practical guide and framework of competencies for the use of PGDs (www.npc.co.uk/publications/pgd/pgd.pdf).

The National electronic Library for Medicines (NeLM) has also developed a website providing support to all healthcare professionals who provide care under PGDs (www.nelm.nhs.uk/PGD/default.aspx). It also provides local examples of PGDs, including some relating to the administration of vaccines.

In Scotland, NHS Quality Improvement Scotland has published a Best Practice Statement concerning PGDs (www.nes.scot.nhs.uk/pgds/documents/22111_NHSQIS_Patient_Group.pdf). In addition, NHS Education for Scotland has developed a website to facilitate the development of PGDs by healthcare professionals (www.nes.scot.nhs.uk/pgds/).

References

NHS Executive (2000) *Patient Group Directions*, HSC 2000/026. Leeds: NHSE.

NHS National Prescribing Centre (2004) *Patient Group Directions: A practical guide and framework of competencies for all professionals using patient group directions* www.npc.co.uk/publications/pgd/pgd.pdf.

The Prescription Only Medicines (Human Use) Amendment Order 2000, SI. 2000/1917. London: The Stationery Office.

6

Contraindications and special considerations

General contraindications to vaccination

Almost all individuals can be safely vaccinated with all vaccines. In very few individuals, vaccination is contraindicated or should be deferred. Where there is doubt, rather than withholding vaccine, advice should be sought from an appropriate consultant paediatrician or physician, the immunisation co-ordinator or consultant in health protection.

All vaccines are contraindicated in those who have had:

- a confirmed anaphylactic reaction to a previous dose of a vaccine containing the same antigens, or
- a confirmed anaphylactic reaction to another component contained in the relevant vaccine, e.g. neomycin, streptomycin or polymyxin B (which may be present in trace amounts in some vaccines).

Live vaccines may be temporarily contraindicated in individuals who are:

- immunosuppressed (see below)
- pregnant.

Specific contraindications

Some vaccines are contraindicated in specific groups. These are outlined in the relevant chapters.

Egg allergy

Individuals with a confirmed anaphylactic reaction to egg should not receive influenza or yellow fever vaccines. MMR vaccine can be safely given to most children with a previous history of allergy after ingestion of egg or egg-containing food, and vaccination with MMR can be performed under normal circumstances. For the small number of individuals who have a history of confirmed anaphylactic reaction after any egg-containing food, specialist advice should be sought with a view to immunisation under controlled conditions.

Pregnancy

There is a theoretical concern that vaccinating pregnant women with live vaccines may infect the foetus. There is no evidence that any live vaccine (including rubella and MMR) causes birth defects. However, since the theoretical possibility of foetal infection exists, live vaccines should generally be delayed until after delivery. Termination of pregnancy following inadvertent immunisation is not recommended.

Since inactivated vaccines cannot replicate they cannot cause infection in either the mother or the foetus. However, inactivated vaccines should be administered to pregnant women only if protection is required without delay.

Immunosuppression

Live vaccines can, in some situations, cause severe or fatal infections in immunosuppressed individuals due to extensive replication of the vaccine strain. For this reason, severely immunosuppressed individuals (see bullet list below) should not be given live vaccines, and vaccination in immunosuppressed individuals should only be conducted in consultation with an appropriate specialist.

Inactivated vaccines cannot replicate and so may be administered to immunosuppressed individuals, although they may elicit a lower response than in immunocompetent individuals.

The following individuals should not receive live vaccines:

- patients with evidence of severe primary immunodeficiency, for example, severe combined immunodeficiency, Wiskott-Aldrich syndrome and other combined immunodeficiency syndromes
- patients currently being treated for malignant disease with immunosuppressive chemotherapy or radiotherapy, or who have terminated such treatment within at least the last six months
- patients who have received a solid organ transplant and are currently on immunosuppressive treatment
- patients who have received a bone marrow transplant, until at least 12 months after finishing all immunosuppressive treatment, or longer where the patient has developed graft-versus-host disease. The decision to vaccinate should depend upon the type of transplant and the immune status of the patient. Further advice can be found in current guidance produced by the European Group for Blood and Marrow Transplantation (www.ebmt.org) and the Royal College of Paediatrics and Child Health (RCPCH) (www.rcpch.ac.uk)

- patients receiving systemic high-dose steroids, until at least three months after treatment has stopped. This would include children who receive prednisolone, orally or rectally, at a daily dose (or its equivalent) of 2mg/kg/day for at least one week, or 1mg/kg/day for one month. For adults, an equivalent dose is harder to define but immunosuppression should be considered in those who receive at least 40mg of prednisolone per day for more than one week. Occasionally, individuals on lower doses of steroids may be immunosuppressed and at increased risk from infections. In those cases, live vaccines should be considered with caution, in discussion with a relevant specialist physician
- patients receiving other types of immunosuppressive drugs (e.g. azathioprine, cyclosporin, methotrexate, cyclophosphamide, leflunomide and the newer cytokine inhibitors) alone or in combination with lower doses of steroids, until at least six months after terminating such treatment. The advice of the physician in charge or immunologist should be sought
- patients with immunosuppression due to human immunodeficiency virus (HIV) infection (see section below).

Other considerations

Many patients with relatively minor immunodeficiencies can, and indeed should, receive all recommended vaccinations, including live vaccines. Where there is doubt or a relatively severe immunodeficiency is present, it is important to obtain individual specialist advice.

Some patients with 22q11 deletion syndromes, including partial DiGeorge syndrome, may be able to receive live vaccines safely provided that they have no evidence of severe immunocompromise (Perez *et al.*, 2003). Specialist advice should be sought.

Non-systemic corticosteroids, such as aerosols or topical or intra-articular preparations, do not cause systemic immunosuppression. Therefore, administration of live vaccines is not contraindicated.

Live vaccines are likely to be safe in those receiving other immunomodulating drugs, for example interferon. However, advice should be sought from the specialist in charge of the therapy to ensure that the patient has not been immunosuppressed by the treatment. Deferral of immunisation may be suggested to avoid side effects of the drugs being confused with reactions to vaccination.

Replacement schedules of corticosteroids for people with adrenal insufficiency do not cause immunosuppression and are not, therefore, contraindications for administration of live vaccines.

For further information, please refer to the RCPCH Best Practice Statement (www.rcpch.ac.uk).

HIV infection

HIV-positive individuals should be given MMR vaccine according to national recommendations unless they have evidence of severe immunosuppression (Table 6.1). For children under 12 months of age, CD4 counts may not be an accurate representation of levels of immunosuppression and immune status should be assessed by an expert using a combination of laboratory and clinical criteria.

Varicella vaccine is contraindicated for HIV-infected individuals with severe immunosuppression (Table 6.1). This guidance may be relaxed in the near future, as evidence is emerging that patients with moderate immunosuppression can be safely vaccinated and will make an adequate response (M Levine, pers. comm., 2005). For HIV-infected individuals with no immunosuppression who are susceptible to varicella, vaccine is indicated to reduce the risk of serious chickenpox or zoster should their condition deteriorate.

Table 6.1 Measure of immunosuppression by CD4 count

CD4 count/μl (% of total lymphocytes)			
Age	1–5 years	6–12 years	>12 years
No suppression	≥1000 (15–24%)	≥500 (≥25%)	≥500 (≥25%)
Moderate suppression	500–999 (15–24%)	200–499 (15–24%)	200–499 (15–24%)
Severe suppression	<500 (<15%)	<200 (<15%)	<200 (<15%)

Because there have been reports of dissemination of Bacillus Calmette-Guérin (BCG) in HIV-positive individuals, such individuals should **not** receive BCG vaccine in the UK (Talbot *et al.*, 1997; Fallo *et al.*, 2005; Langley *et al.*, 2004).

Infants born to HIV-positive mothers where the infant has an indeterminate HIV status may have an increased risk of contracting tuberculosis. Where indicated, BCG vaccine can be given after two appropriately timed negative postnatal PCR blood tests for HIV infection. Unless a mother is known to be at risk of HIV, it is not necessary to test her before giving BCG vaccine to her infant.

Yellow fever vaccine should not be given to HIV-positive individuals. If such individuals intend to visit countries where a yellow fever certificate is required for entry but where there is no risk of exposure, then they should obtain a letter of exemption from a medical practitioner. Fatal myeloencephalitis following yellow fever vaccination has been reported in an individual with severe HIV-induced immunosuppression (Kengsakul *et al.*, 2002). There are limited data, however, suggesting that yellow fever vaccine may be given safely to HIV-infected persons with a CD4 count that is greater than 200 and a suppressed HIV viral load (Receveur *et al.*, 2000; Tattevin *et al.*, 2004). Therefore, if the yellow fever risk is unavoidable, specialist advice should be sought with a view to the vaccination of asymptomatic HIV-infected individuals.

Further guidance is provided by the Royal College of Paediatrics and Child Health (www.rcpch.ac.uk), the British HIV Association (BHIVA) *Immunisation guidelines for HIV-infected adults* (BHIVA, 2006) and the Children's HIV Association of UK and Ireland (CHIVA) immunisation guidelines (www.bhiva.org/chiva).

Deferral of immunisation

There will be very few occasions when deferral of immunisation is required. Minor illnesses without fever or systemic upset are not valid reasons to postpone immunisation. If an individual is acutely unwell, immunisation may be postponed until they have fully recovered. This is to avoid wrongly attributing any new symptom or the progression of symptoms to the vaccine.

In individuals with an evolving neurological condition, immunisation should be deferred until the neurological condition has resolved or stabilised.

Immunoglobulin may interfere with the immune response to live vaccine viruses because it may contain antibodies to measles, varicella and other viruses. Live virus vaccines should therefore be given at least three weeks before or three months after an injection of immunoglobulin. This does not apply to yellow fever vaccine, because immunoglobulin used in the UK is unlikely to contain high levels of antibody to this virus.

The following conditions are NOT contraindications to routine immunisation (in some of these situations, additional precautions may be required – refer to the relevant chapter for further information):

- family history of any adverse reactions following immunisation
- previous history of the disease (with the exception of BCG for people who have evidence of past exposure to tuberculosis)
- contact with an infectious disease
- premature birth

- stable neurological conditions such as cerebral palsy and Down's syndrome
- asthma, eczema or hay fever
- mild self-limiting illness without fever, e.g. runny nose
- treatment with antibiotics or locally acting (e.g. topical or inhaled) steroids
- child's mother or someone in the household being pregnant
- currently breast-feeding or being breast-fed
- history of jaundice after birth
- under a certain weight
- being over the age recommended in the routine childhood immunisation schedule
- personal history of febrile convulsions or epilepsy
- close family history (parent or sibling) of febrile convulsions or epilepsy
- being a sibling or close contact of an immunosuppressed individual
- recent or imminent elective surgery
- imminent general anaesthesia
- unknown or inadequately documented immunisation history.

References

British HIV Association (2006) *Immunisation guidelines for HIV-infected adults:* www.bhiva.org/pdf/2006/Immunisation506.pdf.

Fallo A, De Matteo E, Preciado MV *et al.* (2005) Epstein-Barr virus associated with primary CNS lymphoma and disseminated BCG infection in a child with AIDS. *Int J Infect Dis* **9**(2): 96–103.

Kengsakul K, Sathirapongsasuti K and Punyagupta S (2002) Fatal myeloencephalitis following yellow fever vaccination in a case with HIV infection. *J Med Assoc Thai* **85**(1): 131–4.

Langley J, Ellis E and Deeks S (2004) National Advisory Committee on Immunization; Health Canada First Nations; Inuit Health Branch. Statement on Bacille Calmette-Guérin (BCG) vaccine. *Can Commun Dis Rep* **1**(30): 1–11.

English, French. Erratum in *Can Commun Dis Rep* (2005) Feb 1: **31**(3):40. www.phac-aspc.gc.ca/publicat/ccdr-rmtc/04vol30/acs-dcc-5/index.html

Perez EE, Bokszczanin A, McDonald-McGinn D *et al.* (2003) Safety of live viral vaccines in patients with chromosome 22q11.2 deletion syndrome (DiGeorge syndrome/velocardiofacial syndrome). *Pediatrics* **112**(4): e325.

Receveur MC, Thiebaut R, Vedy S *et al.* (2000) Yellow fever vaccination of human immunodeficiency virus-infected patients: report of two cases. *Clin Infect Dis* **31**(3): E7–8.

Talbot EA, Perkins MD, Silva SF and Frothingham R (1997) Disseminated Bacille Calmette-Guérin disease after vaccination: case report and review. *Clin Infect Dis* **24**(6): 1139–46.

Tattevin P, Depatureaux AG, Chapplain JM *et al.* (2004) Yellow fever vaccine is safe and effective in HIV-infected patients. *AIDS* **18**(5): 825–7.

7

Immunisation of individuals with underlying medical conditions

Introduction

Some medical conditions increase the risk of complications from infectious diseases, and children and adults with such conditions should be immunised as a matter of priority. These groups may also require additional vaccinations or additional doses of vaccines to provide adequate protection.

Immunosuppression

Individuals with immunosuppression and HIV infection (regardless of CD4 count) should be given inactivated vaccines in accordance with national recommendations. However, these individuals may not mount as good an antibody response as immunocompetent individuals. Therefore, wherever possible, immunisation or boosting of HIV-positive individuals should be either carried out before immunosuppression occurs or deferred until an improvement in immunity has been seen.

Further guidance is provided by the Royal College of Paediatrics and Child Health (RCPCH) (www.rcpch.ac.uk), the British HIV Association (BHIVA) *Immunisation guidelines for HIV-infected adults* (BHIVA, 2006) and the Children's HIV Association of UK and Ireland (CHIVA) immunisation guidelines (www.bhiva.org/chiva).

For individuals due to commence immunosuppressive treatments, inactivated vaccines should ideally be administered at least two weeks before commencement. In some cases this will not be possible and therefore vaccination may be carried out at any time and re-immunisation considered after treatment is finished and recovery has occurred. In the case of live vaccines, a longer period before immunosuppression commences may be desirable, but the disadvantages of delaying such treatment are often significant. Specialist advice should be sought from an appropriate physician.

In severely immunosuppressed individuals, re-immunisation should be considered after treatment is finished and/or recovery has occurred.

Specialist advice should be sought. Further guidance is provided by the RCPCH (www.rcpch.ac.uk).

Close contacts of immunosuppressed individuals

Some vaccines are contraindicated in immunosuppressed individuals and such individuals may not respond well to other vaccines. Therefore, to minimise the risk of infection, close contacts of immunosuppressed individuals should be fully immunised according to the UK schedule, as a matter of priority. Close contacts of severely immunosuppressed individuals should also be offered vaccination against varicella and influenza. This will reduce the risk of vulnerable individuals being exposed to the serious consequences of vaccine-preventable infections.

Prematurity

Immune responses in very premature infants (e.g. gestational age under 30 weeks or birthweight below 1500g) may be suboptimal. As these infants may be at high risk from infection, vaccination should not be delayed but given according to the national schedule at the appropriate chronological age. Additional doses of vaccine may need to be considered.

Specific indications for immunisation of other vulnerable groups

Some medical conditions or treatments increase the risk of complications from specific infectious diseases. Individuals who have such conditions or receive such treatments require additional protection, as listed in the appropriate chapters, and so the following vaccines are recommended:

Asplenia or splenic dysfunction

- Hib vaccine (irrespective of age see Chapter 16)
- influenza vaccine (see Chapter 19)
- meningococcal C vaccine (see Chapter 22)
- pneumococcal vaccine (see Chapter 25)

Cochlear implants

- pneumococcal vaccine (see Chapter 25)

Haemodialysis

- hepatitis B vaccine (see Chapter 18)

Haemophilia

- hepatitis A vaccine (see Chapter 17, including advice on route of administration)

- hepatitis B vaccine (see Chapter 18, including advice on route of administration)

Chronic medical conditions (respiratory, heart, renal and liver disease and diabetes)

- influenza vaccine (see Chapter 19)
- pneumococcal vaccine (see Chapter 25)

Immunosuppression

- influenza vaccine (see Chapter 19)
- pneumococcal vaccine (see Chapter 25).

Additionally, individuals who receive bone marrow transplants are likely to lose any natural or immunisation-derived protective antibodies against most vaccine-preventable diseases. It is unclear whether they may acquire the donor's immunity, and therefore all individuals should be considered for a re-immunisation programme. Specialist advice should be sought and is available at: www.rcpch.ac.uk/publications/recent_publications/Immunocomp.pdf (for children) and www.ebmt.org/5workingparties/idwp/wparties-id5.html.

Table 7.1 Immunisation of individuals with asplenia or splenic dysfunction

Suggested schedule for immunisation with conjugate vaccines in individuals with splenic dysfunction and immunosuppression.

Age at which asplenia or splenic dysfunction or immunosuppression is acquired	**Vaccination schedule** Where possible, vaccination course should ideally be started at least two weeks before surgery or commencement of immunosuppressive treatment. If not possible, see advice in pneumo chapter.		
	Month 0	**Month 2**	**Month 4**
Under two years	Routine immunisation schedule should be followed.		
Over two to under five years (fully vaccinated including booster)	Booster dose of Hib/MenC vaccine Booster dose of PCV	Single dose of PPV	None
Over two to under five years (unvaccinated or partially vaccinated)	First dose of Hib/MenC vaccine First dose of PCV	Second dose of Hib/MenC vaccine Second dose of PCV	Single dose of PPV
Five years and older (and previously vaccinated with Hib, MenC, PCV vaccines)	Booster dose of Hib/MenC vaccine Single dose of PPV		
Five years and older (unvaccinated)	First dose of Hib/MenC vaccine Single dose of PPV	Second dose of Hib/MenC vaccine	

PCV = pneumococcal conjugate vaccine, PPV = pneumococcal polysaccharide vaccine

Other methods of protecting vulnerable individuals

Immunosuppressed individuals (as above) can be protected against some infections by the administration of passive antibody. After exposure to measles or chickenpox, such individuals should be considered for an injection of the appropriate preparation of immunoglobulin (varicella zoster immunoglobulin (VZIG) or human normal immunoglobulin (HNIG) – see varicella and measles, Chapters 35 and 22 respectively). Individuals exposed to chickenpox may benefit from prophylactic acyclovir at a dose of 40mg/kg per day in four divided doses (Kumagai *et al.*, 1999). This may be considered in addition to VZIG or as an alternative when VZIG is not indicated. Treatment with acyclovir should be commenced promptly in this group.

Prophylaxis with other antibiotic or antiviral drugs may also be indicated in immunosuppressed individuals exposed to infections such as pertussis or influenza. Advice should be sought from the local health protection unit.

Antibiotic prophylaxis (usually phenoxymethyl penicillin) is advisable for asplenic and hyposplenic patients. Guidelines have been published (Haematology Task Force, 1996) and a patient card and information leaflet are available (details at the end of this chapter).

Resources

To obtain copies of the patient card and leaflet *Splenectomy, information for patients,* contact DH Publications Orderline (Tel: 08701 555 455; e-mail: dh@prolog.uk.com; PO Box 777, London SE1 6XH) or, in Wales, Welsh Assembly Publications Centre (Tel: 029 2082 3683; e-mail: assembly-publications@wales.gsi.gov.uk).

References

British HIV Association (2006) *Immunisation guidelines for HIV-infected adults.* www.bhiva.org/pdf/2006/Immunisation506.pdf.

Haematology Task Force (1996) Guidelines for the prevention and treatment of infection in patients with an absent or dysfunctional spleen. Working Party of the British Committee for Standards in Haematology, Clinical Haematology Task Force. *BMJ* 17;**312**(7028): 430–4.

Kumagai T, Kamada M, Igarashi C *et al.* (1999) Varicella-zoster virus-specific cellular immunity in subjects given acyclovir after household chickenpox exposure. *J Infect Dis* **180**(3): 834–7.

Lin T-Y, Huang Y-C, Ning H-C and Hsueh C (1997) Oral aciclovir prophylaxis of varicella after intimate contact. *Pediatr Infect Dis J* **16**: 1162–5.

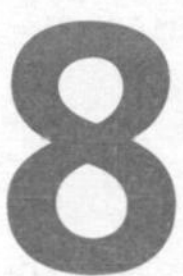

Vaccine safety and the management of adverse events following immunisation

Introduction

Vaccines induce protection by eliciting active immune responses to specific antigens. There may be predictable adverse reactions (side effects): most are mild and resolve quickly. However, it is not always possible to predict individuals who might have a mild or serious reaction to a vaccine. The advice in this chapter uses the World Health Organization (WHO) classification of adverse events following immunisation (AEFIs). It gives an overview of common side effects associated with vaccines and of the management of serious adverse reactions such as anaphylaxis. The process of vaccine safety monitoring in the UK and the reporting of suspected vaccine-induced adverse drug reactions (ADRs) via the Yellow Card scheme are described in Chapter 9.

Adverse events following immunisation

AEFIs may be true adverse reactions that are intrinsic to the vaccine, or may be caused by the way it is administered or be related to an underlying condition in the recipient. Other AEFIs may be coincidental and would have occurred regardless of vaccination.

WHO classifies AEFIs according to four main categories:

- programme-related
- vaccine-induced
- coincidental
- unknown.

Programme-related AEFIs

These are adverse events that result from inappropriate practices in the provision of vaccination. These may include:

- wrong dose of vaccine administered
- vaccines used beyond expiry date
- vaccines used at inappropriate intervals
- inappropriate route, site or technique of administration
- vaccine reconstituted with incorrect diluent
- wrong amount of diluent used
- vaccine prepared incorrectly
- mixing into inappropriate combinations
- drugs substituted for vaccine or diluent
- vaccine or diluent contaminated
- vaccine or diluent stored incorrectly
- contraindications not elicited or ignored
- reconstituted vaccine kept beyond the recommended period.

Some AEFIs can be induced by the vaccination process itself. The administration of the vaccine causes the AEFI, rather than any of the vaccine components: for example fainting in older children and adults during the 1999–2000 meningitis C immunisation campaign (Medicines Control Agency, 2000).

Vaccine-induced AEFIs

These are reactions in individuals specifically caused by a particular vaccine or its component parts. These may be induced, direct effects of the vaccine or one of its components, and/or due to an underlying medical condition or an idiosyncratic response in the recipient.

Direct effects of vaccines include, for example, local reactions and fever within 48 hours of DTaP/IPV/Hib, rash and fever seven to ten days after MMR, and parotitis three weeks after MMR.

An example of an AEFI due to an underlying medical condition is vaccine-associated paralysis which very rarely followed the use of live attenuated oral polio vaccine in a child with previously unrecognised severe combined immune deficiency.

Idiosyncratic responses include idiopathic thrombocytopaenic purpura (ITP) within 30 days of MMR, and anaphylaxis immediately after vaccination. When there has been a confirmed anaphylactic reaction to a previous dose of the same vaccine, then **this contraindicates further vaccinations with the same vaccine or a component of that vaccine**.

This category also includes medical conditions that would have occurred at some point in an individual but are triggered earlier by the vaccination. This may include febrile seizures in a child with a family history of the same, or onset of infantile spasms (Bellman *et al.*, 1983).

Coincidental AEFIs

These are not true adverse reactions to immunisations or vaccines but are only linked because of the timing of their occurrence. When an AEFI is coincidental, the event would have occurred even if the individual had not been immunised. An example would be people who develop a cold with coryzal symptoms following flu vaccination. Flu vaccine does not prevent the common cold and colds are common in the winter when people are receiving flu vaccine.

Unknown AEFIs

Defined as AEFIs which there is insufficient evidence to classify as one of the above.

Common vaccine-induced AEFIs

Common vaccine-induced AEFIs include:

- pain, swelling or redness at the site of injection. These occur commonly after immunisation and should be anticipated
- local adverse reactions that generally start within a few hours of the injection and are usually mild and self-limiting. Although these are often referred to as 'hypersensitivity reactions', they are not allergic in origin, but may be either due to high titres of antibody or a direct effect of the vaccine product, e.g. endotoxin in whole-cell bacterial vaccines. The occurrence or severity of such local reactions **does not contraindicate** further doses of immunisation with the same vaccine or vaccines containing the same antigens
- systemic adverse reactions which include fever, malaise, myalgia, irritability, headache and loss of appetite. The timing of systemic reactions will vary according to the characteristics of the vaccine received, the age of the recipient and the biological response to that vaccine. For example, fever may start within a few hours of tetanus-containing vaccines, but occurs seven to ten days after measles-containing vaccine. The occurrence of such systemic reactions **does not**

contraindicate further doses of the same vaccine or vaccines containing the same antigens.

The types of side effect that are commonly seen after the routine and other childhood immunisations are described in the relevant chapters, along with details of when they are most likely to occur.

Managing common vaccine-induced AEFIs

Parents should be given advice about AEFIs that they can expect and how such events should be managed. The leaflets on vaccinations provided by the Department of Health give information about AEFIs and include advice on their management.

Fevers over 37.5˚C are common in children and are usually mild. Advice on the use and appropriate dose of paracetamol or ibuprofen liquid to prevent or treat a fever should be given at the time of immunisation. Local reactions are usually self-limiting and do not require treatment. If they appear to cause discomfort, then paracetamol or ibuprofen can be given.

Aspirin, or medicines that contain aspirin should never be given to children under 16 years old because of the risk of developing Reye's syndrome.

Rare vaccine-induced AEFIs

Some other AEFIs occur rarely and include those that are neurological or immune-mediated. Examples include seizures, hypotonic-hyporesponsive episodes (HHE), idiopathic thrombocytopaenic purpura (ITP), acute arthropathy, allergic reactions and anaphylaxis.

Anaphylaxis

Anaphylactic reactions to vaccines are extremely rare but have the potential to be fatal. Between 1997 and 2003, there were 130 reports to the Medicines and Healthcare products Regulatory Agency (MHRA) of anaphylaxis or anaphylactic-type reactions following immunisation (excluding the meningitis C campaign), although no deaths as a result of the reaction were reported. In that time, around 117 million doses of all vaccines were supplied to hospitals and GPs. This rate (approximately one per million vaccine doses) is similar to that reported from other countries (Bohlke *et al.,* 2003; Canadian Medical Association, 2002).

Onset of anaphylaxis is rapid, typically within minutes, and its clinical course is unpredictable with variable severity and clinical features. Due to the unpredictable nature of anaphylactic reactions it is not possible to define a particular time period over which all individuals should be observed following immunisation to ensure they do not develop anaphylaxis.

The most serious symptoms of anaphylaxis include cardiovascular collapse, bronchospasm, angioedema (localised oedema of the deeper layers of the skin or subcutaneous tissues), pulmonary oedema, loss of consciousness and urticaria. Asthmatic patients with anaphylaxis often develop bronchospasm. Anaphylaxis generally responds promptly to parenteral adrenaline (epinephrine). Most anaphylactic reactions occur in individuals who have no known risk factors.

Differential diagnosis

All medical and nursing staff involved in immunisation should be able to distinguish an anaphylactic reaction from fainting (syncope) and panic attacks.

Fainting is relatively common when vaccinating adults and adolescents, but infants and children rarely faint. Sudden loss of consciousness in young children should be presumed to be an anaphylactic reaction, particularly if a strong central pulse is absent. A strong central pulse persists during a faint or seizure.

The features listed in Table 8.1 differentiate between anaphylaxis and fainting. If the diagnosis is unclear, anaphylaxis should be presumed and appropriate management given.

There should be rapid recovery from fainting. Although symptoms of malaise may persist, the patient should recover consciousness within a few minutes.

Panic attacks should also be distinguished from anaphylaxis. Some individuals may suffer panic attacks even before immunisation is undertaken. Symptoms include hyperventilation that may lead to paraesthesiae (numbness and tingling) in the arms and legs. There may be an erythematous rash associated with anxiety, although hypotension, pallor or wheezing will not be present.

Management of anaphylaxis

Guidelines on the management of anaphylaxis have been modified to ensure agreement between the Resuscitation Council (UK), the British National Formulary, the Joint Committee on Vaccination and

Table 8.1 Clinical features of fainting and anaphylaxis

	Fainting	Anaphylaxis
Onset	Before, during or within minutes of vaccine administration	Usually within five minutes, but can occur within hours of vaccine administration
Symptoms/signs		
Skin	Generalised pallor, cold clammy skin	Skin itchiness, pallor or flushing of skin, red or pale urticaria (weals) or angioedema
Respiratory	Normal respiration – may be shallow, but not laboured	Cough, wheeze, stridor, or signs of respiratory distress (tachypnoea, cyanosis, rib recession)
Cardiovascular	Bradycardia, but with strong central pulse; hypotension – usually transient and corrects in supine position	Tachycardia, with weak/absent central pulse; hypotension – sustained
Neurological	Sense of light-headedness; loss of consciousness – improves once supine or head down position; transient jerking of the limbs and eye-rolling which may be confused with seizure; incontinence	Sense of severe anxiety and distress; loss of consciousness – no improvement once supine or head down position

Immunisation, and the Royal College of Paediatrics and Child Health (Department of Health, 2001; Resuscitation Council, 2002).

All health professionals responsible for immunisation must be familiar with techniques for resuscitation of a patient with anaphylaxis to prevent disability and loss of life. A protocol for the management of anaphylaxis and an anaphylaxis pack must always be available whenever vaccines are given.

An anaphylaxis pack normally contains two ampoules of adrenaline (epinephrine) 1:1000, four 23G needles and four graduated 1ml syringes, and Laerdal or equivalent masks suitable for children and adults. Packs should be checked regularly to ensure the contents are within their expiry dates. Chlorphenamine (chlorpheniramine) and hydrocortisone are not first-line treatments and do not need to be included in the pack.

Immediate action

1 **Send for additional health professional assistance.**
2 **Send a responsible adult to dial 999 and state that there is a case of suspected anaphylaxis.**
3 **Stay with the patient at all times.**
4 **Lie the patient down, ideally with the legs raised (unless the patient has breathing difficulties).**
5 **Administer oxygen if available.**
6 **If breathing stops, mouth to mouth/mask resuscitation should be performed.**

All patients with clinical signs of shock, airway swelling or definite breathing difficulties should be given adrenaline (epinephrine) 1:1000 administered by intramuscular (IM) injection (never subcutaneously). For information on dosage to be given see below. The preferred site is the mid-point of the anterolateral aspect of the thigh (Simons *et al.*, 1998). If there is no clinical improvement, the dose may be repeated once after five minutes. Further doses of adrenaline can be given if needed.

The use of **intravenous** (IV) adrenaline (epinephrine) is hazardous and should only be considered in extreme emergency in patients with profound shock that is immediately life-threatening. Only dilute adrenaline (at least 1:10,000) should be used, and the injection given slowly.

Because of the possibility of delayed reactions, individuals who have had an anaphylactic reaction should be sent to hospital, even though they may appear to have made a full recovery.

An airway should only be used by properly trained and competent health professionals, and only in unconscious patients.

Adrenaline (epinephrine) dosage

The appropriate dose of adrenaline (epinephrine) 1:1000 (1mg/ml) solution should be administered immediately by IM injection (see Table 8.2). If there is no clinical improvement, the dose given may be repeated after about five minutes.

In some cases, several doses may be needed, particularly if improvement is transient.

Table 8.2 Dose of adrenaline (epinephrine) by age

Age	Dose of adrenaline (epinephrine)
Under 6 months	50μg IM (0.05ml)*
Over 6 months but under 6 years	120μg IM (0.12ml)*
6 to 12 years	250μg IM (0.25ml)
Over 12 years	500μg IM (0.5ml) (250μg IM if patient is small or prepubertal)

* A suitable syringe for small volumes should be used.

Auto-injectors for self-administration of adrenaline should not be used as a substitute for a proper anaphylaxis pack.

Cautions

Patients taking beta-blockers, tricyclic antidepressants or monoamine oxidase inhibitors should receive 50% of the usual dose of adrenaline because of a potentially dangerous drug interaction. Although cocaine may also interact with the action of adrenaline, anaphylaxis is sufficiently rare **not** to recommend either withholding immunisation from known users or undertaking routine questioning about recreational drug use in individuals attending for vaccination. In the unlikely event of collapse in someone who is suspected of having recently taken cocaine, adrenaline should be used only with extreme caution and using half the normal adult dose.

Further management

Antihistamines and/or hydrocortisone are not recommended in the emergency management of anaphylaxis in primary care. They should be considered, however, in the further management of anaphylaxis by appropriately trained staff.

Chlorphenamine

The appropriate dose of chlorphenamine according to age should be administered by IM injection (or by slow IV injection where appropriate) (see Table 8.3)

Table 8.3 Dosage of chlorphenamine by age

Age	Dose of chlorphenamine*
Over 1 month but under 1 year	0.25mg/kg IV
1 to 5 years	2.5–5mg IM
6 to 12 years	5–10mg IM
Over 12 years	10–20 mg IM

* By IM injection or slow IV injection (due to the possibility of drug-induced hypotension).

Chlorphenamine (by slow IV injection) is a useful adjunct to adrenaline in the treatment of anaphylaxis. It may be given after adrenaline and continued for 24 to 48 hours to prevent relapse.

Hydrocortisone

The appropriate dose of hydrocortisone according to age should be administered by IM injection or slow IV injection (see Table 8.4)

Table 8.4 Dose of hydrocortisone by age

Age	Dose of hydrocortisone*
Under 1 year	25mg
1 to 5 years	50mg
6 to 12 years	100mg
Over 12 years	100–500mg

* By slow IV or IM injection

Hydrocortisone should only be given after a severe anaphylactic attack to prevent any late symptoms.

Continuing deterioration requires further treatment, including fluid infusion. A crystalloid solution may be safer than a colloid solution, and should be given in a rapid infusion of 1–2l, or for children 20ml/kg of body weight, with another similar dose if there is no clinical response.

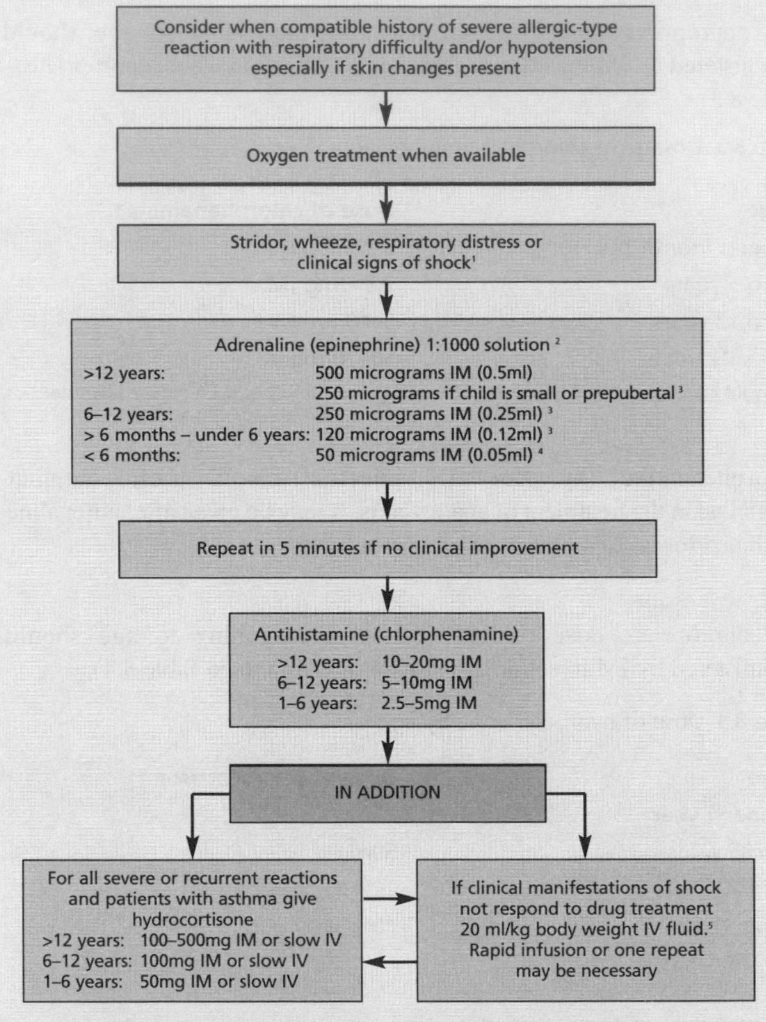

1. An inhaled beta2-agonist such as salbutamol may be used as an adjunctive measure if bronchospasm is severe and does not respond rapidly to other treatment.
2. If profound shock judged **immediately** life threatening give CPR/ALS if necessary. Consider **slow** intravenous (IV) adrenaline (epinephrine) 1:10,000 solution. This is **hazardous** and is recommended only for an experienced practitioner who can also obtain IV access without delay. Note the different strength of adrenaline (epinephrine) that may be required for IV use.
3. For children who have been prescribed Epipen, 150 micrograms can be given instead of 120 micrograms, and 300 micrograms can be given instead of 250 micrograms or 500 micrograms.
4. Absolute accuracy of the small dose is not essential.
5. A crystalloid may be safer than a colloid.

Figure 8.1 Anaphylactic reactions: Treatment algorithm for children by first medical responders (reproduced by kind permission of the Resuscitation Council)

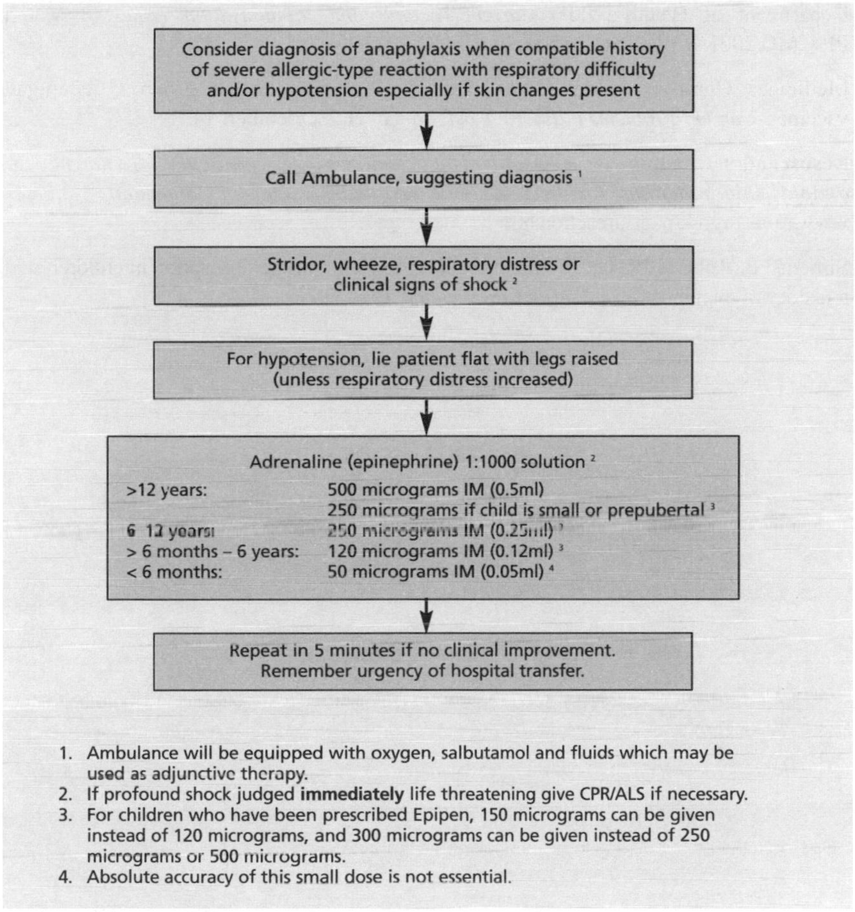

Figure 8.2 Anaphylactic reactions: Treatment algorithm for children in the community (reproduced by kind permission of the Resuscitation Council)

An inhaled bronchodilator such as salbutamol or terbutaline is useful if bronchospasm is a major feature and does not respond rapidly to other treatment.

References

Bellman MH, Ross EM and Miller DL (1983) Infantile spasms and pertussis immunisation. *Lancet* 7: 1031–4.

Bohlke K, David RL, Marcy SH *et al.* (2003) Risk of anaphylaxis after vaccination of children and adolescents. *Pediatrics* **112**: 815–20.

Canadian Medical Association (2002) In: *Canadian Immunisation Guide,* 6th edition. Canadian Medical Association.

Department of Health (2001) *Current Vaccine and Immunisation Issues*, 8 March. PL/CMO/2001/1, PL/CNO/2001/1, PL/CPHO/2001/1.

Medicines Control Agency (2000) Safety of meningococcal group C conjugate vaccines. *Current Problems in Pharmacovigilance*. **26**, September: 14.

Resuscitation Council (2002) *The emergency medical treatment of anaphylactic reactions for first medical responders and for community nurses.* www.resus.org.uk/pages/reaction.htm

Simons FE, Roberts JR, Gu X, Simons KJ (1998) Epinephrine absorption in children with a history of anaphylaxis. *J Allergy Clin Immuno* **101**: 33–7.

9

Surveillance and monitoring for vaccine safety

This chapter describes the process of vaccine safety monitoring in the UK and the reporting of adverse events following immunisation (AEFIs) (see Chapter 8). It also describes the mechanism for the reporting of suspected defects in vaccines or in the devices used for the administration of vaccines.

All vaccines are extensively tested for quality, safety and immunogenicity and/or efficacy before being licensed and used routinely. As not all side effects may have been identified prior to licensing, particularly if they occur very rarely, careful surveillance is required throughout their use. Important information on vaccine safety is routinely collected through the Yellow Card scheme and from other sources, including medical literature, post-marketing safety studies, epidemiological databases and other worldwide organisations.

The Medicines and Healthcare products Regulatory Agency (MHRA) has responsibility for monitoring the safety of all marketed medicines (including vaccines) and medical devices. Suspected adverse events following the use of vaccines, medicines and medical devices should be reported to the MHRA.

The Yellow Card scheme

The Yellow Card scheme is a voluntary reporting system for suspected adverse reactions (ADRs) to medicines, which includes vaccines. AEFIs that are suspected to be vaccine-induced should be reported as ADRs via the Yellow Card scheme. An ADR is an unwanted or harmful reaction following the administration of a medicine, vaccine or combination of vaccines. The ADR may be a known AEFI (see Chapter 8), or it may be previously unrecognised. Spontaneous reports of suspected ADRs are received from UK doctors, pharmacists, dentists, coroners, nurses, midwives, health visitors and patients. There is also a statutory requirement for pharmaceutical companies to report to the MHRA serious suspected ADRs associated with their products.

Reports of suspected ADRs submitted through the Yellow Card scheme are entered onto a computer database operated by the MHRA. The reporter receives an acknowledgement and is supplied with a unique registration number. Reports of suspected ADRs are regularly reviewed, and appropriate investigation and action is initiated if a possible problem is identified. Information relating to the MHRA and the Yellow Card scheme can be found on the MHRA website (www.mhra.gov.uk) and at www.yellowcard.gov.uk. Information on individual patients and reporters submitted to the MHRA is confidential.

The five regional monitoring centres of the Commission on Human Medicines (CHM) work in conjunction with the MHRA in collecting data on ADRs and facilitating local ADR reporting (see end of chapter).

Which ADRs to report

The success of the Yellow Card scheme depends on early, complete and accurate reporting of suspected ADRs. A Yellow Card should be submitted when a causal association is suspected between the product administered and the condition experienced by the patient. The MHRA encourages reporting of suspected ADRs even if there is uncertainty as to whether the vaccine played a causal role.

All suspected ADRs occurring in children should be reported.

Newly licensed vaccine products are subject to enhanced surveillance and are given 'black triangle' status (indicated by an inverted triangle ▼ on the product information). For such products, all serious and non-serious suspected ADRs should be reported, for both adults and children.

For vaccines that have been marketed for two years or more, only serious suspected ADRs should be reported. This applies to all serious reactions, whether or not such reactions have previously been recognised with the suspected vaccine. Serious reactions that should be reported include those that:

- are fatal
- are life-threatening
- are disabling or incapacitating
- result in or prolong hospitalisation
- are medically significant
- lead to congenital abnormalities.

However, a reporter can also state that a case is serious for any reason other than those outlined here.

When submitting a Yellow Card, the vaccine brand name and batch number should be provided. If the brand name is unavailable, the active ingredient or antigen type should be clearly identified, e.g. pneumococcal conjugate vaccine should be clearly distinguished from plain pneumococcal polysaccharide vaccine.

It is important to give as much information as possible about the nature, timing and severity of the suspected ADR, if the patient was hospitalised, what treatment was given and the outcome. Information about other factors, such as immunisation history, concomitant vaccines, underlying disease, allergies or family history, should be provided whenever possible. The provision of additional information, such as test results or relevant hospital correspondence, is always helpful.

Any further information, including where subsequent investigations implicate another possible cause for the condition, should be sent to the MHRA to help in the assessment of the suspected ADR. The Yellow Card registration number, provided to reporters on acknowledgement of receipt of the Yellow Card, should be quoted. The MHRA may also contact the reporter directly if specific information on a suspected ADR is required.

Deciding whether to report a suspected ADR

It is a matter of clinical judgement whether a suspected ADR should be reported or not. Although a reaction might occur in close temporal association with an immunisation, often it can be very difficult to assess whether there is a causal link. If there is any suspicion that the reaction is vaccine-induced, an ADR should be reported. Many suspected ADRs are actually medical conditions that have occurred spontaneously and coincidentally.

The probability that a vaccine has caused an ADR may be increased if there is biological plausibility for the event. For instance, pyrexial illness occurring five to ten days or parotid swelling occurring three weeks after measles, mumps and rubella (MMR) immunisation would be consistent with the incubation periods for measles or mumps viruses. On the other hand, pyrexia occurring less than three days after MMR vaccination is unlikely to be caused by the immunisation, and an underlying infection is a more likely explanation.

Where to get Yellow Cards

Yellow Cards can be downloaded from the MHRA website (www.mhra.gov.uk) and reports can be submitted electronically (www.yellowcard.gov.uk). Yellow Cards are also available in the back of the *British National Formulary* (BNF), the *BNF for Children*, the *Nurse Prescribers' Formulary*, the Association of the British Pharmaceutical Industry *Compendium of Data Sheets and Summaries of Product Characteristics* and *MIMS for Nurses*.

Yellow Cards can also be obtained by calling the national Yellow Card information service (0800 731 6789) or by writing to the MHRA or one of the five regional centres (see contact details at the end of the chapter).

Causality assessment of potential new vaccine safety signals

Yellow Cards are important in generating possible new signals of safety concerns. When assessing whether a signal generated by Yellow Cards or from other sources is vaccine-induced, all of the available evidence is considered.

Causality assessment often depends on factors that include biological plausibility – an excess of events in a specified post-immunisation period compared with background rates and laboratory evidence.

Formal epidemiological studies are required to strengthen or refute an assessment of causality. Where a causal association is demonstrated, the level of risk should be quantified and the risk factors established. For example, by linking computer records of hospital admissions and MMR immunisation, a positive association was found between MMR and idiopathic thrombocytopenic purpura (ITP). One case of ITP, attributable to vaccine, occurs for every 32,000 doses administered (Miller *et al.*, 2001). Using a similar method, the hypothesis that oral live polio vaccine was associated with intussusception was rejected (Andrews *et al.*, 2001).

Matters relating to vaccine safety are kept under constant review. The CHM and the Joint Committee on Vaccination and Immunisation (JCVI) are independent, expert scientific committees that advise the Government. The CHM advises on the safety, quality and efficacy of medicines and vaccines, and the JCVI provides expert advice on immunisation policy. These committees examine carefully any new evidence that relates to vaccine safety, and make recommendations on the subsequent use of a vaccine or the implementation of the immunisation programme.

Action following evidence about vaccine safety

If the available evidence supports a causal association between a vaccine and a reported ADR, the CHM or JCVI may give recommendations for action. These will take into account an assessment of the balance of benefits of vaccination versus the risks.

Regulatory action may be taken by the MHRA on the recommendation of the CHM. This could involve withdrawal of a vaccine but would more often involve an amendment to a vaccine licence (marketing authorisation) in order to ensure that it is used more safely and effectively. Such amendments may include restrictions on usage, refinement of dosage instructions or the introduction of specific recommendations or warnings in the Summary of Product Characteristics (SPC).

Where further evidence to reject a causal association between a vaccine and a condition becomes available, action may include the removal of previous restrictions or a change to the SPC.

Defective vaccines and batch problems

Defects in medicinal products may include errors in the packaging, labels or leaflets, or other product faults, such as particulate contamination of a vaccine. If healthcare professionals suspect that a vaccine is defective, they should not use the product but contact the Defective Medicines Report Centre (DMRC) of the MHRA (see contact details at the end of the chapter). The DMRC assists in the investigation of defective medicines and co-ordinates any action that may need to be taken.

When submitting reports on suspected defective medicinal products to the DMRC, the following information should be provided:

- brand/non-proprietary name
- name of the manufacturer/supplier
- strength and dosage form
- product licence number
- batch number(s)
- expiry date(s)

- nature of the defect
- an account of any action already taken.

Where the defect is noticed after the vaccine has been administered, advice on the management of that patient should be sought from a local immunisation lead or health protection unit.

Adverse reactions to a vaccine may also result from a defective batch of vaccine (programme-related AEFI) and should be reported to the MHRA.

Defective medical devices

Medical devices and equipment are items used for the diagnosis and/or treatment of disease, or for monitoring patients, as well as aids for daily living. This covers a wide range of products used every day in primary and acute care settings, in residential or nursing settings or in the patient's own home, and by school nurses. Examples of devices relevant to the immunisation programme include needles and syringes, vials or ampoules.

Additional information and examples of categories of medical devices can be found on the 'Devices information' part of the MHRA website (www.mhra.gov.uk). The MHRA assesses all reports of adverse incidents involving medical devices and, where appropriate, instigates an investigation, corrective actions and design changes to reduce the risk of recurrence.

Defects in medical devices may occur because of:

- design or manufacture problems
- poor user instructions and training
- inappropriate local modifications
- inadequate maintenance
- unsuitable storage and use conditions.

A defective medical device may cause unexpected or unwanted effects involving the safety of patients, device users or other persons. Any adverse incident involving a medical device should be reported, especially if the incident has led to or could lead to:

- death or serious injury
- medical or surgical intervention or hospitalisation
- unreliable test results (and risk of misdiagnosis).

Minor faults and discrepancies should also be reported, as these can help to demonstrate trends or highlight inadequate manufacturing or supply systems.

Examples of incidents involving immunisation equipment which should be reported include:

- needles that break in use
- needles that leak or disconnect at the hub
- blocked needles
- barbed or blunt needles
- syringe tips, flanges or plungers that break in use
- contaminated products
- missing components
- visible damage (cracked syringe barrels, etc.).

How to report an incident

Defective devices and adverse incidents should be reported at the earliest opportunity, following any local incident-reporting policies. Adverse events involving immunisation equipment (rather than the vaccine itself) should be reported to the medical devices Adverse Incident Centre (AIC) at the MHRA. If in doubt, contact the MHRA about the most appropriate reporting route.

Where possible, reports should be submitted electronically using the medical device online reporting system on the MHRA's website (www.mhra.gov.uk). This provides an immediate acknowledgement and MHRA reference number for each report, and also allows you to e-mail a copy to others within your organisation. However, if necessary, forms may be downloaded from the website or obtained from the AIC and can be e-mailed or faxed to AIC (see contact details at the end of the chapter). Detailed information on reporting adverse incidents with medical devices can be found on the MHRA website, from the AIC or from your local Medical Device Liaison Officer.

Contact details

Yellow Card reports:

Pharmacovigilance Group
Medicines and Healthcare products Regulatory Agency
Market Towers
1 Nine Elms Lane
London SW8 5NQ

Defective medicines:

The Defective Medicines Report Centre
Medicines and Healthcare products Regulatory Agency
Room 1801, Market Towers
1 Nine Elms Lane
London SW8 5NQ
www.mhra.gov.uk

Tel: 020 7084 2574 (weekdays 9am to 5pm)
or 020 7210 3000 (outside normal working hours)

Defective Devices/Adverse Incident Centre:

Adverse Incident Centre
Medicines and Healthcare products Regulatory Agency
2/2G Market Towers
1 Nine Elms Lane
London SW8 5NQ

E-mail: aic@mhra.gsi.gov.uk
Fax: 020 7084 3109
Incident hotline: 020 7084 3080
Text phone: 020 7084 3356

References

Andrews N, Miller E, Waight P *et al.* (2001) Does oral polio vaccine cause intussusception in infants? Evidence from a sequence of three self-controlled cases series studies in the United Kingdom. *Eur J Epidemiol.* **17**(8): 701–6.

BNF for Children www.bnfc.org.

Miller E, Waight P, Farrington CP *et al.* (2001) Idiopathic thrombocytopenic purpura and MMR vaccine. *Arch Dis Child.* **84**(3): 227–9.

10

Vaccine Damage Payment Scheme

Introduction

The Vaccine Damage Payment Scheme (VDPS) provides a single, tax-free payment. A decision to offer vaccine should be based upon the recommendations in the Green Book and must **not** be influenced by vaccine's eligibility for a VDPS settlement. The VDPS payment is provided to people or their families who have suffered severe mental and/or physical disablement as a result of immunisation against one or more of the following diseases:

- diphtheria
- *Haemophilus influenzae* type b (Hib)
- measles
- meningitis C
- mumps
- pertussis
- pneumococcal
- poliomyelitis
- rubella
- tetanus
- tuberculosis (TB)
- smallpox (up to 1 August 1971).

The scheme also covers those found to be severely disabled because their mother was immunised against any of the specified diseases while she was pregnant, or because they have been in close physical contact with a person who has been immunised with oral poliomyelitis vaccine.

The payment is not compensation but is designed to ease the present and future burdens of the vaccine-damaged person and their family. The amount payable is £100,000 for claims made on or after 22 July 2000.

The decision-making process

Decisions on claims are made on the basis of a medical officer's assessment on behalf of the Secretary of State for Work and Pensions. The medical officer assesses the balance of probability that the disability is the result of the immunisation, and the percentage level of disablement attributed to immunisation. If a claim is disallowed, the claimant may, at any time, request an appeal against the decision of the Secretary of State by an independent vaccine damage tribunal.

The claimant may also request a reversal of the decision of the Secretary of State, or that of the vaccine damage tribunal, by writing to the Vaccine Damage Payments Unit giving an explanation of why they believe the decision to be wrong. Such a request must be received within six years of the date of notification of the Secretary of State's determination, or within two years of the date of notification of the decision of the tribunal, whichever is later.

Time and age limits

The disabled person must be over two years of age and must have been immunised in the UK or the Isle of Man. The scheme also applies to individuals or their families if one or any of the immunisations listed above were given as part of the Armed Forces' medical services outside of the UK.

Claimants must have been immunised before their eighteenth birthday, unless the immunisation was against polio, rubella or meningitis C, for which there is no upper age limit. In addition, individuals of any age are eligible if immunised against any of the other listed diseases during an outbreak within the UK or the Isle of Man.

The claim must be made within six years of the date of vaccination, on or before the disabled person's 21st birthday, or, if they have died, the date on which they would have reached 21 years of age – whichever is the later.

Payments are made direct to disabled persons aged 18 or over who are capable of managing their own affairs. In other cases, payment will be made to trustees. If the disabled person lives with their family, the parents may be appointed as trustees. If the disabled person has died, payment will be made to their personal representative.

The percentage disability test

A widely accepted test prescribed in the Industrial Injuries Scheme is used to assess the percentage of disablement. Under this scheme, 60% disablement equates to, for example, lower leg amputation, loss of one hand or deafness where the individual cannot hear a conversational voice beyond a distance of one metre. A vaccine-relevant example would be paralysis of a limb after oral poliomyelitis vaccine.

Doctors who advise on claims under the VDPS have received special training in disability assessment. This enables them to reach a balanced judgement on the claimant's overall level of disability in comparison to the accepted test used to assess the severity of disablement.

How to claim

Claimants can get a claim form from:

Vaccine Damage Payments Unit
Department for Work and Pensions
Palatine House
Lancaster Road
Preston PR1 1HB

Tel: 01772 899944 or 899756

E-mail: CAU-VDPU@dwp.gsi.gov.uk

The claim form is also available for downloading and printing from the website:

www.direct.gov.uk/DisabledPeople/FinancialSupport/OtherBenefitsandSupport/fs/en

Further information

The leaflet *Vaccine damage payments* provides more information about the VDPS. Copies are available from the Vaccine Damage Payments Unit (see 'How to claim' above) or your local benefits office. You can also obtain more information at www.direct.gov.uk.

11

The UK immunisation programme

Routine childhood immunisation programme

The overall aim of the routine childhood immunisation programme is to protect all children against the following preventable childhood infections:

- diphtheria
- tetanus
- pertussis (whooping cough)
- *Haemophilus influenzae* type b (Hib)
- polio
- meningococcal serogroup C (MenC)
- measles
- mumps
- rubella
- pneumococcal.

The immunisation schedule

The schedule for routine immunisations and instructions for how they should be administered are given in Table 11.1.

Primary immunisation with diphtheria, tetanus, pertussis, polio and Hib (DTaP/IPV/Hib) vaccine is given at two, three and four months of age. Pneumococcal vaccine is given at two and four months. MenC vaccine is given at three and four months. This ensures completion of the primary course at an appropriate age to provide protection against infections such as whooping cough, pneumococcal, Hib and meningococcal serogroup C, which are most dangerous for the very young.

Every effort should be made to ensure that all children are immunised, even if they are older than the recommended age range; no opportunity to immunise should be missed.

If any course of immunisation is interrupted, it should be resumed and completed as soon as possible. There is no need to start any course of immunisation again.

Table 11.1 Schedule for the UK's routine childhood immunisations

When to immunise	What vaccine is given	How it is given
Two months old	Diphtheria, tetanus, pertussis (whooping cough), polio and Hib (DTaP/IPV/Hib)	One injection
	Pneumococcal (PCV)	One injection
Three months old	Diphtheria, tetanus, pertussis (whooping cough), polio and Hib (DTaP/IPV/Hib)	One injection
	MenC	One injection
Four months old	Diphtheria, tetanus, pertussis (whooping cough), polio and Hib (DTaP/IPV/Hib)	One injection
	MenC	One injection
	PCV	One injection
Twelve months old	Hib/MenC	One injection
Around 13 months old	Measles, mumps and rubella (MMR)	One injection
	PCV	One injection
Three years four months to five years old	Diphtheria, tetanus, pertussis and polio (DTaP/IPV or dTaP/IPV)	One injection
	Measles, mumps and rubella (MMR)	One injection
Thirteen to 18 years old	Tetanus, diphtheria and polio (Td/IPV)	One injection

Details of immunisation procedures are given in Chapter 4 and in the relevant disease-specific chapters.

Children should have received these vaccines by these ages:

By four months: Three doses of DTaP/IPV/Hib.
Two doses of PCV and MenC.

By 14 months: A booster dose of Hib/MenC and PCV and the first dose of MMR.

By school entry:	Fourth dose of DTaP/IPV or dTaP/IPV and the second dose of MMR.
Before leaving school:	Fifth dose of Td/IPV.

When babies are immunised in special care units, or children are immunised opportunistically in accident and emergency units or inpatient facilities, it is most important that a record of the immunisation is sent to the primary care trust, NHS trust or health board by return of an 'unscheduled immunisation form'.

Vaccination of children with unknown or incomplete immunisation status

For a variety of reasons, some children may not have been immunised or their immunisation history may be unknown. If children coming to the UK are not known to have been completely immunised, they should be assumed to be unimmunised and a full course of immunisations should be planned.

Where a child born in the UK presents with an inadequate immunisation history, every effort should be made to clarify what immunisations they may have had. A child who has not completed the routine childhood programme should have the outstanding doses as described in the relevant chapters.

Children coming to the UK who have a history of completing immunisation in their country of origin may not have been offered protection against all the antigens currently protected against in the UK. For country-specific information, please refer to www.who.int/immunization_monitoring/en/globalsummary/countryprofileselect.cfm.

Children coming from developing countries, from areas of conflict or from hard-to-reach population groups may not have been fully immunised. Where there is no reliable history of previous immunisation, it should be assumed that children are unimmunised and the full UK recommendations should be followed.

Children coming to the UK may have had a fourth dose of a diphtheria/tetanus/pertussis-containing vaccine that is given at around 18 months in some countries. This dose should be discounted, as it may not provide satisfactory protection until the time of the teenage booster. The routine pre-school and subsequent boosters should be given according to the UK schedule.

Premature infants

It is important that premature infants have their immunisations at the appropriate chronological age, according to the schedule. There is no evidence that premature babies are at increased risk of adverse reactions from vaccines (Slack *et al*., 2001).

Selective childhood immunisation programmes

There are a number of selective childhood immunisation programmes that target children at particular risk of certain diseases, such as hepatitis B, tuberculosis, influenza and pneumococcal. For more information please see the relevant chapters.

Adult immunisation programme

Five doses of diphtheria, tetanus and polio vaccines ensure long-term protection through adulthood. Individuals who have not completed the five doses should have their remaining doses at the appropriate interval. Where there is an unclear history of vaccination, adults should be assumed to be unimmunised. A full course of diphtheria, tetanus and polio should be offered in line with advice contained in the relevant chapters.

Older adults (65 years or older) should be routinely offered a single dose of pneumococcal polysaccharide vaccine, if they have not previously received it. Annual influenza vaccination should also be offered.

Selective vaccines should also be considered for young adults unprotected against diseases including measles, mumps, rubella and meningococcal C. Other vaccinations should be considered for any adult with underlying medical conditions and those at higher risk because of their lifestyle. These vaccinations include Hib, MenC, influenza, pneumococcal and hepatitis B. For more information please see the relevant chapters.

Reference

Slack MH, Schapira D, Thwaites RJ *et al.* (2001) Immune response of premature infants to meningococcal serogroup C and combined diphtheria-tetanus toxoids-acellular pertussis-*Haemophilus influenzae* type b conjugate vaccines. *J Infect Dis* **184** (12): 1617–20.

12

Immunisation of healthcare and laboratory staff

Health and safety at work

Under the Health and Safety at Work Act (HSWA) 1974, employers, employees and the self-employed have specific duties to protect, so far as reasonably practicable, those at work and others who may be affected by their work activity, such as contractors, visitors and patients. Central to health and safety legislation is the need for employers to assess the risks to staff and others.

The Control of Substances Hazardous to Health (COSHH) Regulations 2002 require employers to assess the risks from exposure to hazardous substances, including pathogens (called biological agents in COSHH), and to bring into effect the measures necessary to protect workers and others from those risks as far as is reasonably practicable.

Pre-employment health assessment

All new employees should undergo a pre-employment health assessment, which should include a review of immunisation needs. The COSHH risk assessment will indicate which pathogens staff are exposed to in their workplace, and staff considered to be at risk of exposure to pathogens should be offered routine pre-exposure immunisation as appropriate. This decision should also take into account the safety and efficacy of available vaccines. Staff not considered to be at risk need not routinely be offered immunisation, although post-exposure prophylaxis may occasionally be indicated.

Provision of occupational health immunisations

Employers need to be able to demonstrate that an effective employee immunisation programme is in place, and they have an obligation to arrange and pay for this service. It is recommended that immunisation programmes are managed by occupational health services with appropriately qualified specialists. This chapter deals primarily with the immunisation of healthcare and laboratory staff; other occupations are covered in the relevant chapters.

Immunisation of healthcare and laboratory staff

Any vaccine-preventable disease that is transmissible from person to person poses a risk to both healthcare professionals and their patients. Healthcare workers have a duty of care towards their patients which includes taking reasonable precautions to protect them from communicable diseases. Immunisation of healthcare and laboratory workers may therefore:

- protect the individual and their family from an occupationally-acquired infection
- protect patients and service users, including vulnerable patients who may not respond well to their own immunisation
- protect other healthcare and laboratory staff
- allow for the efficient running of services without disruption.

The most effective method for preventing laboratory-acquired infections is the adoption of safe working practices. Immunisation should never be regarded as a substitute for good laboratory practice, although it does provide additional protection. Staff who work mainly with clinical specimens or have patient contact may be exposed to a variety of infections, while staff who mainly work with specific pathogens are only likely to be exposed to those pathogens handled in their laboratory.

Many employers are directly or indirectly involved in the provision of health-care and other patient services. Employees may be working in general practice, in the NHS, nursing homes or private hospitals and clinics. Full- or part-time permanent and agency staff should also have a health assessment.

Further information on pre-employment health assessments for healthcare staff, record-keeping and the exchange of employee records between hospitals can be found in the Association of National Health Occupational Physicians (ANHOPS) guidelines (ANHOPS, 2004). The health assessment for laboratory staff should take into account the local epidemiology of the disease, the nature of material handled (clinical specimens or cultures of pathogens or both), the frequency of contact with infected or potentially infected material, the laboratory facilities (including containment measures), and the nature and frequency of any patient contact. Staff considered to be at risk of exposure to pathogens should be offered pre-exposure immunisation as appropriate.

Following immunisation, the managers of those at risk of occupational exposure to certain infections, as well as the workers themselves, need to have sufficient information about the outcome of the immunisation to allow appropriate decisions to be made about potential work restrictions and about post-exposure prophylaxis following known or suspected exposure.

Recommendations by staff groups

The objective of occupational immunisation of healthcare and laboratory staff is to protect workers at high risk of exposure and their families, to protect patients and other staff from exposure to infected workers, and to sustain the workforce. Potential exposure to pathogens, and therefore the type of immunisation required, may vary from workplace to workplace. Guidance on the types of immunisation that may be appropriate follows.

Staff involved in direct patient care

This includes staff who have regular clinical contact with patients and who are directly involved in patient care. This includes doctors, dentists, midwives and nurses, paramedics and ambulance drivers, occupational therapists, physiotherapists and radiographers. Students and trainees in these disciplines and volunteers who are working with patients must also be included.

Routine vaccination

All staff should be up to date with their routine immunisations, e.g. tetanus, diphtheria, polio and MMR. The MMR vaccine is especially important in the context of the ability of staff to transmit measles or rubella infections to vulnerable groups. While healthcare workers may need MMR vaccination for their own benefit, they should also be immune to measles and rubella in order to assist in protecting patients. Satisfactory evidence of protection would include documentation of having received two doses of MMR or having had positive antibody tests for measles and rubella.

Selected vaccines

BCG

BCG vaccine is recommended for healthcare workers who may have close contact with infectious patients. It is particularly important to test and immunise staff working in maternity and paediatric departments and departments in which the patients are likely to be immunocompromised, e.g. transplant, oncology and HIV units (see Chapter 32 on TB).

Hepatitis B

Hepatitis B vaccination is recommended for healthcare workers who may have direct contact with patients' blood or blood-stained body fluids. This includes any staff who are at risk of injury from blood-contaminated sharp instruments, or of being deliberately injured or bitten by patients. Antibody titres for hepatitis B should be checked one to four months after the completion of a primary course of vaccine. Such information allows appropriate decisions to be made concerning post-exposure prophylaxis following known or suspected exposure to the virus.

Influenza

Influenza immunisation helps to prevent influenza in staff and may also reduce the transmission of influenza to vulnerable patients. Influenza vaccination is therefore recommended for healthcare workers directly involved in patient care, who should be offered influenza immunisation on an annual basis.

Varicella

Varicella vaccine is recommended for susceptible healthcare workers who have direct patient contact. Those with a definite history of chickenpox or herpes zoster can be considered protected. Healthcare workers with a negative or uncertain history of chickenpox or herpes zoster should be serologically tested and vaccine only offered to those without the varicella zoster antibody.

Non-clinical staff in healthcare settings

This includes non-clinical ancillary staff who may have social contact with patients but are not directly involved in patient care. This group includes receptionists, ward clerks, porters and cleaners.

Routine vaccination

All staff should be up to date with their routine immunisations, e.g. tetanus, diphtheria, polio and MMR. The MMR vaccine is especially important in the context of the ability of staff to transmit measles or rubella infections to vulnerable groups. While healthcare workers may need MMR vaccination for their own benefit, they should also be immune to measles and rubella in order to assist in protecting patients. Satisfactory evidence of protection would include documentation of having received two doses of MMR or having had positive antibody tests for measles and rubella.

Selected vaccines

BCG

BCG vaccine is not routinely recommended for non-clinical staff in healthcare settings.

Hepatitis B

Hepatitis B vaccination is recommended for workers who are at risk of injury from blood-contaminated sharp instruments, or of being deliberately injured or bitten by patients. Antibody titres for hepatitis B should be checked one to four months after the completion of a primary course of vaccine. Such information allows appropriate decisions to be made concerning post-exposure prophylaxis following known or suspected exposure to the virus.

Varicella

Varicella vaccine is recommended for susceptible healthcare workers who have regular patient contact but are not necessarily involved in direct patient care. Those with a definite history of chickenpox or herpes zoster can be considered protected. Healthcare workers with a negative or uncertain history of chickenpox or herpes zoster should be serologically tested and vaccine only offered to those without varicella zoster antibody.

Influenza

Influenza vaccination is not routinely recommended in this group.

Laboratory and pathology staff

This includes laboratory and other staff (including mortuary staff) who regularly handle pathogens or potentially infected specimens. In addition to technical staff, this may include cleaners, porters, secretaries and receptionists in laboratories. Staff working in academic or commercial research laboratories who handle clinical specimens or pathogens should also be included.

Routine vaccination

All staff should be up to date with their routine immunisations, e.g. tetanus, diphtheria, polio and MMR. The MMR vaccine is especially important for those who have contact with patients. Satisfactory evidence of protection would include documentation of having received two doses of MMR or having had positive antibody tests for measles and rubella.

In addition to routine vaccination, staff regularly handling faecal specimens who are likely to be exposed to polio viruses should be offered a booster with a polio-containing vaccine every ten years.

Individuals who may be exposed to diphtheria in microbiology laboratories and clinical infectious disease units should be tested and, if necessary, given a booster dose of a diphtheria-containing vaccine. An antibody test should be performed at least three months after immunisation to confirm protective immunity and the individual should be given a booster dose at ten-year intervals thereafter. The cut-off level is 0.01IU/ml for those in routine diagnostic laboratories. For those handling or regularly exposed to toxigenic strains, a level of 0.1IU/ml should be achieved. Where a history of full diphtheria immunisation is not available, the primary course should be completed and an antibody test should be performed at least three months later to confirm protective immunity. Boosters should be given five years later and subsequently at ten-yearly intervals.

Selected vaccines

BCG

BCG is recommended for technical staff in microbiology and pathology departments, attendants in autopsy rooms and any others considered to be at high risk.

Hepatitis B

Hepatitis B vaccination is recommended for laboratory staff who may have direct contact with patients' blood or blood-stained body fluids or with patients' tissues. Antibody titres for hepatitis B should be checked one to four months after the completion of a primary course of vaccine. Such information allows appropriate decisions to be made concerning post-exposure prophylaxis following known or suspected exposure to the virus.

Staff handling specific organisms

For some infections, the probability that clinical specimens and environmental samples of UK origin contain the implicated organism, and therefore present any risk to staff, is extremely low. For these infections, routine immunisation of laboratory workers is not indicated. Staff handling or conducting research on specific organisms and those working in higher risk settings, such as reference laboratories or infectious disease hospitals, may have a level of exposure sufficient to justify vaccination. The following vaccines are recommended for those who work with the relevant organism and should be considered for those working with related organisms, as well as those in reference laboratories or specialist centres:

- hepatitis A
- Japanese encephalitis
- cholera
- meningococcal ACW135Y
- smallpox

- tick-borne encephalitis
- typhoid
- yellow fever
- influenza
- varicella.

Anthrax vaccine is also recommended for those who work with the organism, or those who handle specimens from potentially infected animals.

Rabies vaccination is recommended for those who work with the virus, or handle specimens from imported primates or other animals that may be infected.

Post-exposure management

Specific additional measures may sometimes be required following an incident where exposure to an infected individual, pathogen or contaminated instrument occurs. Advice should be sought from an occupational health department or from the local microbiologist or other appropriate consultant. Some advice on post-exposure management is contained in the relevant chapters or may be found in relevant guidelines (below).

Reference

Association of National Health Occupational Physicians (2004) *Immunisation of Healthcare Workers* (ANHOPS guidelines). www.anhops.org.uk/guidelines.asp

Further reading

Advisory Committee on Dangerous Pathogens (2005) *Biological agents: managing the risks in laboratories and healthcare premises*. Sunbury: HSE Books www.hse.gov.uk/biosafety/biologagents.pdf

Department of Health and Social Security, Welsh Office (1984) *Vaccination and immunisation policy for NHS staff.* London: HMSO.

Department of Health (1993) *Protecting healthcare workers and patients from hepatitis B: HSG(93)40*. London: Department of Health.

Department of Health (1996) *Addendum to HSG(93)40: Protecting healthcare workers and patients from hepatitis B*. London: Department of Health.

Department of Health (2004) *Guidelines on post-exposure prophylaxis for healthcare workers occupationally exposed to HIV*. www.dh.gov.uk, enter 'HIV post-exposure prophylaxis' in search box.

Health and Safety Commission/Advisory Committee on Dangerous Pathogens (1997) *Infection risks to new and expectant mothers in the workplace: A guide for employers.* Sunbury: HSE Books.

Health and Safety Commission's Health Service Advisory Committee (1993) *The management of occupational health services for healthcare staff.* Sunbury: HSE Books.

Health and Safety Executive (2005) *Control of Substances Hazardous to Health (fifth edition). The Control of Substances Hazardous to Health Regulations 2002 (as amended). Approved Code of Practice and Guidance.* Sunbury: HSE Books www.hsebooks.com/Books.

Health and Safety Executive (1998) *The reporting of injuries, diseases and dangerous occurrences regulations 1995: Guidance for employers in the healthcare sector.* Health Services Information Sheet 1. Sunbury: HSE Books.

Joint Tuberculosis Committee of the British Thoracic Society (1994) Control and prevention of tuberculosis in the United Kingdom: Code of Practice. *Thorax* **49**:1193–200.

NHS Executive HSC 2000/020 *Hepatitis B infected healthcare workers.* London: Department of Health.

NHS Executive HSC 2000/020 *Guidance on implementation of HSC 2000/020.* London: Department of Health.

NHS Executive HSC 2000/020 *Further background information for occupational health departments.* London: Department of Health.

UK Health Departments (1998) *Guidance for clinical health care workers: protection against infection with blood-borne viruses. Recommendations of the Expert Advisory Group on AIDS and the Advisory Group on Hepatitis.* London: Department of Health.

Part 2

The diseases, vaccinations and vaccines

13

Anthrax

NOTIFIABLE

The disease

Anthrax is a bacterial disease which primarily affects herbivorous animals, although all mammals are susceptible to infection. In humans, anthrax can affect the skin and, rarely, the respiratory or gastro-intestinal tract. It is caused by the aerobic bacillus, *Bacillus anthracis,* and is spread by spores. Spores can be found in animal products such as wool, hair, hides, skins, bones, bonemeal and in the carcasses of infected animals. The spores can also contaminate soil and may survive for many years.

The incubation period is usually 48 hours but can be up to seven days. In cutaneous anthrax, a lesion appears on the skin and develops into a characteristic ulcer with a black centre. Inhalational anthrax begins with a flu-like illness and is followed by respiratory compromise and shock around two to six days later. Intestinal anthrax results in severe abdominal pain, fever and bloody diarrhoea.

Anthrax can be treated effectively with antibiotics if identified early. If untreated, the infection can cause septicaemia, toxaemia or meningitis, and is fatal in around 5% of cases.

In the UK, human anthrax is rare, and is almost entirely an occupational disease affecting those handling imported infected animal products or working with infected animals (see Table 13.1). Prevention depends on controlling anthrax in livestock and on disinfecting, washing and scouring imported animal products. Processing of hides, wool and bone by tanning, dyeing, carbonising or acid treatment also reduces the risk of infection. Bonemeal used as horticultural fertiliser may rarely contain anthrax spores when not correctly treated in the country of origin; a certificate of sterilisation should accompany any consignment on entry to the UK. Those handling bonemeal in bulk should wear impervious gloves that should be destroyed after use.

Table 13.1 Anthrax: reported cases by occupation 1975–96

Occupations	Number of cases
Slaughterhouse/abattoir worker	7
Tannery/leather worker	5
Farmer/farm worker	2
Butcher	2
Engineer	1
Textile worker	1
Bonemeal worker	1

Source: Health and Safety Executive, 1997.

Anthrax spores have been used as biological weapons, most recently reported in the USA (Plotkin and Orenstein, 2004). Guidance on assessment and management of this type of risk is not included in this chapter and can be found elsewhere (www.hpa.org.uk).

History and epidemiology of the disease

Anthrax is well documented in ancient historical texts and has been a notifiable disease in the UK since 1895. Vaccination for UK workers at risk was first introduced in 1965 and limited studies suggest that vaccination provides good protection against occupationally acquired infection (Plotkin and Orenstein, 2004). In the period 1961–80, there was a decrease in the number of reported cases. Human anthrax is uncommon in the UK with only a handful of cases being notified over the last decade.

Human infections occur in countries where the disease is common in animals including those in the Southern and Central Americas, Southern and Eastern Europe, Asia and Africa.

The anthrax vaccination

The vaccine is made from antigens found in the sterile filtrate from cultures of the Sterne strain of *B. anthracis*. These antigens are adsorbed onto an aluminium adjuvant to improve their immunogenicity and are preserved with thiomersal.

The vaccine is inactivated, does not contain live organisms and cannot cause the disease against which it protects.

There have been no formal efficacy trials with the UK vaccine. In 1958, the introduction of vaccine successfully controlled cutaneous anthrax at a government wool-disinfecting station in Liverpool (Hambleton *et al.*, 1984). A controlled clinical trial was carried out in the 1950s among workers in goat-hair mills in New Hampshire, USA, using a vaccine similar to that currently licensed in the USA and the UK (Brachman *et al.*, 1962). Although the study did not have sufficient power to accurately measure protection against pulmonary anthrax, no cases occurred in the vaccinated group compared with five in the unvaccinated.

There have been no recorded cases of anthrax infection in individuals vaccinated in the UK.

Storage

Vaccines should be stored in the original packaging at +2˚C to +8˚C and protected from light. All vaccines are sensitive to some extent to heat and cold. Heat speeds up the decline in potency of most vaccines, thus reducing their shelf life. Effectiveness cannot be guaranteed for vaccines unless they have been stored at the correct temperature. Freezing may cause increased reactogenicity and loss of potency for some vaccines. It can also cause hairline cracks in the container, leading to contamination of the contents.

Presentation

Anthrax vaccine is presented as a suspension ready for injection, which should be shaken before administration.

Dosage and schedule

- First dose of 0.5ml on day 0.
- Second dose of 0.5ml, at least three weeks after the first dose.
- Third dose of 0.5ml at least three weeks after the second dose.
- Fourth dose of 0.5ml at least six months after the third dose.

Administration

The vaccine is given by intramuscular injection, preferably into the upper arm. However, individuals with a bleeding disorder should be given the vaccine by deep subcutaneous injection to reduce the risk of bleeding.

Anthrax vaccine can be given at the same time as other vaccines. The vaccines should be given at separate sites, preferably in a different limb. If given in the same limb, they should be given at least 2.5cm apart (American Academy of Pediatrics, 2003). The site at which each vaccine is given and the batch numbers of the vaccines should be recorded in the individual's records. It is recommended that the employer keeps a vaccination record.

Disposal

Equipment used for vaccination, including used vials or ampoules, should be disposed of at the end of a session by sealing in a proper, puncture-resistant 'sharps' box (UN-approved, BS 7320).

Recommendations for the use of the vaccine

The objective of the anthrax vaccination is to provide a minimum of four doses at appropriate intervals for individuals at high risk of occupational exposure.

Occupations dealing with infected animals

Workers dealing with infected animals where there may be a risk of occupationally acquired anthrax include:

- farm workers, e.g. livestock breeders/keepers, shepherds, dairy workers – from skin contact with, or inhalation of, spores from diseased animals, or during disposal of infected carcasses and slurry
- veterinary surgeons – from treatment of infected animals
- local authority workers – from disposal of infected carcasses
- zoo keepers – as above
- abattoir workers/butchers – from exposure to anthrax spores during preparation of animals for food and food products
- construction workers – people working in old buildings may be exposed to animal material, e.g. hair containing anthrax spores
- laboratory workers – people working in laboratories that handle specimens from infected animals and/or humans.

Occupations involving processing of infected animal material

A variety of industrial processes present situations where workers may be at risk of acquiring anthrax. These include those who work with/in:

- certain textiles, e.g. goat hair, wool
- leather, e.g. importers, tanners
- rendering, e.g. glue, gelatin, tallow, bone processing
- storage and distribution, e.g. docks, warehousing or transport of any of the above.

Guidance on the risk of occupational exposure to infected animals or animal products is available from the Health and Safety Executive (1997).

Primary immunisation

The primary course of anthrax vaccination consists of four doses. Three doses of 0.5ml are given with an interval of three weeks between each dose. The fourth dose is given six months after the third dose.

Reinforcing immunisation

A reinforcing dose of 0.5ml should be given annually to those at continued risk.

Contraindications

There are very few individuals who cannot receive anthrax vaccine. Where there is doubt and there is clear risk of infection, further advice can be obtained from the Health Protection Agency, Porton Down. The vaccine should not be given to those who have had:

- a confirmed anaphylactic reaction to a previous dose of anthrax vaccine, or
- a confirmed anaphylactic reaction to any of the components of the vaccine.

With the exception of confirmed anaphylaxis, it may be possible to continue the immunisation course where there is a history of other allergic reactions (such as rashes). Non-allergic local or general reactions to a previous dose of vaccine do not contraindicate further doses. Specialist advice must be sought from the Health Protection Agency, Porton Down.

Precautions

Minor illnesses without fever or systemic upset are not valid reasons to postpone immunisation.

Unless protection is needed urgently, immunisation may be postponed in acutely unwell individuals until they have fully recovered. This is to avoid wrongly attributing any new symptom or the progression of symptoms to the vaccine.

Pregnancy and breast-feeding

Anthrax vaccine may be given to pregnant women when clinically indicated. There is no evidence of risk from vaccinating pregnant women or those who are breast-feeding with inactivated viral or bacterial vaccines or toxoids (Plotkin and Orenstein, 2004).

Immunosuppression and HIV infection

Individuals with immunosuppression and HIV infection (regardless of CD4 count) should be given anthrax vaccine if indicated. These individuals may not make a full antibody response. Specialist advice may be required.

Further guidance is provided by the Royal College of Paediatrics and Child Health (www.rcpch.ac.uk), the British HIV Association (BHIVA) *Immunisation guidelines for HIV-infected adults* (BHIVA, 2006) and the Children's HIV Association of UK and Ireland (CHIVA) immunisation guidelines (www.bhiva.org/chiva).

Adverse reactions

Pain, swelling or redness at the injection site are common and may last for two or more days. Such reactions have been reported to occur at the site of a previous anthrax injection. Regional lymphadenopathy, mild febrile reactions, flu-like symptoms, urticaria or other allergic reactions occur less commonly. Local or general reactions to the first injection are not good predictors of reactions to second or subsequent doses.

All serious suspected adverse reactions to vaccines in adults should be reported to the Commission on Human Medicines through the Yellow Card scheme.

Management of suspected cases and exposure

All cases of anthrax must be notified. An attempt should be made to confirm the diagnosis bacteriologically and the source of infection should be investigated. Transmission from person to person is very rare and, therefore, neither quarantine nor vaccination are used to control spread. Ciprofloxacin is the treatment of choice. Skin lesions should be covered; any discharge or soiled articles should be disinfected.

Guidance on exposure to potentially infected material is available on the Health Protection Agency website. Antibiotic prophylaxis and post-exposure vaccination may be recommended (www.hpa.org.uk/infections/topics_az/anthrax/menu.htm).

Supplies

Anthrax vaccine is available from:
Health Protection Agency (Porton Down) (Tel: 01980 612100).

Scotland:
Borders General Hospital (Tel: 01896 826000).
Hairmyres Hospital (Tel: 01355 585000).

Northern Ireland:
Public Health Laboratory, Belfast City Hospital (Tel: 028 9026 3765).

References

American Academy of Pediatrics (2003) Active immunization. In: Pickering LK (ed.) *Red Book: 2003 Report of the Committee on Infectious Diseases,* 26th edition. Elk Grove Village, IL: American Academy of Pediatrics, p 33.

Brachman PS, Gold H, Plotkin SA *et al.* (1962) Field evaluation of a human anthrax vaccine. *Am J Public Health* **52**: 632–45.

British HIV Association (2006) *Immunisation guidelines for HIV-infected adults:* www.bhiva.org/pdf/2006/Immunisation506.pdf.

Hambleton P, Carman A and Melling K (1984) Anthrax: the disease in relation to vaccines. *Vaccine* **2**: 125–32.

Health and Safety Executive (1997) *Anthrax. Safe working and the prevention of infection, HSG174.* Available from HSE Books at www.hsebooks.com or 01787 881165.

Plotkin SA and Orenstein WA (eds) (2004) *Vaccines,* 4th edition. Philadelphia: WB Saunders Company.

14

Cholera

NOTIFIABLE

The disease

Cholera is an acute diarrhoeal illness caused by the gram-negative bacterium *Vibrio cholerae*. Following colonisation of the small bowel, *V. cholerae* produces an enterotoxin that causes secretion of fluid and electrolytes and leads to painless, watery diarrhoea. Cholera is characterised by the sudden onset of profuse, watery stools with occasional vomiting. In severe disease, dehydration, metabolic acidosis and circulatory collapse may follow rapidly. Untreated, over 50% of the most severe cases die within a few hours of onset; with prompt, correct treatment, mortality is less than 1%. Mild cases with only moderate diarrhoea also occur and asymptomatic infection is common. The incubation period is usually between two and five days but may be only a few hours.

The disease is mainly water-borne through ingestion of faecally contaminated water or shellfish and other foods. Person-to-person spread may occur through the faecal–oral route. The risk to travellers even in infected areas is very small.

Cholera serogroup O1 is classified by biotype (classical or El Tor) and is further divided into subtypes (Ogawa or Inaba). Worldwide, *V. cholerae* El Tor is currently the predominant biotype and Ogawa the predominant subtype.

History and epidemiology of the disease

The last indigenous case of cholera in England and Wales was reported in 1893. Occasional imported cases occur, but the risk of an outbreak is very small in countries with modern sanitation and water supplies, and high standards of food hygiene. In England, Wales and Northern Ireland, 126 laboratory notifications of cholera from 1990 through to 2001 were reported (Lawrence and Jones, 2004). Of these, 64% were imported from the Indian subcontinent. Cholera due to the classical biotype of *V. cholerae* was endemic in the Ganges Delta of West Bengal and Bangladesh during the last two centuries and caused epidemics and global pandemics. The seventh global pandemic, which started in 1961, is due to the El Tor biotype and is now widespread in Asia and Africa; Central and South America were affected in the early and mid-1990s but have largely brought the disease under control. A new serogroup of *V. cholerae* (O139), which produces similar symptoms, emerged in the Bay of Bengal in the early 1990s, is present in South-East Asia and China, and is responsible for about 15% of reported cholera cases in these regions (World Health Organization, 2004).

In 2003, 45 countries officially reported to the World Health Organization (WHO) 111,575 cases of cholera and 1,894 deaths (WHO, 2004), an overall case–fatality ratio (CFR) of 1.7%. In certain vulnerable groups and high-risk areas, the CFR reached as high as 41%. These reports of cases and deaths are considered to grossly underestimate the actual numbers due to under-reporting and the limitations of surveillance systems. Countries in Africa (particularly the Democratic Republic of Congo, Liberia, Mozambique, Somalia and Uganda) accounted for 96% of reported cases in 2003.

Prevention of cholera depends primarily on improving sanitation and water supplies in endemic areas and on scrupulous personal and food and water hygiene. While new oral cholera vaccines can provide individual protection against *V. cholerae* O1, their role in endemic and outbreak conditions is not yet defined (WHO, 2004). Since 1973, when the WHO removed cholera vaccination from the International Health Regulations, there has been no requirement for cholera vaccination for travel between countries (WHO, 1983).

The only cholera vaccine licensed in the UK since May 2004 is Dukoral®, a killed *V. cholerae* whole-cell (WC) vaccine with recombinant B subunit of cholera toxin (rCTB), administered orally. Intramuscular cholera vaccines are no longer recommended for use.

The whole-cell, B subunit vaccine (WC-rCTB, which used purified cholera toxin prior to the development of recombinant cholera toxin) has been evaluated for protective efficacy in trials in Bangladesh and Peru. In the trials in Bangladesh, three doses of vaccine demonstrated 85% protective efficacy (95% confidence interval 56%–94%) at six months in children aged two to 15 years and in women over the age of 15 (Clemens *et al.*, 1986; Clemens *et al.*, 1990).

The protective efficacy of the vaccine when given to children aged two to five years waned rapidly so that, by 36 months after administration, the cumulative protective efficacy was 26%, compared with children and adults over the age of five years in whom it was 63%. From this data, adults require two doses of vaccine and a reinforcing dose after two years. Young children require three doses of vaccine to establish effective immunity (Clemens *et al.*, 1987) with a reinforcing dose after six months.

A trial in Peru using two doses of vaccine (WC-rCTB) in young adult military recruits demonstrated 86% protective efficacy (95% confidence interval, 36%–97%) at about four months (Sánchez *et al.*, 1994). This trial followed an earlier trial in Peru which did not reach as high a level of protection (Taylor *et al.*, 2000). In a challenge study with North American volunteers, three doses of WC-rCTB provided 64% protection (Black *et al.*, 1987).

The cholera vaccination

Oral, killed cholera vaccine (Dukoral®) is the only licensed cholera vaccine available in the UK. It contains 1mg of recombinant cholera toxin B (rCTB) in a liquid suspension of four strains of killed *V. cholerae* O1, representing subtypes Inaba and Ogawa and biotypes El Tor and classical (25×10^9 bacteria in each batch). This suspension is mixed with buffer and water as indicated below.

The vaccine is thiomersal-free. It is inactivated, does not contain live organisms and cannot cause the disease against which it protects. It does not contain the A subunit of the cholera toxin which is responsible for the pathogenicity of the toxin.

Storage

Vaccines should be stored in the original packaging at +2°C to +8°C and protected from light. All vaccines are sensitive to some extent to heat and cold. Heat speeds up the decline in potency of most vaccines, thus reducing their shelf life. Effectiveness cannot be guaranteed for vaccines unless they have been stored at the correct temperature. Freezing may cause increased reactogenicity and loss of potency for some vaccines. It can also cause hairline cracks in the container, leading to contamination of the contents.

Presentation

Oral cholera vaccine is supplied as approximately 3ml of a whitish suspension in a glass vial. A sachet of sodium hydrogen carbonate as white granules is also supplied and should be mixed with water as described below (see Figure 14.1).

Dosage and schedule

Adults and children over six years of age

- First dose of vaccine on day 0.
- Second dose between one and six weeks after the first dose.

Each dose of vaccine should be dissolved in 150ml of the prepared buffer solution.

For continuous protection, a booster dose should be given at the appropriate interval (see page 105).

Children two to six years of age

- First dose of vaccine on day 0.
- Second dose between one and six weeks after the first dose.
- Third dose between one and six weeks after the second dose.

Each dose of vaccine should be dissolved in 75ml of the prepared buffer solution.

Administration

Food and drink should be avoided for one hour before and one hour after vaccination. Oral administration of other medicinal products should be avoided within one hour before and after administration of the vaccine.

The buffer of sodium hydrogen carbonate is supplied as effervescent granules, which should be dissolved in approximately 150ml of cool water in a disposable plastic cup. For children aged two to six years, half of the buffer solution should then be discarded. For children over six years of age and adults, the whole 150ml of buffer solution should be used (see Figure 14.1).

The appropriate volume of the solution should then be mixed with the whitish vaccine suspension to obtain a colourless, slightly opalescent fluid. The vaccine must be drunk within two hours of reconstitution.

Cholera vaccine can be given at the same time as injected vaccines.

Disposal

Equipment used for vaccination, including used vials or ampoules, should be disposed of at the end of a session by sealing in a proper, puncture-resistant 'sharps' box (UN-approved, BS 7320). The plastic cup can be disposed of in a yellow, clinical waste bag.

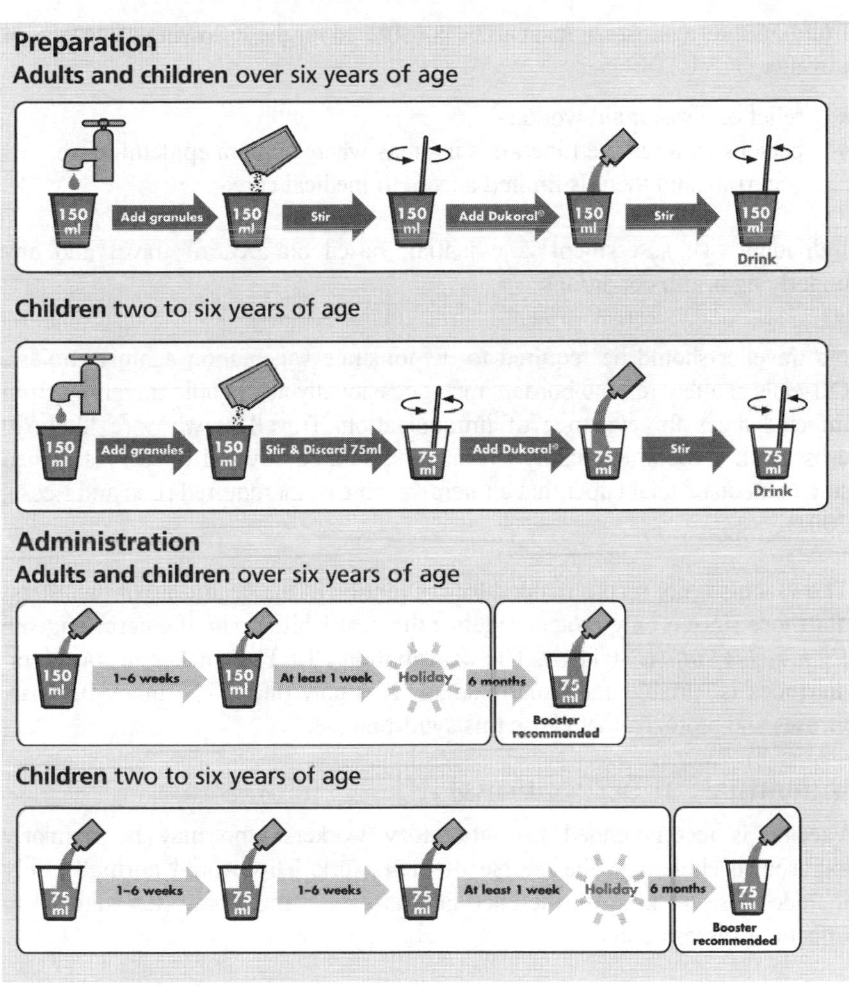

Figure 14.1 Preparation and administration of oral cholera vaccine

Recommendations for the use of the vaccine

The objective of the cholera immunisation programme is to protect those who are most at risk of serious illness or death from the disease. Cholera vaccine is indicated for active immunisation against disease caused by *V. cholerae* serogroup O1 in adults and child travellers from two years of age who are considered at risk for cholera. General estimates of travellers' risk of cholera based on imported cases into Europe and North America are in the order of two to three per million travellers (Mahon *et al.*, 1996; Morger *et al.*, 1983; Wittlinger *et al.*, 1995; Sánchez and Taylor, 1997).

Immunisation against cholera can be considered for the following categories of traveller (JCVI, 2004):

- relief or disaster aid workers
- persons with remote itineraries in areas where cholera epidemics are occurring and there is limited access to medical care.

Individual risk assessment is essential, based on area of travel and any underlying health conditions.

No traveller should be required to demonstrate vaccination against cholera. Officials at a few remote borders may occasionally ask people travelling from infected areas for evidence of immunisation. Travellers who are likely to cross such borders, especially overland, should be advised to carry a signed statement on official paper that cholera vaccine is not required (Lea and Leese, 2001).

The vaccine is not recommended for prevention of the syndrome of travellers' diarrhoea since it only protects against the heat-labile toxin of enterotoxigenic *Escherichia coli* (LT-ETEC). The contribution LT-ETEC makes in travellers' diarrhoea is variable and usually small. It is only one of the many bacteria, viruses and protozoa that cause this syndrome.

Individuals at occupational risk

Vaccine is recommended for laboratory workers who may be regularly exposed to cholera in the course of their work. This would normally only include those working in reference laboratories or in laboratories attached to infectious disease units.

Primary immunisation

The primary course of the immunisation must be restarted if more than six weeks have elapsed between the first and second doses or if more than two years have elapsed since the last vaccination. These recommendations are unique to this vaccine.

Adults and children over six years of age

The standard primary course of vaccination with this vaccine against cholera consists of two doses with an interval of at least one week but less than six weeks between doses.

Children two to six years of age

The standard primary course of vaccination with this vaccine against cholera consists of three doses with an interval of at least one week but less than six weeks between doses.

If more than six weeks have elapsed between doses, the primary immunisation course should be restarted.

Immunisation should be completed at least one week prior to potential exposure to *V. cholerae* O1.

Children under two years of age

The protective efficacy of this cholera vaccine in children between one and two years of age has not been studied. Therefore, cholera vaccine is not recommended for children under two years of age.

Reinforcing immunisation

For continuous protection against cholera, a single booster dose is recommended two years after completing the primary course for adults and children over six years of age, and after six months for children aged two to six years. No clinical efficacy data have been generated on repeat booster dosing.

If more than two years have elapsed since the last vaccination, the primary course should be repeated. The need to repeat a primary course of the immunisation is unique to this vaccine.

No clinical data are available on the protective efficacy of this vaccine against cholera after administration of booster doses.

Contraindications

There are very few individuals who cannot receive oral cholera vaccine when it is recommended. Where there is doubt, appropriate advice should be sought from a travel health specialist.

The vaccine should not be given to those who have had:

- a confirmed anaphylactic reaction to a previous dose of oral cholera vaccine, or
- a confirmed anaphylactic reaction to formaldehyde or any of the components of the vaccine.

Precautions

Minor illnesses without fever or systemic upset are not valid reasons to postpone immunisation.

If an individual is acutely unwell, immunisation may be postponed until they have fully recovered. This is to avoid confusing the differential diagnosis of any acute illness by wrongly attributing any signs or symptoms to the adverse effects of the vaccine.

Cholera vaccine confers protection specific to *V. cholerae* serogroup O1. Immunisation does not protect against *V. cholerae* serogroup O139 or other species of *Vibrio*. Vaccination is not a substitute for adhering to standard protective hygiene measures to avoid cholera.

Vaccination should be delayed in individuals suffering from acute gastro-intestinal illness. Pre-existing gastro-intestinal disorders are not a contraindication to giving the vaccine.

Pregnancy and breast-feeding

No data are available on the safety of oral cholera vaccine in pregnant or breast-feeding women. There is no evidence of risk from vaccinating pregnant women or those who are breast-feeding with inactivated viral or bacterial vaccines or toxoids (Plotkin and Orenstein, 2004). If the risk of cholera is high then the vaccine should be considered in these circumstances.

Immunosuppression and HIV infection

Individuals with immunosuppression or with HIV infection (regardless of CD4 counts) should be considered for cholera vaccination in accordance with the recommendations above. However, these individuals may not develop a full antibody response if they are immunosuppressed, and vaccine protective efficacy has not been studied. Specialist advice may be required.

Further guidance is provided by the Royal College of Paediatrics and Child Health (www.rcpch.ac.uk), the British HIV Association (BHIVA) *Immunisation guidelines for HIV-infected adults* (BHIVA, 2006) and the Children's HIV Association of UK and Ireland (CHIVA) immunisation guidelines (www.bhiva.org/chiva).

Adverse reactions

Adverse events described in trials comparing individuals taking oral cholera vaccine with those ingesting buffer without the vaccine were comparable and in the range of 11% to 14% (Sánchez *et al.*, 1997).

More than 1 million doses of this vaccine have been sold in Sweden and Norway. Based on passive reporting from clinical trials and post-marketing surveillance, mild gastro-intestinal symptoms (abdominal pain, cramping, diarrhoea, nausea) are the most commonly reported symptoms occurring at a frequency of 0.1% to 1%. Serious adverse events, including a flu-like syndrome, rash, arthralgia and paraesthesiae are rare, occurring in fewer than one per 10,000 doses distributed (Summary of Product Characteristics, 2004).

Management of cases, contacts and outbreaks

As cholera is a notifiable disease in the UK, for public health management of cases, contacts and outbreaks, all suspected cases should be notified to the local health protection unit immediately. Sources of infection should be identified and treated appropriately. Contacts of patients with cholera should maintain high standards of personal hygiene to avoid becoming infected. In the UK, cholera vaccine has no role in the management of contacts of cases or in controlling the spread of infection; control of the disease depends on public health measures.

Supplies

Dukoral® oral, killed cholera vaccine is supplied by Novartis Vaccines (Tel: 08457 451500).

References

Black RE, Levine MM, Clements ML *et al.* (1987) Protective efficacy in humans of killed whole-vibrio oral cholera vaccine with and without the B subunit of cholera toxin. *Infect Immun* **55**: 1116–20.

British HIV Association (2006) *Immunisation guidelines for HIV-infected adults:* www.bhiva.org/pdf/2006/Immunisation506.pdf.

Clemens JD, Sack DA, Harris JR *et al.* (1986) Field trial of oral cholera vaccines in Bangladesh. *Lancet* **2**: 124–7.

Clemens JD, Stanton BF, Chakraborty J *et al.* (1987) B subunit-whole-cell and whole-cell-only oral vaccines against cholera: studies on reactogenicity and immunogenicity. *J Infect Dis* **155**: 79–85.

Clemens JD, Sack DA, Harris JR *et al.* (1990) Field trial of oral cholera vaccines in Bangladesh: results from three-year follow-up. *Lancet* **1**: 270–3.

Joint Committee on Vaccination and Immunisation. Minutes from the Joint Committee of Vaccination and Immunisation meeting: 4 June 2004. (www.advisorybodies.doh.gov.uk/jcvi/mins040604.htm).

Lawrence J and Jones J (eds) (2004) *Illness in England, Wales, and Northern Ireland associated with foreign travel.* London: Health Protection Agency.

Lea G and Leese J (eds) (2001) *Health information for overseas travel.* London: The Stationery Office.

Mahon BE, Mintz ED, Greene KD *et al.*, (1996) Reported cholera in the United States, 1992–1994. *JAMA* **276**: 307–12.

Morger H, Steffen R and Schär M (1983) Epidemiology of cholera in travellers, and conclusions for vaccination recommendations. *BMJ* **286**: 184–6.

Novartis Vaccines (2004) *Summary of Product Characteristics.* Dukoral®. Oxford: Novartis Vaccines.

Plotkin SA and Orenstein WA (eds) (2004) *Vaccines,* 4th edition. Philadelphia: WB Saunders Company.

Sánchez JL, Trofa AF, Taylor DN *et al.* (1993) Safety and immunogenicity of the oral, whole-cell/recombinant-B-subunit cholera vaccine in North American volunteers. *J Infect Dis* **167**: 1446–9.

Sánchez JL, Vasquez B, Begue RE *et al.* (1994) Protective efficacy of oral whole-cell/recombinant-B-subunit cholera vaccine in Peruvian military recruits. *Lancet* **344**: 1273–6.

Sánchez JL and Taylor DN (1997) Cholera. *Lancet* **349**: 1825–30.

Taylor DN, Cardenas V, Sánchez JL *et al.* (2000) Two-year study of the protective efficacy of the oral whole-cell plus recombinant-B-subunit cholera vaccine in Peru. *J Infect Dis* **181**: 1667–73.

Wittlinger F, Steffen R, Watanabe H and Handszuh H (1995) Risk of cholera among Western and Japanese travelers. *Journal of Travel Medicine* **2**: 154–8.

World Health Organization (1983) *International health regulations 1969.* Geneva: WHO.

WHO (2004) Cholera, 2003. *Weekly Epidemiological Record* 2004; **79**: 281–8.

15

Diphtheria

NOTIFIABLE

The disease

Diphtheria is an acute infectious disease affecting the upper respiratory tract, and occasionally the skin, caused by the action of diphtheria toxin produced by toxigenic *Corynebacterium diphtheriae* or by *Corynebacterium ulcerans*. The most characteristic features of diphtheria affecting the upper respiratory tract are a membranous pharyngitis (often referred to as a pseudo-membrane) with fever, enlarged anterior cervical lymph nodes and oedema of soft tissue giving a 'bull neck' appearance. The pseudo-membrane may cause respiratory obstruction. In the UK, the classical disease is now very rare and clinicians may not recognise it. Milder infections (without toxin production) resemble streptococcal pharyngitis and the pseudo-membrane may not develop, particularly in vaccinated individuals. Carriers may be asymptomatic. Diphtheria toxin affects the myocardium, nervous and adrenal tissues, causing paralysis and cardiac failure.

The incubation period is from two to five days. Patients with untreated disease may be infectious for up to four weeks, but carriers may potentially transmit the infection for longer. Transmission of the infection is by droplet and through contact with articles (such as clothing or bed linen) soiled by infected persons.

In countries where hygiene is poor, cutaneous diphtheria is the predominant clinical manifestation and source of infection. The normal reservoir of *C. ulcerans* is cattle. Infections in humans are associated with the consumption of raw dairy products and contact with animals. Person-to-person spread cannot be ruled out, although it is probably uncommon (Bonnet and Begg, 1999).

There is little likelihood of developing natural immunity from sub-clinical infection acquired in the UK. Based on sero-surveillance studies, approximately 50% of UK adults over 30 years are susceptible to diphtheria. The proportion susceptible increases to over 70% in older age cohorts (Edmunds *et al.*, 2000). High immunisation uptake must be maintained in order to prevent the resurgence of disease which could follow the introduction of cases or carriers of toxigenic strains from overseas.

History and epidemiology of the disease

Prior to the 1940s, diphtheria was a common disease in the UK. The introduction of immunisation against diphtheria on a national scale during the 1940s resulted in a dramatic fall in the number of notified cases and deaths from the disease. In 1940, more than 61,000 cases with 3,283 deaths were notified in the UK, compared with 38 cases and six deaths in 1957 (see Figure 15.1).

From 1986 to 2002, 56 isolates of toxigenic *C. diphtheriae* and 47 isolates of toxigenic *C. ulcerans* were identified in England and Wales by the Health Protection Agency (HPA) Streptococcus and Diphtheria Reference Unit (formerly the Public Health Laboratory Service). Of these, eight patients with *C. diphtheriae* infection and six patients with *C. ulcerans* presented with classical pharyngeal diphtheria: the remainder had mild pharyngitis or were asymptomatic. Two deaths from diphtheria occurred between 1986 and 2002: in 1994 an unvaccinated 14-year-old died with a *C. diphtheriae* infection following a visit to Pakistan, and in 2000 an elderly woman died with a *C. ulcerans* infection acquired in the UK.

An increase in notifications of diphtheria since 1992 has been due to a rise in isolations of non-toxigenic strains of *C. diphtheriae* which do not cause classical diphtheria disease (Reacher *et al.*, 2000). These may be associated with a mild sore throat without signs of toxicity.

Diphtheria cases continue to be reported in South-East Asia, South America, Africa and India. A large number of UK citizens travel to and from these regions, maintaining the possibility of the reintroduction of *C. diphtheriae* into the UK. Most cases of diphtheria that have occurred in recent years in the UK have been imported from the Indian subcontinent or from Africa; four cases of cutaneous diphtheria were reported in travellers returning in 2002 (De Benoist *et al.*, 2004). Secondary cases are rare but do occur in the UK.

There was a resurgence of diphtheria in the former Soviet Union, starting with an initial peak in the 1980s and followed by a larger epidemic from 1990 (Dittmann *et al.*, 2000). The epidemic rapidly disseminated, affecting all newly independent states, and peaked in 1994–95. From 1990 to 1998, more than 157,000 cases and 5000 deaths had been reported to the World Health Organization (WHO) (Dittmann *et al.*, 2000). This epidemic was caused by low immunisation coverage in young children, waning immunity in adults and large-scale population movements. Several importations of diphtheria occurred from former Soviet Union countries into Western Europe, including one case into the UK in 1997 (CDR, 1997).

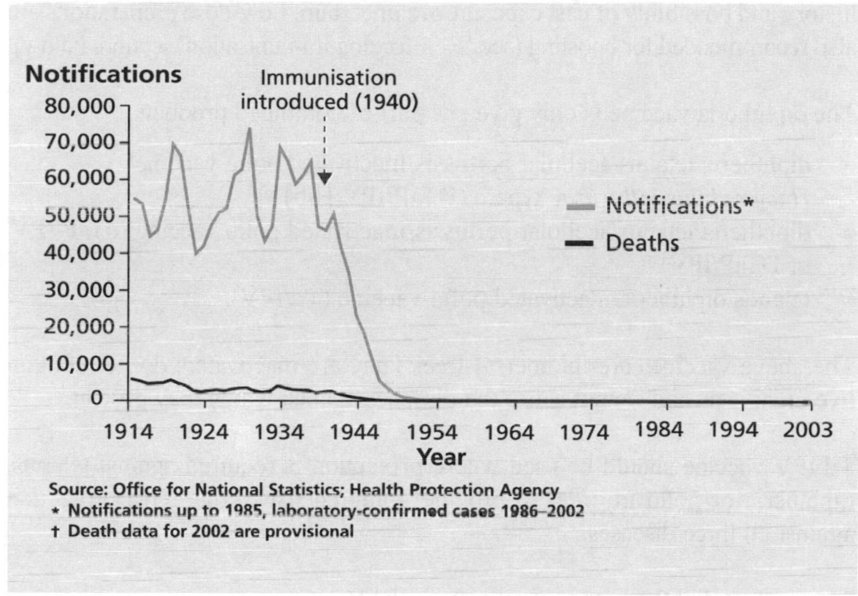

Figure 15.1 Diphtheria cases and deaths, England and Wales (1914–2003)

The diphtheria vaccination

The vaccine is made from a cell-free purified toxin extracted from a strain of *C. diphtheriae*. This is treated with formaldehyde, which converts it into diphtheria toxoid. This is adsorbed on to an adjuvant – either aluminium phosphate or aluminium hydroxide – to improve its immunogenicity.

Diphtheria vaccines are produced in two strengths according to the diphtheria toxoid content:

- vaccines containing the higher dose of diphtheria toxoid (abbreviated to 'D') contain not less than 30IU
- vaccines containing the lower dose of diphtheria toxoid (abbreviated to 'd') contain approximately 2IU.

Vaccines containing the higher dose of diphtheria toxoid (D) are used to achieve satisfactory primary immunisation of children under ten years of age. Vaccines containing the lower dose of diphtheria toxoid (d) should be used for primary immunisation in individuals aged ten years or over, where they provide a satisfactory immune response and the risk of reactions is minimised. This precautionary advice is particularly pertinent when the early immunisation history and possibility of past exposure are uncertain. Low-dose preparations are also recommended for boosting (see 'Reinforcing immunisation' section, below).

The diphtheria vaccine is only given as part of combined products:

- diphtheria/tetanus/acellular pertussis/inactivated polio vaccine/ *Haemophilus influenzae* type b (DTaP/IPV/Hib)
- diphtheria/tetanus/acellular pertussis/inactivated polio vaccine (dTaP/IPV or DTaP/IPV)
- tetanus/diphtheria/inactivated polio vaccine (Td/IPV).

The above vaccines are thiomersal-free. They are inactivated, do not contain live organisms and cannot cause the diseases against which they protect.

Td/IPV vaccine should be used where protection is required against tetanus, diphtheria or polio in order to provide comprehensive long-term protection against all three diseases.

Monovalent diphtheria vaccine is not available.

Storage

Vaccines should be stored in the original packaging at +2˚C to +8˚C and protected from light. All vaccines are sensitive to some extent to heat and cold. Heat speeds up the decline in potency of most vaccines, thus reducing their shelf life. Effectiveness cannot be guaranteed for vaccines unless they have been stored at the correct temperature. Freezing may cause increased reactogenicity and loss of potency for some vaccines. It can also cause hairline cracks in the container, leading to contamination of the contents.

Presentation

Diphtheria vaccine is only available as part of combined products. It is supplied as a cloudy white suspension, either in a single dose ampoule or pre-filled syringe. The suspension may settle during storage, so the vaccine should be shaken to distribute the suspension uniformly before administration.

Dosage and schedule

- First dose of 0.5ml of a diphtheria-containing vaccine.
- Second dose of 0.5ml, one month after the first dose.
- Third dose of 0.5ml, one month after the second dose.
- Fourth and fifth doses of 0.5ml should be given at the recommended intervals (see below).

Administration

Vaccines are routinely given intramuscularly into the upper arm or anterolateral thigh. This is to reduce the risk of localised reactions, which are more common when vaccines are given subcutaneously (Mark *et al.*, 1999, Diggle and Deeks, 2000; Zuckerman, 2000). However, for individuals with a bleeding disorder, vaccines should be given by deep subcutaneous injection to reduce the risk of bleeding.

Diphtheria-containing vaccines can be given at the same time as other vaccines such as MMR, MenC and hepatitis B. The vaccines should be given at a separate site, preferably in a different limb. If given in the same limb, they should be given at least 2.5cm apart (American Academy of Pediatrics, 2003). The site at which each vaccine was given should be noted in the individual's records.

Disposal

Equipment used for vaccination, including used vials or ampoules, should be disposed of at the end of a session by sealing in a proper, puncture-resistant 'sharps' box (UN-approved, BS 7320).

Recommendations for the use of the vaccine

The objective of the immunisation programme is to provide a minimum of five doses of a diphtheria-containing vaccine at appropriate intervals for all individuals. For most circumstances, a total of five doses of vaccine at the appropriate intervals are considered to give satisfactory long-term protection.

To fulfil this objective, the appropriate vaccine for each age group is also determined by the need to protect individuals against tetanus, pertussis, Hib and polio.

Primary immunisation

Infants and children under ten years of age

The primary course of diphtheria vaccination consists of three doses of a D-containing product. DTaP/IPV/Hib is recommended to be given at two, three and four months of age but can be given at any stage from two months to ten years of age. If the primary course is interrupted it should be resumed but not repeated, allowing an interval of one month between the remaining doses.

Children aged ten years or over, and adults

The primary course of diphtheria vaccination consists of three doses of a d-containing product with an interval of one month between each dose. Td/IPV is recommended for all individuals aged ten years or over. If the primary course is interrupted it should be resumed but not repeated, allowing an interval of one month between the remaining doses.

Reinforcing immunisation

Children under ten years should receive the first diphtheria booster combined with tetanus, pertussis and polio vaccines. The first booster of a diphtheria-containing vaccine should ideally be given three years after completion of the primary course, normally when the child is between three-and-a-half and five years of age. When primary vaccination has been delayed, this first booster dose may be given at the scheduled visit – provided it is one year since the third primary dose. This will re-establish the child on the routine schedule. DTaP/IPV or dTaP/IPV should be used in this age group. Td/IPV should not be used routinely for this purpose in this age group because it does not contain pertussis and has not been shown to give an equivalent diphtheria antitoxin response compared with other recommended preparations.

Individuals aged ten years or over who have only had three doses of a diphtheria-containing vaccine should receive the first diphtheria booster combined with tetanus and polio vaccines (Td/IPV).

The second booster dose of Td/IPV should ideally be given to all individuals ten years after the first booster dose. Where the previous doses have been delayed, the second booster should be given at the school session or scheduled appointment – provided a minimum of five years have elapsed between the first and second boosters. This will be the last scheduled opportunity to ensure long-term protection.

If a person attends for a routine booster dose and has a history of receiving a vaccine following a tetanus-prone wound, attempts should be made to identify which vaccine was given. If the vaccine given at the time of the injury was the same as that due at the current visit and given after an appropriate interval, then the routine booster dose is not required. Otherwise, the dose given at the time of injury should be discounted as it may not provide long-term protection against all antigens, and the scheduled immunisation should be given. Such additional doses are unlikely to produce an unacceptable rate of reactions (Ramsay *et al.*, 1997).

Vaccination of children with unknown or incomplete immunisation status

Where a child born in the UK presents with an inadequate immunisation history, every effort should be made to clarify what immunisations they may have had (see Chapter 11). A child who has not completed the primary course should have the outstanding doses at monthly intervals. Children may receive the first booster dose as early as one year after the third primary dose to re-establish them on the routine schedule. The second booster should be given at the time of school leaving to ensure long-term protection at this time. Wherever possible, a minimum of five years should be left between the first and second boosters.

Children coming to the UK who have a history of completing immunisation in their country of origin may not have been offered protection against all the antigens currently used in the UK. They will probably have received diphtheria-containing vaccines in their country of origin. For country-specific information, please refer to www.who.int/immunization_monitoring/en/globalsummary/countryprofileselect.cfm.

Children coming from developing countries, from areas of conflict, or from hard-to-reach population groups may not have been fully immunised. Where there is no reliable history of previous immunisation, it should be assumed that they are unimmunised and the full UK recommendations should be followed (see Chapter 11 on vaccine schedules).

Children coming to the UK may have had a fourth dose of a diphtheria-containing vaccine that is given at around 18 months in some countries. This dose should be discounted as it may not provide satisfactory protection until the time of the teenage booster. The routine pre-school and subsequent boosters should be given according to the UK schedule.

Travellers and those going to live abroad

All travellers to epidemic or endemic areas should ensure that they are fully immunised according to the UK schedule. Additional doses of vaccines may be required according to the destination and the nature of travel intended, for example for those who are going to live or work with local people in epidemic or endemic areas (Department of Health, 2001). Where tetanus, diphtheria or polio protection is required and the final dose of the relevant antigen was received more than ten years ago, Td/IPV should be given.

Diphtheria vaccination in laboratory and healthcare workers

Individuals who may be exposed to diphtheria in the course of their work, in microbiology laboratories and clinical infectious disease units, are at risk and must be protected (see Chapter 12).

Contraindications

There are very few individuals who cannot receive diphtheria-containing vaccines. When there is doubt, appropriate advice should be sought from a consultant paediatrician, immunisation co-ordinator or consultant in communicable disease control, rather than withholding the vaccine.

The vaccine should not be given to those who have had:

- a confirmed anaphylactic reaction to a previous dose of a diphtheria-containing vaccine, or
- a confirmed anaphylactic reaction to any of the components of the vaccine.

Confirmed anaphylaxis occurs extremely rarely. Data from the UK, Canada and the US point to rates of 0.65 to 3 anaphylaxis events per million doses of vaccine given (Bohlke *et al.*, 2003; Canadian Medical Association, 2002). Other allergic conditions may occur more commonly and are not contraindications to further immunisation. A careful history of the event will often distinguish between anaphylaxis and other events that are either not due to the vaccine or are not life-threatening. In the latter circumstance, it may be possible to continue the immunisation course. Specialist advice must be sought on the vaccines and circumstances in which they could be given. The risk to the individual of not being immunised must be taken into account.

Precautions

Minor illnesses without fever or systemic upset are not valid reasons to postpone immunisation. If an individual is acutely unwell, immunisation may be postponed until they have fully recovered. This is to avoid confusing the differential diagnosis of any acute illness by wrongly attributing any signs or symptoms to the adverse effects of the vaccine.

Systemic and local reactions following a previous immunisation

This section gives advice on the immunisation of children with a history of a severe or mild systemic or local reaction within 72 hours of a preceding vaccine. Immunisation with diphtheria-containing vaccine **should** continue following a history of:

- fever, irrespective of its severity
- hypotonic-hyporesponsive episodes (HHEs)
- persistent crying or screaming for more than three hours
- severe local reaction, irrespective of extent.

Children who have had severe reactions as above have continued and completed immunisation with diphtheria-containing vaccines without recurrence (Vermeer-de Bondt *et al.*, 1998; Gold *et al.*, 2000).

In Canada, a severe general or local reaction to DTaP/IPV/Hib is not a contraindication to further doses of the vaccine (Canadian Medical Association, 1998). Adverse events after childhood immunisation are carefully monitored in Canada (Le Saux *et al.*, 2003), and experience there suggests that further doses were not associated with recurrence or worsening of the preceding events (S Halperin and R Pless, pers. comm., 2003).

Pregnancy and breast-feeding

Diphtheria-containing vaccines may be given to pregnant women when the need for protection is required without delay. There is no evidence of risk from vaccinating pregnant women or those who are breast-feeding with inactivated viral or bacterial vaccines or toxoids (Plotkin and Orenstein, 2004).

Premature infants

It is important that premature infants have their immunisations at the appropriate chronological age, according to the schedule. There is no evidence that premature babies are at an increased risk of adverse reactions from vaccines (Slack *et al.,* 2001).

Immunosuppression and HIV infection

Individuals with immunosuppression or with HIV infection (regardless of CD4 counts) should be considered for diphtheria-containing vaccines in accordance with the recommendations above. However, these individuals may not develop a full antibody response if they are immunosuppressed, and vaccine protective efficacy has not been studied. Re-immunisation should be considered after treatment is finished and recovery has occurred. Specialist advice may be required.

Further guidance is provided by the Royal College of Paediatrics and Child Health (www.rcpch.ac.uk), the British HIV Association (BHIVA) *Immunisation guidelines for HIV-infected adults* (BHIVA, 2006) and the

Children's HIV Association of UK and Ireland (CHIVA) immunisation guidelines (www.bhiva.org/chiva).

Neurological conditions

Pre-existing neurological conditions

The presence of a neurological condition is not a contraindication to immunisation. Where there is evidence of a neurological condition in a child, the advice given in the flow chart in Figure 15.2 should be followed.

If a child has a stable pre-existing neurological abnormality such as spina bifida, congenital abnormality of the brain or perinatal hypoxic-ischaemic encephalopathy, they should be immunised according to the recommended schedule. When there has been a documented history of cerebral damage in the neonatal period, immunisation should be carried out unless there is evidence of an evolving neurological abnormality.

If there is evidence of current neurological deterioration, including poorly controlled epilepsy, immunisation should be deferred and the child should be referred to a child specialist for investigation to see if an underlying cause can be identified. If a cause is not identified, immunisation should be deferred until the condition has stabilised. If a cause is identified, immunisation should proceed as normal.

A family history of seizures is not a contraindication to immunisation. When there is a personal or family history of febrile seizures, there is an increased risk of these occurring after any fever, including that caused by immunisation. Seizures associated with fever are rare in the first six months of life, and most common in the second year of life. After this age the frequency falls, and they are rare after five years of age.

When a child has had a seizure associated with fever in the past, with no evidence of neurological deterioration, immunisation should proceed as recommended. Advice on the prevention and management of fever should be given before immunisation.

When a child has had a seizure that is not associated with fever, and there is no evidence of neurological deterioration, immunisation should proceed as recommended. When immunised with DTP vaccine, children with a family or personal history of seizures had no significant adverse events and their developmental progress was normal (Ramsay *et al.,* 1994).

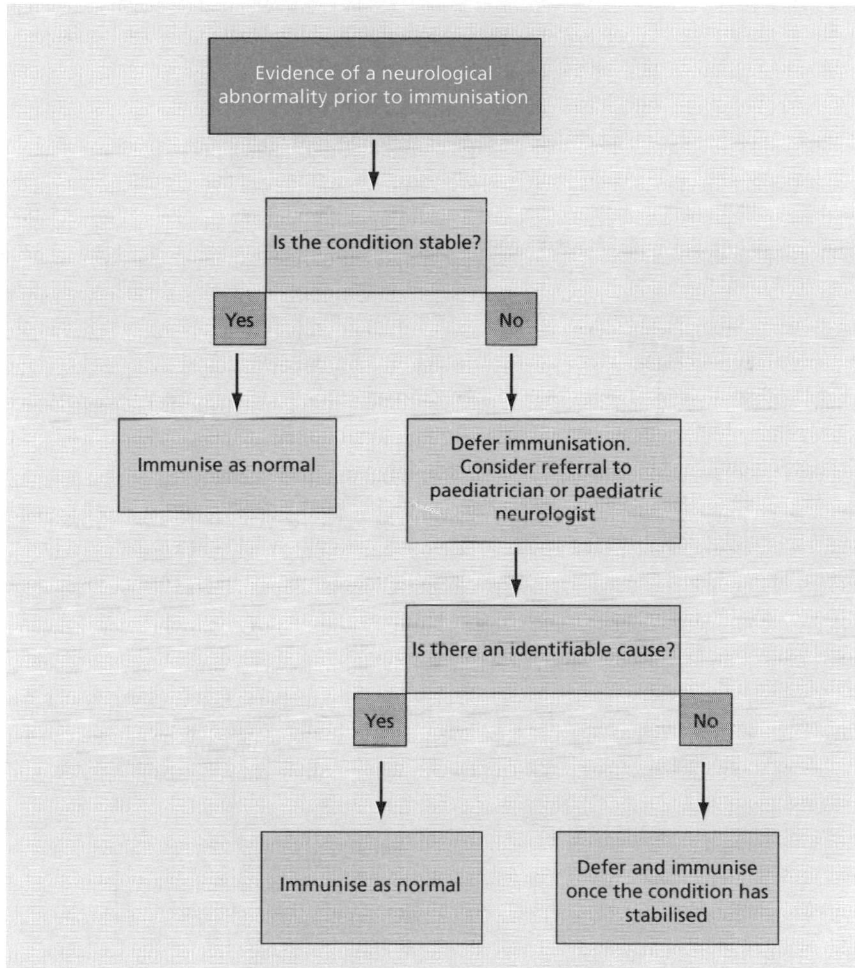

Figure 15.2 Flow chart for immunisation procedure if there is evidence of a neurological condition before immunisation

Neurological abnormalities following immunisation

If a child experiences encephalopathy or encephalitis within seven days of immunisation, the advice in the flow chart in Figure 15.3 should be followed. It is unlikely that these conditions will have been caused by the vaccine, and they should be investigated by a specialist. Immunisation should be deferred until the condition has stabilised in children where no underlying cause was found, **and** the child did not recover completely within seven days. If a cause is identified or the child recovers within seven days, immunisation should proceed as recommended.

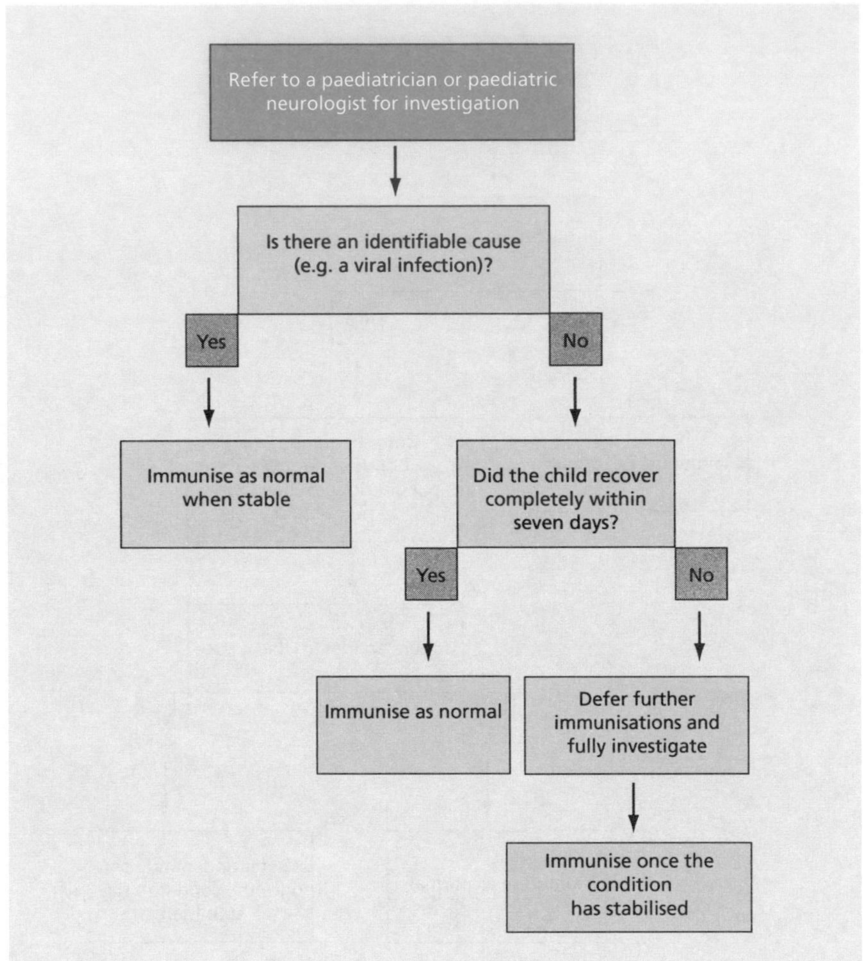

Figure 15.3 Flow chart for encephalitis or encephalopathy occurring within seven days of immunisation

If a seizure associated with a fever occurs within 72 hours of an immunisation, further immunisation should be deferred if no underlying cause has been found **and** the child did not recover completely within 24 hours, until the condition is stable. If a cause is identified or the child recovers within 24 hours, immunisation should continue as recommended.

Deferral of immunisation

There will be very few occasions when deferral of immunisation is required (see above). Deferral leaves the child unprotected; the period of deferral should be minimised so that immunisation can commence as soon as possible. If a specialist recommends deferral, this should be clearly communicated to the general practitioner and he or she must be informed as soon as the child is fit for immunisation.

Adverse reactions

Pain, swelling or redness at the injection site are common and may occur more frequently following subsequent doses. A small, painless nodule may form at the injection site; this usually disappears and is of no consequence. The incidence of local reactions is lower with diphtheria vaccines combined with acellular pertussis vaccines than with whole-cell pertussis vaccines, and similar to that after DT vaccine (Miller, 1999; Tozzi and Olin, 1997).

Fever, convulsions, high-pitched screaming, and episodes of pallor, cyanosis and limpness (HHE) occur rarely but with equal frequency after both DTaP and DT vaccines (Tozzi and Olin, 1997).

Confirmed anaphylaxis occurs extremely rarely. Data from the UK, Canada and the US point to rates of 0.65 to 3 anaphylaxis events per million doses of vaccine given (Bohlke *et al.*, 2003; Canadian Medical Association, 2002). Other allergic conditions may occur more commonly and are not contraindications to further immunisation.

All suspected adverse reactions to vaccines occurring in children, or in individuals of any age after vaccines labelled with a black triangle (▼), should be reported to the Commission on Human Medicines using the Yellow Card scheme. Serious suspected adverse reactions to vaccines in adults should also be reported through the Yellow Card scheme.

Management of cases, contacts, carriers and outbreaks

As diphtheria is a notifiable disease in the UK, for public health management of cases, contacts and outbreaks, all suspected cases should be notified to the local health protection unit immediately.

Management of cases

Diphtheria antitoxin is only used in suspected cases of diphtheria in a hospital setting. Tests to exclude hypersensitivity to horse serum should be carried out. Diphtheria antitoxin should be given without waiting for bacteriological confirmation. It should be given according to the manufacturer's instructions, the dosage depending on the clinical condition of the patient.

Diphtheria antitoxin is based on horse serum and therefore severe, immediate anaphylaxis occurs more commonly than with human immunoglobulin products. If anaphylaxis occurs, adrenaline (0.5ml or 1ml aliquots) should be administered immediately by either intramuscular (0.5ml of 1:1000 solution) or intravenous (1ml of 1:10,000 solution) injection. This advice differs from that for treatment of anaphylaxis after immunisation because the antitoxin is being administered in the hospital setting.

In most cutaneous infections, large-scale toxin absorption is unlikely and therefore the risk of giving antitoxin is usually considered substantially greater than any benefit. Nevertheless, if the ulcer in cutaneous diphtheria infection were sufficiently large (i.e. more than $2cm^2$) and especially if it were membranous, then larger doses of antitoxin would be justified.

Antibiotic treatment is needed to eliminate the organism and to prevent spread. The antibiotics of choice are erythromycin, azithromycin, clarithromycin or penicillin (Bonnet and Begg, 1999).

The immunisation history of cases of toxigenic diphtheria should be established. Partially or unimmunised individuals should complete immunisation according to the UK schedule. Completely immunised individuals should receive a single reinforcing dose of a diphtheria-containing vaccine according to their age.

Management of contacts

Contacts of a case or carrier of toxigenic diphtheria should be promptly investigated, kept under surveillance and given antibiotic prophylaxis and vaccine. The immunisation history of all individuals exposed to toxigenic diphtheria should be established. Partially immunised or unimmunised individuals should complete immunisation according to the UK schedule (see above). Completely immunised individuals should receive a single reinforcing dose of a diphtheria-containing vaccine according to their age.

Contacts of a case or carrier of toxigenic diphtheria should be given a prophylactic course of erythromycin or penicillin. Contacts of cases of toxigenic *C. ulcerans* do require prophylaxis as, although it is rare, person-to-person transmission cannot be ruled out (Bonnet and Begg, 1999).

Supplies

Vaccines

- Pediacel (diphtheria/tetanus/5-component acellular pertussis/inactivated polio vaccine/*Haemophilus influenzae* type b (DTaP/IPV/Hib) – manufactured by Sanofi Pasteur MSD.

- Repevax (diphtheria/tetanus/5-component acellular pertussis/inactivated polio vaccine (dTaP/IPV)) – manufactured by Sanofi Pasteur MSD.

- Infanrix IPV (diphtheria/tetanus/3-component acellular pertussis/ inactivated polio vaccine (DTaP/IPV)) – manufactured by GlaxoSmithKline.

- Revaxis (tetanus/diphtheria/inactivated polio vaccine (Td/IPV)) – manufactured by Sanofi Pasteur MSD.

These vaccines are supplied by Healthcare Logistics (Tel: 0870 871 1890) as part of the national childhood immunisation programme.

In Scotland, supplies should be obtained from local childhood vaccine holding centres. Details of these are available from Scottish Healthcare Supplies (Tel: 0141 282 2240).

Diphtheria antitoxin is supplied by the Butantan Institute, in 10ml vials containing 10,000IU. It is distributed in the UK by the Health Protection Agency, Centre for Infections, Immunisation Department (Tel: 020 8200 6868).

References

American Academy of Pediatrics (2003) Active immunization. In: Pickering LK (ed.) *Red Book: 2003 Report of the Committee on Infectious Diseases*, 26th edition. Elk Grove Village, IL: American Academy of Pediatrics, p 33.

Bohlke K, Davis RL, Marcy SH *et al.* (2003) Risk of anaphylaxis after vaccination of children and adolescents. *Pediatrics* **112**: 815–20.

Bonnet JM and Begg NT (1999) Control of diphtheria: guidance for consultants in communicable disease control. *CDPH* **2**: 242–9.

British HIV Association (2006) *Immunisation guidelines for HIV-infected adults:* www.bhiva.org/pdf/2006/Immunisation506.pdf.

Canadian Medical Association (1998) Pertussis vaccine. In: *Canadian Immunisation Guide*, 5th edition. Canadian Medical Association, p 133.

Canadian Medical Association (2002) – General considerations. In: *Canadian Immunisation Guide,* 6th edition. Canadian Medical Association, p 14.

CDR (1997) Diphtheria acquired during a cruise in the Baltic sea: update. *Communicable Disease Report* 7: 219.

De Benoist AC, White JM, Efstratiou A *et al.* (2004) Cutaneous diphtheria, United Kingdom. *Emerging Infectious Diseases* **10**: 511–13.

Department of Health (2001) *Health information for overseas travel*, second edition. London: TSO.

Diggle L and Deeks J (2000) Effect of needle length on incidence of local reactions to routine immunisation in infants aged 4 months: randomised controlled trial. *BMJ* **321**: 931– 3.

Dittmann S, Wharton M, Vitek C *et al.* (2000) Successful control of epidemic diphtheria in the states of the Former Union of Soviet Socialist Republics: lessons learned. *JID* **181** (Suppl 1): S10 –22.

Edmunds WJ, Pebody RG, Aggerback H *et al.* (2000) The sero-epidemiology of diphtheria in Western Europe. *Epidemiol Infect* **125**: 113–25.

Gold M, Goodwin H, Botham S *et al.* (2000) Re-vaccination of 421 children with a past history of an adverse reaction in a specialised service. *Arch Dis Child* **83**: 128–31.

Mark A, Carlsson RM and Granstrom M (1999) Subcutaneous versus intramuscular injection for booster DT vaccination in adolescents. *Vaccine* **17**: 2067–72

Miller E (1999) Overview of recent clinical trials of acellular pertussis vaccines. *Biologicals* **27**: 79–86.

Plotkin SA and Orenstein WA (eds) (2004) *Vaccines,* 4th edition. Philadelphia: WB Saunders Company, Chapter 8.

Ramsay M, Begg N, Holland B and Dalphinis J (1994) Pertussis immunisation in children with a family or personal history of convulsions: a review of children referred for specialist advice. *Health Trends* **26**: 23–4.

Ramsay M, Joce R and Whalley J (1997) Adverse events after school leavers received combined tetanus and low-dose diphtheria vaccine. *CDR Review* **5**: R65–7.

Reacher M, Ramsay M, White J *et al.* (2000) Nontoxigenic *Corynebacterium diphtheriae*: an emerging pathogen in England and Wales? *Emerg Infect Diseases* **6**: 640–5.

Le Saux N, Barrowman NJ, Moore DL *et al.* (2003) Canadian Paediatric Society/Health Canada Immunization Monitoring Program – Active (IMPACT). Decrease in hospital admissions for febrile seizures and reports of hypotonic-hyporesponsive episodes presenting to hospital emergency departments since switching to acellular pertussis vaccine in Canada: a report from IMPACT. *Pediatrics* **112**(5): e348.

Slack MH, Schapira D, Thwaites RJ *et al.* (2001) Immune response of premature infants to meningococcal serogroup C and combined diphtheria-tetanus toxoids-acellular pertussis-*Haemophilus influenzae* type b conjugate vaccines. *J Infect Dis* **184** (12): 1617–20.

Tozzi AE and Olin P (1997) Common side effects in the Italian and Stockholm 1 Trials. *Dev Biol Stand.* **89**: 105–8.

Vermeer-de Bondt PE, Labadie J and Rümke HC (1998) Rate of recurrent collapse after vaccination with whole-cell pertussis vaccine: follow-up study. *BMJ* **316**: 902.

Zuckerman JN (2000) The importance of injecting vaccines into muscle. *BMJ* **321**: 1237–8.

16

Haemophilus influenzae type b (Hib)

H. INFLUENZAE MENINGITIS NOTIFIABLE (EXCEPT IN SCOTLAND)

The disease

Haemophilus influenzae can cause serious invasive disease, especially in young children. Invasive disease is usually caused by encapsulated strains of the organism. Six typeable capsular serotypes (a–f) are known to cause disease; non-typeable encapsulated strains can occasionally cause invasive disease. Before the introduction of vaccination, type b (Hib) was the prevalent strain. The proportion of typeable to non-typeable strains depends largely on the prevalence of the type b strain. Non-encapsulated strains are mainly associated with respiratory infections such as exacerbation of chronic bronchitis and otitis media.

The most common presentation of invasive Hib disease is meningitis, frequently accompanied by bacteraemia. This presentation accounts for approximately 60% of all cases (Anderson *et al.*, 1995). Fifteen per cent of cases present with epiglottitis, a potentially dangerous condition that presents with airway obstruction. Bacteraemia, without any other concomitant infection, occurs in 10% of cases. The remainder is made up of cases of septic arthritis, osteomyelitis, cellulitis, pneumonia and pericarditis. The sequelae following Hib meningitis may include deafness, seizures, and intellectual impairment. In studies conducted in Wales and Oxford, 8 to 11% had permanent neurological sequelae (Howard *et al.*, 1991; Tudor-Williams *et al.*, 1989). The case fatality rate from Hib meningitis is 4–5%.

Individuals can carry Hib bacteria in their nose and throat without showing signs of the disease. Before Hib vaccine was introduced, about four in every 100 pre-school children carried the Hib organism; after the vaccine was introduced, carriage rates fell below the level of detection (McVernon *et al.*, 2004). Hib is spread through coughing, sneezing or close contact with a carrier or an infected person.

History and epidemiology of the disease

Before the introduction of Hib immunisation, the estimated annual incidence of invasive Hib disease was 34 per 100,000 children under five years of age. One in every 600 children developed some form of invasive Hib disease before their fifth birthday (Booy *et al.*, 1994). The disease was rare in children under three months of age, but the incidence rose progressively during the first year, reaching a peak between 10 and 11 months of age. Thereafter, the incidence declined steadily to four years of age after which infection was uncommon.

Vaccines against Hib were first produced in the early 1970s and they contained purified capsular polysaccharide. These vaccines were effective in children over 18 months of age, but failed to protect younger children, in whom the risk of disease was highest. The development of conjugate Hib vaccines overcame this problem. In conjugate vaccines, the capsular polysaccharides were linked to proteins, improving the vaccine's immunogenicity, particularly in children less than one year of age. In 1992, Hib conjugate vaccine was introduced into the routine UK immunisation schedule. Hib conjugate vaccine was originally administered as a separate vaccine. In 1996, combination vaccines (DTwP/Hib) were introduced, and in 2004, Hib vaccine combined with DTaP and IPV (DTaP/IPV/Hib) became available.

The efficacy and safety of the conjugate Hib vaccines have been demonstrated in large field trials in Finland, the United States and in the UK, where efficacy ranged from 83 to 100% (Black *et al.*, 1991a; Black *et al.*, 1991b; Eskola *et al.*, 1990). Studies comparing different vaccines, using the present UK primary schedule, have shown that 90 to 99% of children developed protective levels of antibodies following three doses of vaccine (Booy *et al.*, 1994). Cases of invasive disease in fully vaccinated children (vaccine failures) have been reported from some countries, including the UK (Heath and McVernon, 2002). A small proportion of such cases have underlying conditions, such as immunoglobulin deficiency, predisposing the child to vaccine failure.

Since the introduction of Hib immunisation in the UK, disease incidence has fallen (see Figure 16.1). In 1998, only 21 cases of invasive Hib were reported in England and Wales in children under five years of age (0.65 per 100,000) compared with 803 in 1991 (20.5 per 100,000). In infants under one year of age, the highest risk age group for disease, reported cases fell by over 95% (from 300 to 7). Notifications of *H. influenzae* meningitis for the same period declined from 485 to 29. In 1998, coverage by the second birthday was 95%.

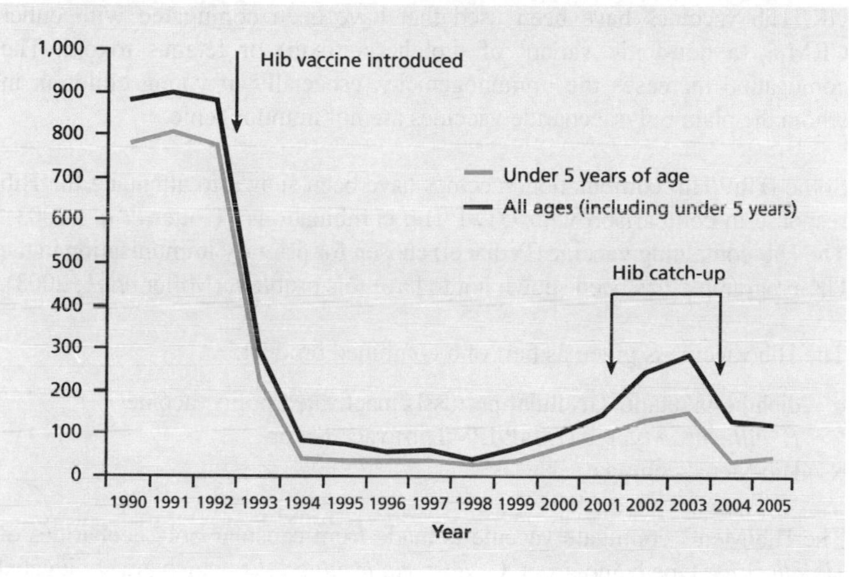

Figure 16.1 Laboratory reports of Hib disease in England and Wales (1990–2005)

From 1999, there was a small but gradual increase in the number of cases of Hib disease reported, mostly in children less than four years of age. However, this increase was most notable among children born in 2000 and 2001 (McVernon *et al.*, 2003). Reasons for this increase in vaccine failures are thought to include an effect of the DTaP/Hib combination vaccine which was in use at that time and a waning of the impact of the catch-up programme when the vaccine was introduced. In this latter group, who were immunised at an older age, the efficacy was higher than in children vaccinated routinely as infants.

In 2003, a booster campaign was implemented with call-back of children aged six months to four years (Chief Medical Officer *et al.*, 2004). Following the campaign, cases have begun to return to the low levels achieved previously (see Figure 16.1). In 2006, following studies that showed that protection against Hib waned during the second year of life (Trotter *et al.*, 2003), a booster dose (combined with MenC as Hib/MenC) was introduced.

The Hib vaccination

Hib-containing vaccines are made from capsular polysaccharide that has been extracted from cultures of Hib bacteria. The polysaccharide is linked (conjugated) to a protein, according to the manufacturer's methodology. In the

UK, Hib vaccines have been used that have been conjugated with either CRM_{197} (a non-toxic variant of diphtheria toxin) or tetanus toxoid. The conjugation increases the immunogenicity, especially in young children, in whom the plain polysaccharide vaccines are not immunogenic.

Some DTaP/Hib combination vaccines have been shown to attenuate the Hib response in comparison with DTwP/Hib combinations (Trotter *et al.*, 2003). The Hib-containing vaccine (Pediacel) chosen for primary immunisation in the UK programme has been shown not to have this problem (Miller *et al.*, 2003).

The Hib vaccine is given as part of a combined product:

- diphtheria/tetanus/acellular pertussis/inactivated polio vaccine/ *H. influenzae* type b (DTaP/IPV/Hib) vaccine, or
- Hib/MenC conjugate.

The Hib/MenC conjugate vaccine is made from capsular polysaccharides of *H. influenzae* type b and group C *Neisseria meningitidis*, which are conjugated to tetanus toxoid. The vaccine has been shown to elicit booster responses to both Hib and MenC when given in the second year of life to children who were primed in infancy with Hib and MenC conjugate vaccines.

The above vaccines are thiomersal-free. They are inactivated, do not contain live organisms and cannot cause the diseases against which they protect.

Storage

Vaccines should be stored in the original packaging at +2˚C to +8˚C and protected from light. All vaccines are sensitive to some extent to heat and cold. Heat speeds up the decline in potency of most vaccines, thus reducing their shelf life. Effectiveness cannot be guaranteed for vaccines unless they have been stored at the correct temperature. Freezing may cause increased reactogenicity and loss of potency for some vaccines. It can also cause hairline cracks in the container, leading to contamination of the contents.

Presentation

Hib vaccines are available as part of combined products DTaP/IPV/Hib or Hib/MenC. The combined product, DTaP/IPV/Hib is supplied as a cloudy white suspension either in a single dose ampoule or pre-filled syringe. The suspension may sediment during storage and should be shaken to distribute the suspension uniformly before administration.

Hib/MenC is supplied as a vial of white powder and 0.5ml of solvent in a pre-filled syringe. The vaccine must be reconstituted by adding the entire contents of the pre-filled syringe to the vial containing the powder. After addition of the solvent, the mixture should be shaken well until the powder is completely dissolved. After reconstitution, the vaccine should be administered promptly, or allowed to stand between +2°C and +8°C and used within 24 hours.

Dosage and schedule

For children under one year of age:

- First dose of 0.5ml of a Hib-containing vaccine.
- Second dose of 0.5ml, one month after the first dose.
- Third dose of 0.5ml, one month after the second dose.
- A fourth booster dose of 0.5ml of a Hib-containing vaccine should be given at the recommended interval (see below).

For children over one year of age and under ten years of age who have either not been immunised or not completed a primary course of diphtheria, tetanus, pertussis or polio, DTaP/IPV/Hib vaccination should be used. Children over one year and under ten years of age who have completed a primary course of diphtheria, tetanus, pertussis or polio should have Hib/MenC.

Administration

Vaccines are routinely given intramuscularly into the upper arm or anterolateral thigh. This is to reduce the risk of localised reactions, which are more common when vaccines are given subcutaneously (Mark *et al.*, 1999; Diggle and Deeks, 2000; Zuckerman, 2000). However, for individuals with a bleeding disorder, vaccines should be given by deep subcutaneous injection to reduce the risk of bleeding.

Hib-containing vaccines can be given at the same time as other vaccines such as MMR, MenC and hepatitis B. The vaccines should be given at a separate site, preferably in a different limb. If given in the same limb, they should be given at least 2.5cm apart (American Academy of Pediatrics, 2003). The site at which each vaccine was given should be noted in the patient's records.

At the moment, there are no data on the administration of Hib/MenC vaccine at the same time as pneumococcal conjugate vaccine (PCV). Although there is no reason to think that this would cause any safety concerns, there is a theoretical possibility of reduced response to one or other vaccine. Therefore, as a precautionary measure, Hib/MenC should not be given routinely at the same time as the booster of PCV. However, where rapid protection is required, the two can be given on the same day or at any interval. As more data accumulates, this advice may be modified.

Disposal

Equipment used for vaccination, including used vials or ampoules, should be disposed of at the end of a session by sealing in a proper, puncture-resistant 'sharps' box (UN-approved, BS 7320).

Recommendations for the use of the vaccine

The objective of the immunisation programme is to protect individuals under ten years of age, and individuals older than this who may be at elevated risk from invasive Hib disease.

To fulfil this objective, the appropriate vaccine for each age group is determined also by the need to protect individuals against diphtheria, tetanus, pertussis, Hib and polio.

Primary immunisation

Infants and children under ten years of age

The primary course of Hib vaccination in infants consists of three doses of a Hib-containing product with an interval of one month between each dose. DTaP/IPV/Hib is recommended for all children from two months up to ten years of age. Although one dose of Hib vaccine is effective from one year of age, three doses of DTaP/IPV/Hib should be given to children who have either not been immunised or who have not completed a primary course, in order to be fully protected against diphtheria, tetanus, pertussis and polio. If the primary course is interrupted it should be resumed but not repeated, allowing an interval of one month between the remaining doses.

Children of one to ten years of age who have completed a primary course of diphtheria, tetanus, pertussis and polio but have not received Hib-containing vaccines, should receive a single dose of Hib/MenC vaccine.

Reinforcing immunisation

A reinforcing (booster) dose of Hib/MenC is recommended at 12 months for children who have received a complete primary course of three Hib-containing vaccine injections. It should be given one month before pneumococcal conjugate and MMR vaccines.

Vaccination of children with unknown or incomplete immunisation status

Where a child born in the UK presents with an inadequate immunisation history, every effort should be made to clarify what immunisations they may have had (see Chapter 11, on immunisation schedule). A child who has not completed the primary course should have the outstanding doses at monthly intervals.

Children coming to the UK who have a history of completing immunisation in their country of origin may not have been offered protection against all the antigens currently used in the UK. They may not have received Hib-containing vaccines in their country of origin (www-nt.who.int/immunization_monitoring/en/globalsummary/countryprofileselect.cfm).

Children coming from developing countries, from areas of conflict, or from hard-to-reach population groups may not have been fully immunised. Where there is no reliable history of previous immunisation, it should be assumed that they are unimmunised and the full UK recommendations should be followed (see Chapter 11).

Children and adults with asplenia or splenic dysfunction

Children and adults with asplenia or splenic dysfunction may be at increased risk of invasive Hib infection. It is important that such children under ten years of age complete the primary immunisation schedule. Unimmunised individuals aged ten years or over should receive two doses of combined Hib/MenC vaccine, two months apart.

Children and adults who have been fully immunised with Hib as part of the routine programme who then develop splenic dysfunction, should be offered an additional dose of Hib (usually as combined Hib/MenC vaccine).

Contraindications

There are very few individuals who cannot receive Hib-containing vaccines. Where there is doubt, appropriate advice should be sought from a consultant paediatrician, immunisation co-ordinator or consultant in communicable disease control rather than withhold vaccine.

The vaccines should not be given to those who have had:

- a confirmed anaphylactic reaction to a previous dose of a Hib-containing vaccine, or

- a confirmed anaphylactic reaction to any components of the vaccine.

Confirmed anaphylaxis occurs extremely rarely. Data from the UK, Canada and the US point to rates of 0.65 to 3 anaphylaxis events per million doses of vaccine given (Bohlke *et al.*, 2003; Canadian Medical Association, 2002). Other allergic conditions may occur more commonly and are not contraindications to further immunisation. A careful history of the event will often distinguish between anaphylaxis and other events that are either not due to the vaccine or are not life-threatening. In the latter circumstance, it may be possible to continue the immunisation course. Specialist advice must be sought on the vaccines and circumstances in which they could be given. The risk to the individual of not being immunised must be taken into account.

Precautions

Minor illnesses without fever or systemic upset are not valid reasons to postpone immunisation. If an individual is acutely unwell, immunisation may be postponed until they have recovered. This is to avoid confusing the differential diagnosis of any acute illness by wrongly attributing any signs or symptoms to the adverse effects of the vaccine.

Systemic and local reactions following a previous immunisation

This section gives advice on the immunisation of children with a history of a severe or mild systemic or local reaction within 72 hours of a preceding vaccine. Immunisation with Hib-containing vaccine should continue following a history of:

- fever, irrespective of its severity
- hypotonic-hyporesponsive episodes (HHE)
- persistent crying or screaming for more than three hours, or
- severe local reaction, irrespective of extent.

In Canada, a severe general or local reaction to DTaP/IPV/Hib is not a contraindication to further doses of the vaccine (Canadian Medical Association, 1998). Adverse events after childhood immunisation are carefully monitored in Canada (Le Saux *et al.*, 2003) and their experience suggests that further doses were not associated with recurrence or worsening of the preceding events (S Halperin and R Pless, pers. comm., 2003).

Pregnancy and breast-feeding

Hib-containing vaccines may be given to pregnant women when protection is required without delay. There is no evidence of risk from vaccinating pregnant women or those who are breast-feeding with inactivated viral or bacterial vaccines or toxoids (Plotkin and Orenstein, 2004).

Premature infants

It is important that premature infants have their immunisations at the appropriate chronological age, according to the schedule. There is no evidence that premature babies are at an increased risk of adverse reactions from vaccines (Slack *et al.,* 2001).

Immunosuppression and HIV infection

Individuals with immunosuppression and HIV infection (regardless of CD4 count) should be given Hib-containing vaccines in accordance with the recommendations above. These individuals may not make a full antibody response. Re-immunisation should be considered after treatment is finished and recovery has occurred. Specialist advice may be required.

Further guidance is provided by the Royal College of Paediatrics and Child Health (RCPCH) (www.rcpch.ac.uk), the British HIV Association (BHIVA) *Immunisation guidelines for HIV-infected adults* (BHIVA, 2006) and the Children's HIV Association of UK and Ireland (CHIVA) immunisation guidelines (www.bhiva.org/chiva).

Neurological conditions

Pre-existing neurological conditions

The presence of a neurological condition is not a contraindication to immunisation. Where there is evidence of a neurological condition in a child, the advice given in the flow chart in Figure 16.2 should be followed.

If a child has a stable pre-existing neurological abnormality such as spina bifida, congenital abnormality of the brain or perinatal hypoxic-ischaemic encephalopathy, they should be immunised according to the recommended schedule. When there has been a documented history of cerebral damage in the neonatal period, immunisation should be carried out unless there is evidence of an evolving neurological abnormality.

If there is evidence of current neurological deterioration, including poorly controlled epilepsy, immunisation should be deferred and the child should be

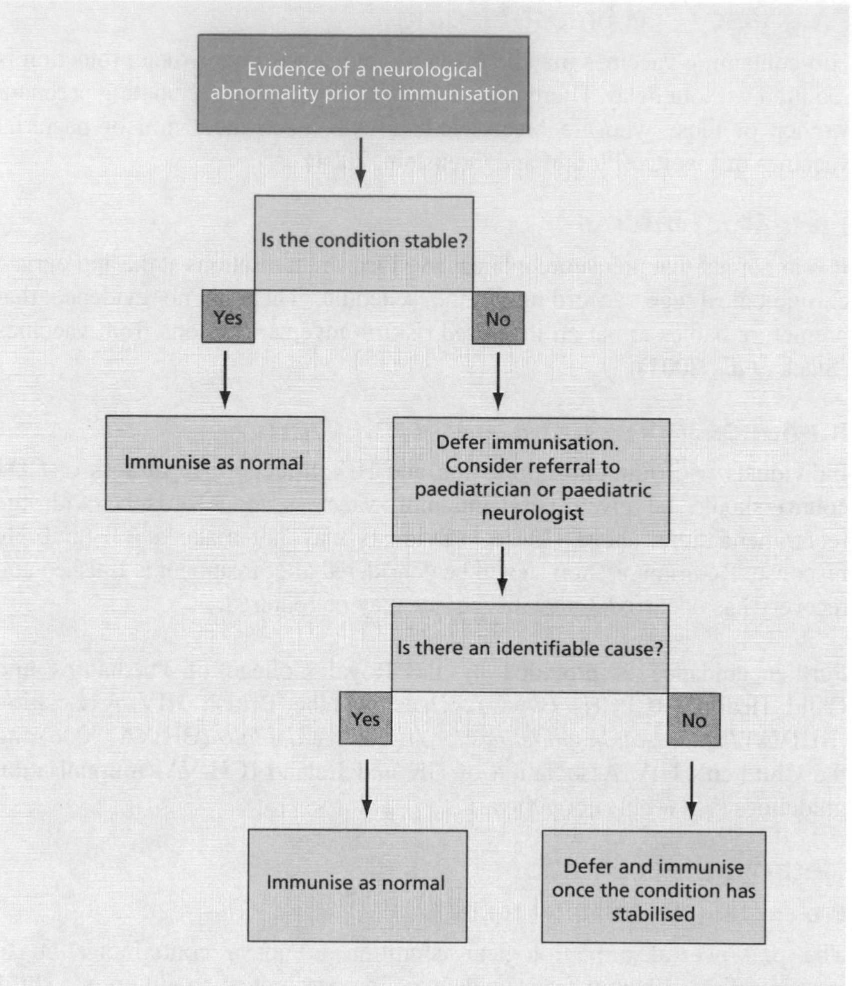

Figure 16.2 Flow chart for immunisation procedure if there is evidence of a neurological condition before immunisation

referred to a child specialist for investigation to see if an underlying cause can be identified. If a cause is not identified, immunisation should be deferred until the condition has stabilised. If a cause is identified, immunisation should proceed as normal.

A family history of seizures is not a contraindication to immunisation. When there is a personal or family history of febrile seizures, there is an increased risk of these occurring after any fever, including that caused by immunisation. Seizures associated with fever are rare in the first six months of life and most common in the second year of life. After this age, the frequency falls and they are rare after five years of age.

When a child has had a seizure associated with fever in the past, with no evidence of neurological deterioration, immunisation should proceed as recommended. Advice on the prevention and management of fever should be given before immunisation.

When a child has had a seizure that is not associated with fever, and there is no evidence of neurological deterioration, immunisation should proceed as recommended. When immunised with DTP vaccine, children with a family or personal history of seizures had no significant adverse events and their developmental progress was normal (Ramsay *et al.,* 1994).

Neurological abnormalities following immunisation

If a child experiences encephalopathy or encephalitis within seven days of immunisation, the advice in the flow chart in Figure 16.3 should be followed. It is unlikely that these conditions will have been caused by the vaccine and should be investigated by a specialist. Immunisation should be deferred in children where no underlying cause is found and the child does not recover completely within seven days, until the condition has stabilised. If a cause is identified or the child recovers within seven days, immunisation should proceed as recommended.

If a seizure associated with a fever occurs within 72 hours of an immunisation, further immunisation should be deferred until the condition is stable if no underlying cause has been found and the child does not recover completely within 24 hours. If a cause is identified or the child recovers within 24 hours, immunisation should continue as recommended.

Deferral of immunisation

There will be very few occasions when deferral of immunisation is required (see above). Deferral leaves the child unprotected; the period of deferral should be minimised so that immunisation can commence as soon as possible. If a specialist recommends deferral, this should be clearly communicated to the general practitioner and he or she must be informed as soon as the child is fit for immunisation.

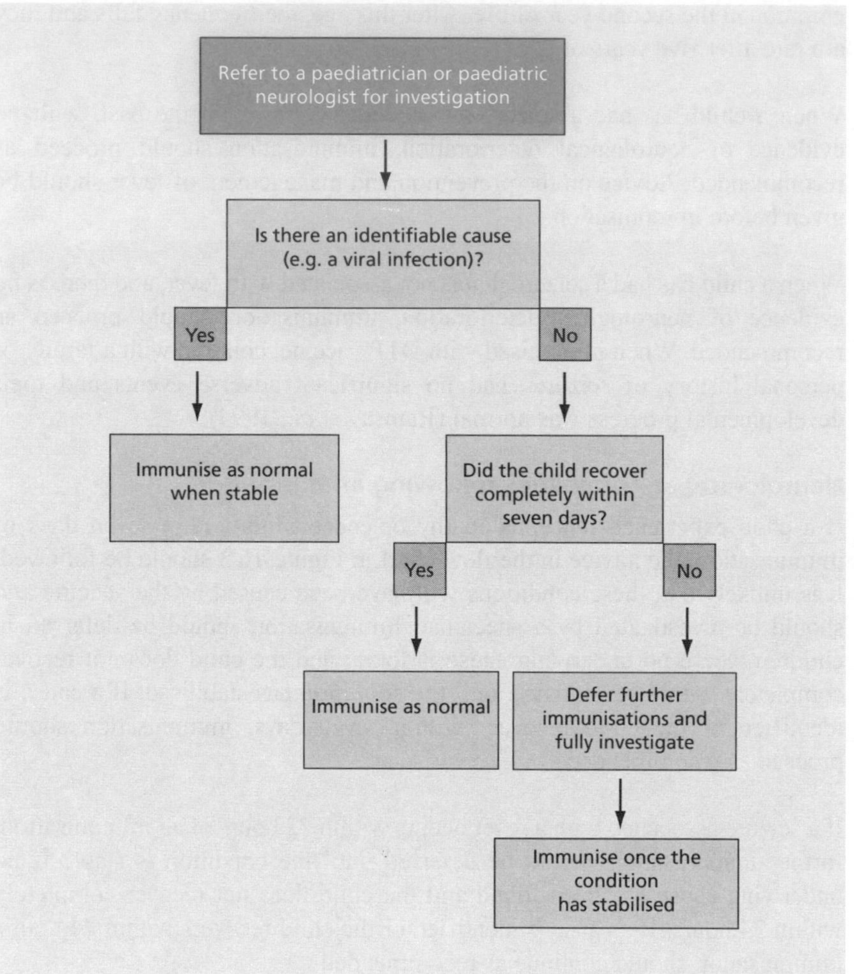

Figure 16.3 Flow chart for encephalitis or encephalopathy occurring within seven days of immunisation

Adverse reactions

Pain, swelling or redness at the injection site are common and may occur more frequently following subsequent doses. A small, painless nodule may form at the injection site; this usually disappears and is of no consequence. The incidence of local reactions is lower with tetanus vaccines combined with acellular pertussis vaccines than with whole-cell pertussis vaccines, and similar to that after diphtheria (DT) vaccine (Miller, 1999; Tozzi and Olin, 1997).

Fever, convulsions, high-pitched screaming, and episodes of pallor, cyanosis and limpness (HHE) occur with equal frequency after both DTaP and DT vaccines (Tozzi and Olin, 1997).

Confirmed anaphylaxis occurs extremely rarely. Data from the UK, Canada and the US point to rates of 0.65 to 3 anaphylaxis events per million doses of vaccine given (Bohlke *et al.*, 2003; Canadian Medical Association, 2002). Other allergic conditions may occur more commonly and are not contraindications to further immunisation.

Hib/MenC conjugate vaccine

Mild side effects such as irritability, loss of appetite, pain, swelling, redness at the site of the injection and slightly raised temperature commonly occur. Less commonly crying, diarrhoea, vomiting, atopic dermatitis, malaise and fever over 39.5°C have been reported.

All suspected adverse reactions to vaccines occurring in children, or in individuals of any age after vaccines labelled with a black triangle (▼), should be reported to the Commission on Human Medicines using the Yellow Card scheme. Serious suspected adverse reactions to vaccines in adults should be reported through the Yellow Card scheme.

Management of cases and contacts

Unimmunised cases up to the age of ten years should be immunised because recurrence of Hib infection can occur. Individuals who have been vaccinated against Hib, but who later acquire Hib infection, should have their convalescent antibody levels measured, and booster vaccination may be advised. Where antibody testing is not possible, an additional dose of Hib-containing vaccine should be given.

Household contacts of a case of invasive Hib disease have an increased risk of contracting the disease. Unimmunised children under four years of age are at substantial risk, and older, unimmunised children and even fully immunised children may be vulnerable. Contacts of cases should be managed following the advice of the local health protection unit, as follows:

- Children who have never received any immunisations should receive three doses of DTaP/IPV/Hib vaccine if below ten years of age.
- Children who have never received Hib vaccine, but who have been immunised against diphtheria, tetanus, pertussis and polio, should

receive three doses of Hib/MenC vaccine if under one year, and one dose if aged between one and ten years.

- Where there is any individual in the household of a case who is also at risk, the index case and all household contacts should be given rifampicin prophylaxis. Those at risk in the household include all children under four years of age and vulnerable individuals of any age (e.g. those who are immunosuppressed or asplenic) regardless of their immunisation status. The purpose of this recommendation is to prevent transmission of Hib to vulnerable individuals within a household. The recommended dose is 20mg/kg body weight (up to a maximum of 600mg) once a day for four days.

When a case occurs in a playgroup, nursery, crèche or school, the opportunity should be taken to identify and vaccinate any unimmunised children under ten years of age. When two or more cases of Hib disease have occurred in a playgroup, nursery, crèche or school within 120 days, chemoprophylaxis should be offered to all room contacts – teachers and children. This is a precautionary measure as there is little evidence that children in such settings are at significantly higher risk of Hib disease than the general population of the same age.

Supplies

Vaccines

- Pediacel (diphtheria/tetanus/5-component acellular pertussis/inactivated polio vaccine/*H. influenzae* type b (DTaP/IPV/Hib) – manufactured by Sanofi Pasteur MSD.
- Menitorix (Hib/MenC) – manufactured by GlaxoSmithKline.

These vaccines are supplied by Healthcare Logistics (Tel: 0870 871 1890) as part of the national childhood immunisation programme.

In Scotland, supplies should be obtained from local childhood vaccine holding centres. Details of these are available from Scottish Healthcare Supplies (Tel: 0141 282 2240).

References

American Academy of Pediatrics (2003) Active immunization. In: Pickering LK (ed.) *Red Book: 2003 Report of the Committee on Infectious Diseases,* 26th edition. Elk Grove Village, IL: American Academy of Pediatrics, p 33.

Anderson EC, Begg NT, Crawshaw SC *et al.* (1995) Epidemiology of invasive *Haemophilus influenzae* infections in England and Wales in the pre-vaccination era (1990–2). *Epidemiol Infect* **115**: 89–100.

British HIV Association (2006) *Immunisation guidelines for HIV-infected adults:* www.bhiva.org/pdf/2006/Immunisation506.pdf.

Black SB, Shinefield HR, Fireman B *et al.* (1991a) Efficacy in infancy of oligosaccharide conjugate *Haemophilus influenzae* type b (HbOC) vaccine in a United States population of 61,080 children. *Pediatr Infect Dis J* **10**: 97–104.

Black SB, Shinefield H, Lampert D *et al.* (1991b) Safety and immunogenicity of oligosaccharide conjugate *Haemophilus influenzae* type b (HbOC) vaccine in infancy. *Pediatr Infect Dis J* **10**: 2.

Bohlke K, Davis RL, Marcy SH *et al.* (2003) Risk of anaphylaxis after vaccination of children and adolescents. *Pediatrics* **112**: 815–20.

Booy R, Hodgson S, Carpenter L *et al.* (1994) Efficacy of *Haemophilus influenzae* type b conjugate vaccine PRP-T. *Lancet* **344** (8919): 362–6.

Canadian Medical Association (1998) Pertussis vaccine. In: *Canadian Immunization Guide*. 5th edition. Canadian Medical Association, p 133.

Canadian Medical Association (2002) General considerations. In: *Canadian Immunization Guide*, 6th edition. Canadian Medical Association, p 14.

Chief Medical Officer, Chief Nursing Officer and Chief Pharmaceutical Officer (2004) Planned Hib vaccination catch-up campaign – further information. www.dh.gov.uk/cmo/letters/cmo0302.htm

Department of Health (2001) *Health information for overseas travel*, 2nd edition. London: The Stationery Office.

Diggle L and Deeks J (2000) Effect of needle length on incidence of local reactions to routine immunisation in infants aged 4 months: randomised controlled trial. *BMJ* **321**: 931–3.

Eskola J, Kayhty H, Takala AK *et al.* (1990) A randomised, prospective field trial of a conjugate vaccine in the protection of infants and young children against invasive *Haemophilus influenzae* type b disease. *NEJM* **323** (20): 1381–7.

Heath PT and McVernon J (2002) The UK Hib vaccine experience. *Arch Dis Child* **86**: 396–9.

Howard AJ, Dunkin KT, Musser JM and Palmer SR (1991) Epidemiology of *Haemophilus influenzae* type b invasive disease in Wales. *BMJ* **303**: 441–5.

Le Saux N, Barrowman NJ, Moore D *et al.* (2003) Canadian Paediatric Society/Health Canada Immunization Monitoring Program – Active (IMPACT). Decrease in hospital admissions for febrile seizures and reports of hypotonic-hyporesponsive episodes presenting to hospital emergency departments since switching to acellular pertussis vaccine in Canada: a report from IMPACT. *Pediatrics* **112** (5): e348.

McVernon J, Andrews N, Slack MPE and Ramsay ME (2003) Risk of vaccine failure after *Haemophilus influenzae* type b (Hib) combination vaccines with acellular pertussis. *Lancet* **361**: 1521–3.

McVernon J, Howard AJ, Slack MP and Ramsay ME (2004) Long-term impact of vaccination on *Haemophilus influenzae* type b (Hib) carriage in the United Kingdom. *Epidemiol Infect* **132** (4): 765–7.

Mark A, Carlsson RM and Granstrom M (1999) Subcutaneous versus intramuscular injection for booster DT vaccination in adolescents. *Vaccine* **17**: 2067–72

Miller E (1999) Overview of recent clinical trials of acellular pertussis vaccines. *Biologicals* **27**: 79–86.

Miller E, Southern J, Kitchin N *et al.* (2003) Interaction between different meningococcal C conjugate vaccines and the Hib component of concomitantly administered diphtheria/tetanus/pertussis/Hib vaccines with either whole-cell or acellular pertussis antigens. 21st Annual Meeting of the European Society for Paediatric Infectious Diseases, Sicily.

Plotkin SA and Orenstein WA (eds) (2004) *Vaccines,* 4th edition. Philadelphia: WB Saunders Company, Chapter 8.

Ramsay M, Begg N, Holland B and Dalphinis J (1994) Pertussis immunisation in children with a family or personal history of convulsions: a review of children referred for specialist advice. *Health Trends* **26**: 23–4.

Slack MH, Schapira D, Thwaites RJ *et al.* (2001) Immune response of premature infants to meningococcal serogroup C and combined diphtheria-tetanus toxoids-acellular pertussis-*Haemophilus influenzae* type b conjugate vaccines. *J Infect Dis* **184** (12): 1617–20.

Tozzi AE and Olin P (1997) Common side effects in the Italian and Stockholm 1 Trials. *Dev Biol Stand* **89**: 105–8.

Trotter CL, Ramsay ME and Slack MPE (2003) Rising incidence of *Haemophilus influenzae* type b disease in England and Wales indicates a need for a second catch-up vaccination campaign. *Commun Dis Public Health* **6**: 55–8.

Tudor-Williams G, Frankland J, Isaacs D *et al.* (1989) *Haemophilus influenzae* type b disease in the Oxford region. *Arch Dis Child* **64**: 517–19.

Zuckerman JN (2000) The importance of injecting vaccines into muscle. *BMJ* **321**: 1237–8.

17

Hepatitis A

NOTIFIABLE

The disease

Hepatitis A is an infection of the liver caused by hepatitis A virus. The disease is generally mild, but severity tends to increase with age. Asymptomatic disease is common in children. Jaundice may occur in 70–80% of those infected as adults. Fulminant hepatitis can occur but is rare. The overall case–fatality ratio is low but is greater in older patients and those with pre-existing liver disease. There is no chronic carrier state and chronic liver damage does not occur.

The virus is usually transmitted by the faecal–oral route through person-to-person spread or contaminated food or drink. Foodborne outbreaks have been reported following ingestion of certain shellfish (bivalve molluscs such as mussels, oysters and clams that feed by filtering large volumes of sewage-polluted waters) and salad vegetables. Transmission of hepatitis A has been associated with the use of factor VIII and factor IX concentrates where viral inactivation procedures did not destroy hepatitis A virus. The incubation period is usually around 28–30 days but may occasionally be as little as 15 or as much as 50 days.

History and epidemiology of the disease

Improved standards of living and hygiene have led to a marked fall in the incidence of hepatitis A infection. In the UK, this has resulted in high susceptibility levels in adults, with the typical age of infection shifting from children to older age groups. In 1996, the overall seroprevalence of hepatitis A in England and Wales was estimated to be 31%, and was 11% among those aged 10–19 years (Morris *et al.*, 2002). Therefore, the majority of adolescents and adults remain susceptible to hepatitis A infection and will remain so throughout life, with the potential for outbreaks to occur.

Hepatitis A infection acquired in the UK may either present as sporadic cases, as community-wide outbreaks resulting from person-to-person transmission or, uncommonly, as point of source outbreaks related to contaminated food. Previously, the incidence of hepatitis A showed a cyclical pattern in the UK. However, there has been no peak in incidence since 1990 when 7545 cases

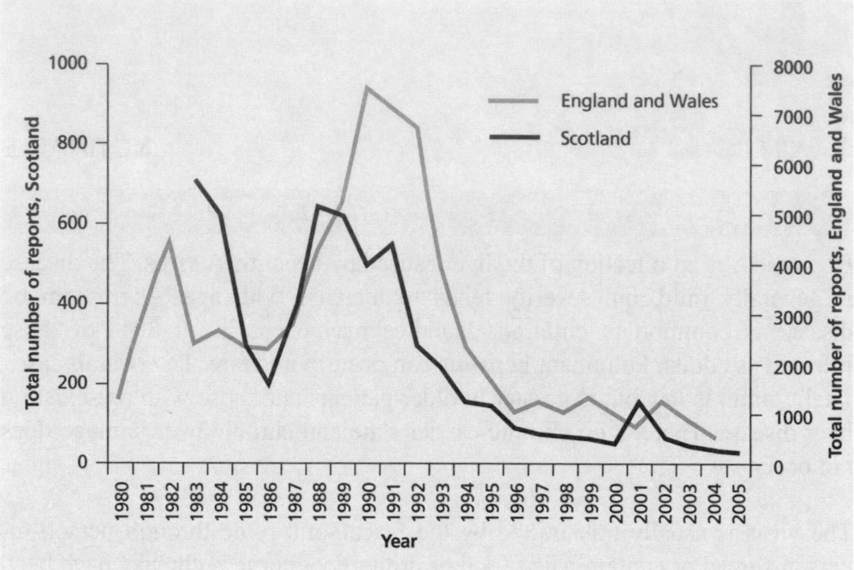

Figure 17.1 Number of laboratory-confirmed hepatitis A reports in England and Wales (1980–2004) and Scotland (1983–2005)

were reported for England and Wales. There were 669 reports in 2004 (HPA, 2005). In Scotland, 26 cases of hepatitis A infection were reported to Health Protection Scotland (formerly the Scottish Centre for Infection and Environmental Health (SCIEH)) in 2005. This is the lowest annual number of acute cases ever recorded. Acute hepatitis A infection had been observed to decrease steadily in Scotland from 1993 (241 cases) to 2000 (50 cases).

In recent decades in the UK, there has been a number of outbreaks of hepatitis A among men who have sex with men (MSM). Similarly, outbreaks have also been documented in a number of other European countries. Transmission appears to be by the faecal–oral route. Some studies have shown associations with multiple anonymous sexual contacts, particularly in 'darkrooms' or clubs (Reintjes *et al.*, 1999; Bell *et al.*, 2001).

Outbreaks of hepatitis A have also been documented among injecting drug users in several countries. An outbreak among injecting drug users in Aberdeen (Roy *et al.*, 2004) contributed to a major increase in the number of cases in Scotland in 2001 (148 cases). Recently, outbreaks of hepatitis A in other parts of the UK have involved a high proportion of individuals with a history of injecting and homeless people living together in hostels and shelters (O'Donovan *et al.*, 2001; Syed *et al.*, 2003; Perrett *et al.*, 2003). Close contact and poor standards of personal hygiene among these groups, with possible faecal contamination of shared injecting equipment or drugs, appears to be the most likely mode of transmission (Hutin *et al.*, 2000; Roy *et al.*, 2004).

Hepatitis A is more common in countries outside Northern and Western Europe, North America, Australia and New Zealand. Travel abroad is a common factor in sporadic cases in the UK. The highest risk areas for UK travellers are the Indian subcontinent and the Far East, but the risk extends to Eastern Europe.

The hepatitis A vaccination

There are two products for immunisation against hepatitis A. An immunoglobulin provides rapid but temporary immunity. The vaccine confers active immunity but response is not immediate. Vaccines are available as either monovalent, or combined with either typhoid or hepatitis B.

Hepatitis A monovalent vaccines and those combined with either typhoid or hepatitis B do not contain thiomersal. The vaccines are inactivated, do not contain live organisms and cannot cause the diseases against which they protect.

Monovalent vaccines

Four monovalent vaccines are currently available, prepared from different strains of the hepatitis A virus; all are grown in human diploid cells (MRC5). Three (Havrix®, Vaqta® and Avaxim®) are adsorbed onto an aluminium hydroxide adjuvant. The fourth, Epaxal® vaccine, contains formalin-inactivated hepatitis A particles attached to phospholipid vesicles together with influenza virus haemagglutinin derived from inactivated influenza virus H1N1 (Gluck *et al.*, 1992; Loutan *et al.*, 1994). These vaccines can be used interchangeably (Bryan *et al.*, 2000; Clarke *et al.*, 2001; Beck *et al.*, 2004).

Combined hepatitis A and hepatitis B vaccine

A combined vaccine containing purified inactivated hepatitis A virus and purified recombinant hepatitis B surface antigen (Twinrix®), adsorbed onto aluminium hydroxide and aluminium phosphate respectively, may be used when protection against both hepatitis A and hepatitis B infections is required. If rapid protection against hepatitis A is required, for example following exposure or during outbreaks, then a single dose of monovalent vaccine is preferred as this may provide protection more quickly than the two courses of combined vaccine.

Combined hepatitis A and typhoid vaccine

Combined vaccines containing purified inactivated hepatitis A virus adsorbed onto aluminium hydroxide and purified Vi capsular polysaccharide typhoid vaccine (Hepatyrix® or ViATIM®) may be used where protection against hepatitis A and typhoid fever is required (see also Chapter 34 on typhoid).

Human normal immunoglobulin

Human normal immunoglobulin (HNIG) is prepared from pooled plasma derived from blood donations. Use of HNIG should be limited to situations where it may have a definite advantage over vaccine. HNIG can provide immediate protection, although antibody levels are lower than those eventually produced by hepatitis A vaccine. There have been no studies directly comparing the efficacy of HNIG with vaccine for prophylaxis in contacts of cases. HNIG licensed for use for prophylaxis must have a hepatitis A antibody level of at least 100IU/ml.*

Because of a theoretical risk of transmission of vCJD from plasma products, HNIG used in the UK is now prepared from plasma sourced from outside the UK, and supplies are scarce. All donors are screened for HIV, hepatitis B and C, and all plasma pools are tested for the presence of RNA from these viruses. A solvent detergent inactivation step for envelope viruses is included in the production process.

Storage

Vaccines should be stored in the original packaging at +2°C to +8°C and protected from light. All vaccines are sensitive to some extent to heat and cold. Heat speeds up the decline in potency of most vaccines, thus reducing their shelf life. Effectiveness cannot be guaranteed for vaccines unless they have been stored at the correct temperature. Freezing may cause increased reactogenicity and loss of potency for some vaccines. It can also cause hairline cracks in the container, leading to contamination of the contents.

HNIG should be stored in the original packaging in a refrigerator at +2°C to +8°C. These products are tolerant to higher ambient temperatures for up to one week. They can be distributed in sturdy packaging outside the cold chain, if needed.

* HNIG for hepatitis A prophylaxis is in short supply and, from time to time, alternative products and doses may need to be used. For the latest advice, please check with the Health Protection Agency (www.hpa.org.uk) or Health Protection Scotland (www.hps.scot.nhs.uk).

Presentation

Vaccine	Product	Pharmaceutical presentation	Instructions on handling before use
Monovalent hepatitis A vaccines	Havrix Monodose® Avaxim® Vaqta® Vaqta Paediatric® Havrix Junior Monodose®	Suspension for injection	Shake well to produce a slightly opaque, white suspension
	Epaxal®	Emulsion for injection	Check for any particulate matter
Combined hepatitis A and B vaccine	Twinrix Adult® Twinrix Paediatric®	Suspension for injection	Shake the vaccine well to obtain a slightly opaque, white suspension
Combined hepatitis A and typhoid vaccine	ViATIM®	A dual-chamber syringe containing a cloudy, white suspension and a clear, colourless solution	Shake to ensure suspension is fully mixed. The contents of the two compartments are mixed as the vaccines are injected
	Hepatyrix®	Slightly opaque white suspension for injection	Shake the container well

Dosage and schedule

The immunisation regimes for hepatitis A vaccine and for combined hepatitis A and typhoid vaccine consist of a single dose. The standard schedule for the combined hepatitis A and hepatitis B vaccine consists of three doses, the first on the elected date, the second one month later and the third six months after the first dose. An accelerated schedule of combined hepatitis A and B vaccine at 0, 7 and 21 days may be used when early protection against hepatitis B is required (e.g. for travellers departing within one month).

Dosage for monovalent hepatitis A immunisation

Vaccine product	Ages	Dose	Volume
Havrix Monodose®	16 years or over	1440 ELISA units	1.0ml
Havrix Junior Monodose®	One to 15 years	720 ELISA units	0.5ml
Avaxim®	16 years or over	160 antigen units	0.5ml
Vaqta Paediatric®	One to 17 years	~25 units	0.5ml
Epaxal®	One year or over	500 RIA units	0.5ml

Dosage of combined hepatitis A and typhoid vaccines

Vaccine product	Ages	Dose HAV	Dose Vi P Ty	Volume
Hepatyrix®	15 years or over	1440 ELISA units	25μg	1.0ml
ViATIM®	16 years or over	160 antigen units	25μg	1.0ml

Dosage of combined hepatitis A and hepatitis B vaccines

Vaccine product	Ages	Dose HAV	Dose HBV	Volume
Twinrix Adult®	16 years or over	720 ELISA units	20μg	1.0ml
Twinrix Paediatric®	1 to 15 years	360 ELISA units	10μg	0.5ml

Dosage of HNIG

- 250mg for children under ten years.
- 500mg for those aged ten years or older.

Administration

Vaccines are routinely given into the upper arm or anterolateral thigh. However, for individuals with a bleeding disorder, vaccines should be given by deep subcutaneous injection to reduce the risk of bleeding.

Hepatitis A-containing vaccines can be given at the same time as other vaccines such as hepatitis B, MMR, MenC, Td/IPV and other travel vaccines. The vaccines should be given at a separate site, preferably in a different limb. If given in the same limb, they should be given at least 2.5cm apart (American Academy of Pediatrics, 2003). The site at which each vaccine was given should be noted in the individual's records.

HNIG can be administered in the upper outer quadrant of the buttock or anterolateral thigh (see Chapter 4). If more than 3ml is to be given to young children and infants, or more than 5ml to older children and adults, the immunoglobulin should be divided into smaller amounts and administered at different sites. HNIG may be administered, at a different site, at the same time as hepatitis A vaccine.

Disposal

Equipment used for vaccination, including used vials or ampoules, should be disposed of at the end of a session by sealing in a proper, puncture-resistant 'sharps' box (UN-approved, BS 7320).

Recommendations for the use of the vaccine

Pre-exposure vaccination

The objective of the immunisation programme is to provide two doses of a hepatitis A-containing vaccine at appropriate intervals for all individuals at high risk of exposure to the virus or of complications from the disease.

Groups recommended to receive pre-exposure vaccination

People travelling to or going to reside in areas of high or intermediate prevalence

Immunisation with hepatitis A vaccine is recommended for those aged one year and over travelling to areas of moderate or high endemicity, such as the Indian subcontinent, for prolonged periods, particularly if sanitation and food hygiene is likely to be poor. Vaccine is also recommended for all individuals going to reside in or likely to be posted for long periods to hepatitis A virus-endemic countries.

Although hepatitis A is usually sub-clinical in children, it can be severe and require hospitalisation. Even children who acquire mild or sub-clinical hepatitis A may be a source of infection to others. The risks of disease for children under one year old are low, and vaccines are not licensed for their use at this age. Care should be taken to prevent exposure to hepatitis A infection through food and water.

For travellers, vaccine should preferably be given at least two weeks before departure, but can be given up to the day of departure. Although antibodies may not be detectable for 12–15 days following administration of monovalent hepatitis A vaccine, the vaccine may provide some protection before antibodies can be detected using current assays.

Immunisation is not considered necessary for individuals travelling to or going to reside in Northern or Western Europe (including Spain, Portugal and Italy), or North America, Australia or New Zealand. HNIG is no longer recommended for travel prophylaxis. Country-by-country recommendations for hepatitis A and other travel vaccines are given in *Health information for overseas travel* (www.nathnac.org).

Patients with chronic liver disease

Although patients with chronic liver disease may be at no greater risk of acquiring hepatitis A infection, it can produce a more serious illness in these patients (Akriviadis and Redeker, 1989; Keefe, 1995). Immunisation against hepatitis A is therefore recommended for patients with severe liver disease of whatever cause. Vaccine should also be considered for individuals with chronic hepatitis B or C infection and for those with milder forms of liver disease.

Patients with haemophilia

As standard viral inactivation processes may not be effective against hepatitis A, patients with haemophilia who are receiving plasma-derived clotting factors should be immunised against hepatitis A. Patients with haemophilia should be immunised subcutaneously.

Men who have sex with men

MSM with multiple sexual partners need to be informed about the risks of hepatitis A, and about the need to maintain high standards of personal hygiene. Immunisation should be offered to such individuals, particularly during periods when outbreaks are occurring.

Injecting drug users

Hepatitis A immunisation is recommended for injecting drug users and can be given at the same time as hepatitis B vaccine, as separate or combined preparations.

Individuals at occupational risk

Hepatitis A vaccination is recommended for the following groups:

- **laboratory workers:** individuals who may be exposed to hepatitis A in the course of their work, in microbiology laboratories and clinical infectious disease units, are at risk and must be protected.
- **staff of some large residential institutions:** outbreaks of hepatitis A have been associated with large residential institutions for those with learning difficulties. Transmission can occur more readily in such institutions and immunisation of staff and residents is appropriate. Similar considerations apply in other institutions where standards of personal hygiene among clients or patients may be poor.
- **sewage workers:** raw, untreated sewage is frequently contaminated with hepatitis A. A UK study to evaluate this risk showed that frequent occupational exposure to raw sewage was an independent risk factor for hepatitis A infection (Brugha *et al.*, 1998). Immunisation is, therefore, recommended for workers at risk of repeated exposure to raw sewage, who should be identified following a local risk assessment.
- **people who work with primates:** vaccination is recommended for those who work with primates that are susceptible to hepatitis A infection.

Hepatitis A vaccination may be considered under certain circumstances for:

- **food packagers and handlers:** food packagers or food handlers in the UK have not been associated with transmission of hepatitis A sufficiently often to justify their immunisation as a routine measure. Where a case or outbreak occurs, advice should be sought from the local health protection unit (HPU)
- **staff in day-care facilities:** infection in young children is likely to be sub-clinical, and those working in day-care centres and other settings with children who are not yet toilet trained may be at increased risk (Severo *et al.*, 1997). Under normal circumstances, the risk of transmission to staff and children can be minimised by careful attention to personal hygiene. However, in the case of a well-defined community outbreak, such as in a pre-school nursery, the need for immunisation of staff and children should be discussed with the local HPU
- **healthcare workers:** most healthcare workers are not at increased risk of hepatitis A and routine immunisation is not indicated.

Post-exposure immunisation

Either passive or active immunisation, or a combination of the two, is available for the management of contacts of cases and for outbreak control.

There have been no trials directly comparing the efficacy of hepatitis A vaccine alone against HNIG in the management of contacts. HNIG is preferred when protection is required in a shorter time than it takes for a protective antibody response to the vaccine. Vaccine and HNIG may be given at the same time, but in different sites, when both rapid and prolonged protection is required. A single dose of monovalent hepatitis A vaccine will provide more rapid protection than the combined preparations where more than one dose is required.

HNIG has a proven record in providing prophylaxis for contacts of cases of acute hepatitis A. HNIG will protect against hepatitis A infection if administered within 14 days of exposure, and may modify disease if given after that time (Winokur and Stapleton, 1992). Protection lasts for four to six months.

There is some evidence that vaccine may be effective in preventing infection in contacts of cases, provided it can be given soon enough after the onset of symptoms in the index case. A study in Naples (Sagliocca *et al.*, 1999) showed hepatitis A vaccine had a 79% protective efficacy in household contacts of people with sporadic infection, where 56% of contacts received vaccine within four days of onset of symptoms in the index cases, and all within eight days. If vaccine is to be used in preference to HNIG for prophylaxis of contacts, cases of acute hepatitis A will need to be diagnosed and reported to public health officials quickly enough to allow administration of vaccine within one week of onset.

Contacts of cases of hepatitis A infection

Hepatitis A vaccine should be given to previously unvaccinated contacts of cases of hepatitis A with onset of jaundice within the last week. When the interval is longer, HNIG should be used, particularly for older people, given the greater severity of disease in this age group. Further guidance on the management of contacts is available in 'Guidelines for the control of hepatitis A virus infection' (Crowcroft *et al.*, 2001).

Prophylaxis restricted to household and close contacts may be relatively ineffective in controlling further spread. If given to a wider social group of recent household visitors (kissing contacts and those who have eaten food prepared by an index case), spread may be prevented more effectively.

If a food handler develops acute jaundice or is diagnosed clinically or serologically with hepatitis A infection, the local HPU should be immediately informed by telephone. This will allow a timely risk assessment of whether other food handlers in the same food preparation area could have been exposed and should be considered for post-exposure prophylaxis. Rapid serological confirmation and notification of hepatitis A infection will allow an assessment of the possible risks to any customers who can be traced and offered prophylaxis.

Further prophylaxis will not be required in immunocompetent contacts who have previously received hepatitis A vaccine.

If a contact is at ongoing risk of hepatitis A infection because of their lifestyle or any other reason, then they should be offered vaccine irrespective of whether they are offered HNIG.

Outbreaks

Active immunisation with monovalent hepatitis A vaccine provides longer duration of protection, and will be more effective in prolonged outbreaks, such as those that may occur among MSM or injecting drug users, where transmissions may continue after the protective effects of HNIG have ceased.

The appropriate approach to the management of outbreaks of hepatitis A infection with HNIG and/or hepatitis A vaccine should be discussed with the local HPU. Further guidance on the management of outbreaks is available in 'Guidelines for the control of hepatitis A virus infection' (Crowcroft *et al.*, 2001).

Primary immunisation

The immunisation regimes for hepatitis A vaccine and for combined hepatitis A and typhoid vaccine consist of a single dose, whereas the combined hepatitis A and B vaccine consists of three doses. Antibodies persist for at least one year.

Reinforcing immunisation

A booster dose of hepatitis A vaccine should be given at six to 12 months after the initial dose. This results in a substantial increase in the antibody titre and will give immunity beyond ten years. Until further evidence is available on persistence of protective immunity, a further booster at 20 years is indicated for those at ongoing risk (Van Damme, 2003).

Where a combined hepatitis A and typhoid vaccine has been used to initiate immunisation, a dose of single antigen hepatitis A vaccine will be required six to 12 months later in order to provide prolonged protection against hepatitis A infection. Booster doses of the typhoid component will be required at three years.

For individuals who have received combined hepatitis A and B vaccine in an accelerated schedule, a booster dose is required at one year.

Delayed administration of the booster dose

Ideally, the manufacturers' recommended timing for the administration of the booster dose of hepatitis A vaccine should be followed. In practice, and particularly in infrequent travellers, there may be a delay in accessing this injection. Studies have shown that successful boosting can occur even when the second dose is delayed for several years (Landry *et al.*, 2001; Beck *et al.*, 2003), so a course does not need to be re-started.

Contraindications

There are very few individuals who cannot receive hepatitis A-containing vaccines. When there is doubt, appropriate advice should be sought from a consultant paediatrician, immunisation co-ordinator or local HPU rather than withholding vaccine.

The vaccine should not be given to those who have had:

- a confirmed anaphylactic reaction to a previous dose of a hepatitis A-containing vaccine, or
- a confirmed anaphylactic reaction to any component of the vaccine.

Epaxal should not be given to those who have had a confirmed anaphylactic hypersensitivity to egg products as a component of the vaccine is prepared on hens' eggs.

Precautions

Minor illnesses without fever or systemic upset are not valid reasons to postpone immunisation.

If an individual is acutely unwell, immunisation may be postponed until they have fully recovered. This is to avoid confusing the differential diagnosis of any acute illness by wrongly attributing any signs or symptoms to the adverse effects of the vaccine.

HNIG

When HNIG is being used for prevention of hepatitis A, it must be remembered that it may interfere with the subsequent development of active immunity from live virus vaccines. If immunoglobulin has been administered first, then an interval of three months should be observed before administering a live virus vaccine. If immunoglobulin has been given within three weeks of administering a live vaccine, then the vaccine should be repeated three months later. This does not apply to yellow fever vaccine since HNIG does not contain significant amounts of antibodies to this virus.

Pregnancy and breast-feeding

Hepatitis A-containing vaccines may be given to pregnant women when clinically indicated. There is no evidence of risk from vaccinating pregnant women or those who are breast-feeding with inactivated viral or bacterial vaccines or toxoids (Plotkin and Orenstein, 2004).

Immunosuppression and HIV infection

Individuals with immunosuppression and HIV infection can be given hepatitis A-containing vaccines (Bodsworth *et al.*, 1997; Kemper *et al.*, 2003) although seroconversion rates and antibody titre may be lower and appear to be related to the individual's CD4 count at the time of immunisation (Neilsen *et al.*, 1997; Kemper *et al.*, 2003). Re-immunisation should be considered and specialist advice may be required.

Further guidance is provided by the Royal College of Paediatrics and Child Health (www.rcpch.ac.uk), the British HIV Association (BHIVA) *Immunisation guidelines for HIV-infected adults* (BHIVA, 2006) and the Children's HIV Association of UK and Ireland (CHIVA) immunisation guidelines (www.bhiva.org/chiva).

Adverse reactions

Adverse reactions to hepatitis A vaccines are usually mild and confined to the first few days after immunisation. The most common reactions are mild, transient soreness, erythema and induration at the injection site. A small, painless nodule may form at the injection site; this usually disappears and is of no consequence.

General symptoms such as fever, malaise, fatigue, headache, nausea and loss of appetite are also reported less frequently.

HNIG is well tolerated. Very rarely, anaphylactoid reactions occur in individuals with hypogammaglobulinaemia who have IgA antibodies, or those who have had an atypical reaction to blood transfusion.

Serious, suspected adverse reactions to vaccines should be reported through the Yellow Card scheme.

No cases of blood-borne infection acquired through immunoglobulin preparations designed for intramuscular use have been documented in any country.

Supplies

Hepatitis A vaccine

- Avaxim® (adolescents and adults aged 16 years or over)
- Vaqta Paediatric® (children and adolescents from one up to 17 years)

These vaccines are available from Sanofi Pasteur MSD
(Tel: 0800 0855511).

- Havrix Monodose® (adults aged 16 years or over)
- Havrix Junior Monodose® (children and adolescents from one up to 15 years)

These vaccines are available from GlaxoSmithKline
(Tel: 0808 1009997).

- Epaxal® (adults and children from one year of age)

This vaccine is available from MASTA
(Tel: 0113 238 7555).

Combined vaccines

- ViATIM® (adults and adolescents aged 16 years or over) (with typhoid)

This vaccine is available from Sanofi Pasteur MSD.

- Twinrix Adult® (aged 16 years or over) (with hepatitis B)
- Twinrix Paediatric® (children/adolescents aged one to 15 years) (with hepatitis B)
- Hepatyrix® (adults and adolescents aged 15 years or over) (with typhoid)

These vaccines are available from GlaxoSmithKline.

Immunoglobulin

HNIG is available **for contacts of cases and control of outbreaks only** from:

England and Wales:
Health Protection Agency
Centre for Infections
(Tel: 020 8200 6868).

Scotland:

Health Protection Scotland
Glasgow
(Tel: 0141 300 1100).

Northern Ireland:

Northern Ireland Public Health Laboratory
Belfast City Hospital
(Tel: 02890 329241).

HNIG is produced by the Scottish National Blood Transfusion Service

(Tel: 0131 536 5797 or 5763).

References

Akriviadis EA and Redeker AG (1989) Fulminant hepatitis A in intravenous drug users with chronic liver disease. *Ann Intern Med* **110**: 838–9.

American Academy of Pediatrics (2003) Active immunization. In: Pickering LK (ed.) *Red Book: 2003 Report of the Committee on Infectious Diseases,* 26th edition. Elk Grove Village, IL: American Academy of Pediatrics, p. 33.

Beck BR, Hatz C, Bronnimann R *et al.* (2003) Successful booster antibody response up to 54 months after single primary vaccination with virosome-formulated, aluminium-free hepatitis A vaccine. *Clin Infect Dis* **37**: 126–8.

Beck BR, Hatz CFR, Loutan L *et al.* (2004) Immunogenicity of booster vaccination with a virosomal hepatitis A vaccine after primary immunisation with an aluminium-adsorbed hepatitis A vaccine. *J Travel Med* **11**: 201–207.

Bell A, Ncube F, Hansell A *et al.* (2001) An outbreak of hepatitis A among young men associated with having sex in public places. *Commun Dis Public Health* **4**(3): 163–70.

Bodsworth NJ, Neilson GA and Donovan B (1997) The effect of immunisation with inactivated hepatitis A vaccine on the clinical course of HIV-1 infection: one-year follow-up. *AIDS* **11**: 747–9.

British HIV Association (2006) *Immunisation guidelines for HIV-infected adults.* www.bhiva.org/pdf/2006/Immunisation506.pdf

Brugha R, Heptonstall J, Farrington P *et al.* (1998) Risk of hepatitis A infection in sewage workers. *Occup Environ Med* **55**: 567–9.

Bryan JP, Henry CH, Hoffman AG *et al.* (2000) Randomized, cross-over, controlled comparison of two inactivated hepatitis A vaccines. *Vaccine* **19**: 743–50.

Clarke P, Kitchin N and Souverbie F (2001) A randomised comparison of two inactivated hepatitis A vaccines, Avaxim and Vaqta, given as a booster to subjects primed with Avaxim. *Vaccine* **19**: 4429–33.

Crowcroft NS, Walsh B, Davison KL *et al.* (2001) Guidelines for the control of hepatitis A infection. *Commun Dis Public Health* **4**: 213–27.

Department of Health (2001) *Health information for overseas travel*, 2nd edition. London: TSO.

Gluck R, Mischler R, Brantschen S *et al.* (1992) Immunopotentiating reconstructed influenza virus virosome (IRIV) vaccine delivery system for immunisation against hepatitis A. *J Clin Invest* **90**: 2491–5.

Health Protection Agency (2005) Laboratory reports of hepatitis A in England and Wales: 2004. *Commun Dis Rep CDR Wkly* [serial online] **15** (34). www.hpa.org.uk/cdr/archives/2005/cdr3405.pdf.

Henning KJ, Bell E, Braun J and Barkers ND (1995) A community-wide outbreak of hepatitis A: risk factors for infection among homosexual and bisexual men. *Am J Med* **99**: 132–6.

Hutin YJ, Sabin KM, Hutwager LC *et al.* (2000) Multiple modes of hepatitis A virus transmission among methamphetamine users. *Am J Epidemiol* **152**: 186–92.

Keefe EB (1995) Is hepatitis A more severe in patients with chronic hepatitis B and other chronic liver diseases? *Am J Gastroenterol* **90**: 201–5.

Kemper CA, Haubrich R, Frank I *et al.* (2003) Safety and immunogenicity of hepatitis A vaccine in human immunodeficiency virus-infected patients: a double blind, randomised, placebo-controlled trial. *J Infect Dis* **187**: 1327–31.

Landry P, Tremblay S, Darioli R *et al.* (2001) Inactivated hepatitis A vaccine booster given at or after 24 months after the primary dose. *Vaccine* **19**: 399–402.

Loutan L, Bovier P, Althaus B *et al.* (1994) Inactivated virosome hepatitis A vaccine. *Lancet* **343**: 322–4.

Mele A, Sagliocca L, Palumbo F *et al.* (1991) Travel-associated hepatitis A: effect of place of residence and country visited. *J Public Health Med* **13**: 256–9.

Morris MC, Gay NJ, Hesketh LM *et al.* (2002) The changing epidemiological pattern of hepatitis A in England and Wales. *Epidemiol Infect.* **128**: 457–63.

Neilsen GA, Bodsworth NJ and Watts N (1997) Response to hepatitis A vaccination in human immunodeficiency virus-infected and -uninfected homosexual men. *J Infect Dis* **176**: 1064–7.

O'Donovan D, Cooke RPD, Joce R *et al.* (2001) An outbreak of hepatitis A among injecting drug users. *Epidemiol Infect* **127**: 469–73.

Perrett K, Granerod J, Crowcroft N *et al.* (2003) Changing epidemiology of hepatitis A: should we be doing more to vaccinate injecting drug users? *Commun Dis Public Health* **6**: 97–100.

Plotkin SA and Orenstein WA (eds) (2004) *Vaccines*, 4th edition. Philadelphia: WB Saunders Company.

Reid TM and Robinson HG (1987) Frozen raspberries and hepatitis A. *Epidemiol Infect* **98**: 109–12.

Reintjes R, Bosman A, de Zwart O *et al.* (1999) Outbreak of hepatitis A in Rotterdam associated with visits to 'darkrooms' in gay bars. *Commun Dis Public Health* **2**(1): 43–6.

Roy K, Howie H, Sweeney C *et al.* (2004) Hepatitis A virus and injecting drug misuse in Aberdeen, Scotland: a case-control study. *J Viral Hepat* **11**: 277–82.

Sagliocca L, Amoroso P, Stroffolini T *et al.* (1999) Efficacy of hepatitis A vaccine in prevention of secondary hepatitis A infection: a randomised trial. *Lancet* **353**: 1136–9.

Severo CA, Abensur P, Buisson Y *et al.* (1997) An outbreak of hepatitis A in a French day-care center and efforts to combat it. *Eur J Epidemiol* **13**: 139–44.

Syed NA, Hearing SD, Shaw IS *et al.* (2003) Outbreak of hepatitis A in the injecting drug user and homeless populations in Bristol: control by a targeted vaccination programme and possible parenteral transmission. *Eur J Gastroenterol Hepatol* **15**: 901–6.

Van Damme P, Banatvala J, Fay O *et al.* (2003) Hepatitis A booster vaccination: is there a need? *Lancet* **362**: 1065–71.

Winokur PL and Stapleton JT (1992) Immunoglobulin prophylaxis for hepatitis A. *Clin Infect Dis* **14**: 580–6.

18

Hepatitis B

NOTIFIABLE

The disease

Hepatitis B is an infection of the liver caused by the hepatitis B virus (HBV). Many new infections with hepatitis B are sub-clinical or may have a flu-like illness. Jaundice only occurs in about 10% of younger children and in 30 to 50% of adults. Acute infection may occasionally lead to fulminant hepatic necrosis, which is often fatal.

The illness usually starts insidiously – with anorexia and nausea and an ache in the right upper abdomen. Fever, when present, is usually mild. Malaise may be profound, with disinclination to smoke or to drink alcohol. As jaundice develops, there is progressive darkening of the urine and lightening of the faeces. In patients who do not develop symptoms suggestive of hepatitis, the illness will only be detected by abnormal liver function tests and/or the presence of serological markers of hepatitis B infection (e.g. hepatitis B surface antigen (HBsAg), antiHBc IgM).

The virus is transmitted by parenteral exposure to infected blood or body fluids. Transmission mostly occurs:

- through vaginal or anal intercourse
- as a result of blood-to-blood contact (e.g. sharing of needles and other equipment by injecting drug users (IDUs), 'needlestick' injuries)
- through perinatal transmission from mother to child.

Transmission has also followed bites from infected persons, although this is rare. Transfusion-associated infection is now rare in the UK as blood donations are screened. Viral inactivation of blood products has eliminated these as a source of infection in this country.

The incubation period ranges from 40 to 160 days, with an average of 60 to 90 days. Current infection can be detected by the presence of HBsAg in the serum. Blood and body fluids from these individuals should be considered to be infectious. In most individuals, infection will resolve and HBsAg disappears from the serum, but the virus persists in some patients who become chronically infected with hepatitis B.

Chronic hepatitis B infection is defined as persistence of HBsAg in the serum for six months or longer. Individuals with chronic infection are sometimes referred to as chronic carriers. Among those who are HBsAg positive, those in whom hepatitis B e-antigen (HBeAg) is also detected in the serum are the most infectious. Those who are HBsAg positive and HBeAg negative (usually anti-HBe positive) are infectious but generally of lower infectivity. Recent evidence suggests that a proportion of chronically infected people who are HBeAg negative will have high HBV DNA levels, and may be more infectious.

The risk of developing chronic hepatitis B infection depends on the age at which infection is acquired. Chronic infection occurs in 90% of those infected perinatally but is less frequent in those infected as children (e.g. 20 to 50% in children between one and five years of age). About 5% or less of previously healthy people, infected as adults, become chronically infected (Hyams, 1995). The risk is increased in those whose immunity is impaired.

Around 20 to 25% of individuals with chronic HBV infection worldwide have progressive liver disease, leading to cirrhosis in some patients. The risk of progression is related to the level of active viral replication in the liver. Individuals with chronic hepatitis B infection – particularly those with an active inflammation and/or cirrhosis, where there is rapid cell turnover – are at increased risk of developing hepatocellular carcinoma.

History and epidemiology of the disease

The World Health Organization (WHO) has estimated that over 350 million people worldwide are chronically infected with HBV. The WHO has categorised countries based upon the prevalence of HBsAg into high (more than 8%), intermediate (2 to 8%) and low (less than 2%) endemicity countries. In many high-prevalence countries, 10% or more of the population have chronic hepatitis B infection. High-prevalence regions include sub-Saharan Africa, most of Asia and the Pacific islands. Intermediate-prevalence regions include the Amazon, southern parts of Eastern and Central Europe, the Middle East and the Indian sub-continent. Low-prevalence regions include most of Western Europe and North America (see Figure 18.1).

The importance of the various modes of transmission varies according to the prevalence in a particular country. In areas of high prevalence, infection is acquired predominantly in childhood – by perinatal transmission or by horizontal transmission among young children. In low-endemicity countries, most infections are acquired in adulthood, where sexual transmission or sharing of blood-contaminated needles and equipment by injecting drug users

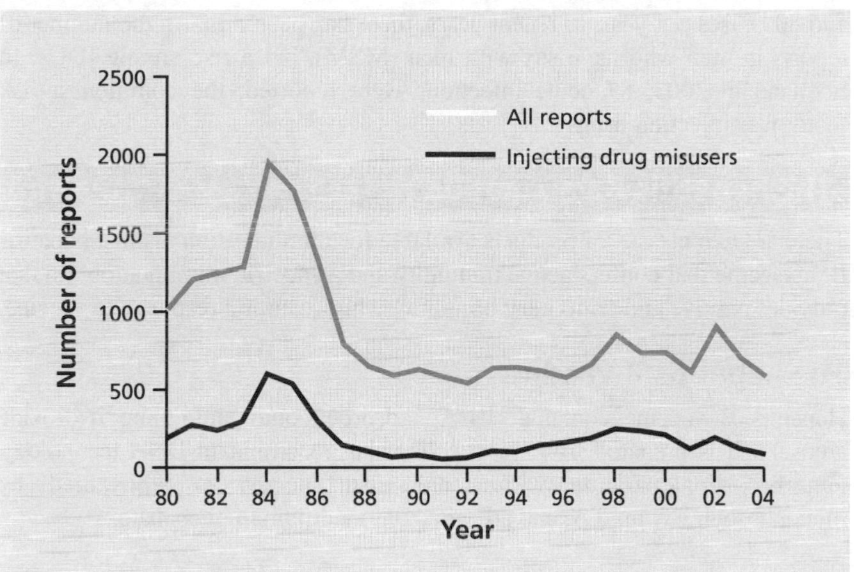

Figure 18.1 Laboratory reports of confirmed acute hepatitis B, England and Wales

accounts for a significant proportion of new infections. In areas of intermediate endemicity, the pattern of perinatal, childhood and adult infection is mixed, and nosocomial infection may be important.

The UK is a very low-prevalence country, but prevalence of HBsAg varies across the country. It is higher in those born in high-endemicity countries, many of whom will have acquired infection at birth or in early childhood (Boxall *et al.*,1994; Aweis *et al.*, 2001). This is reflected in the prevalence rates found in antenatal women, which vary from 0.05 to 0.08% in some rural areas but rise to 1% or more in certain inner city areas. Overall, the prevalence in antenatal women in the UK is around 0.14%.

The incidence of acute infection is high among those with certain lifestyle or occupational risk factors. Most reports of acute infection in the UK occur as a result of injecting drug use or sexual exposure.

Laboratory reports of acute hepatitis B to the Health Protection Agency fell from a peak of just below 2000 reports from England and Wales in 1984 to 531 reports in 1992, mainly due to a decline in cases in IDUs. The decrease was also seen in other risk groups, most probably linked to a modification of risk behaviours in response to the HIV/AIDS epidemic. Since then there has been no further fall; reports have fluctuated between around 600 and 800 cases per year. In recent years, there has been a fall in the number of reports in men who have sex with men (MSM), but a rise among IDUs. In Scotland in 2003, 87 acute infections were reported; the commonest risk factor was injecting drugs.

The hepatitis B vaccination

There are two classes of products available for immunisation against hepatitis B: a vaccine that confers active immunity and a specific immunoglobulin that provides passive and temporary immunity while awaiting response to vaccine.

The hepatitis B vaccine

Hepatitis B vaccine contains HBsAg adsorbed onto aluminium hydroxide adjuvant. It is prepared from yeast cells using recombinant DNA technology. Fendrix®, for patients with renal insufficiency, is adjuvanted by monophosophoryl lipid A, and adsorbed onto aluminium phosphate.

A combined vaccine containing purified inactivated hepatitis A virus (HAV) and purified recombinant HBsAg, separately adsorbed onto aluminium hydroxide and aluminium phosphate, is also available where protection against both hepatitis A and hepatitis B infections is required.

Thiomersal is not used as a preservative in hepatitis B vaccines available in the UK. Thiomersal is still used in the production process for Engerix B®, Twinrix® and Fendrix® and, therefore, residues are present in the final product.

Hepatitis B-containing vaccines are inactivated, do not contain live organisms and cannot cause the diseases against which they protect.

There are vaccines that are effective in preventing infection in individuals who produce specific antibodies to HBsAg (anti-HBs). However, it is important that immunisation against hepatitis B does not encourage relaxation of other measures designed to prevent exposure to the virus, for example condom use and needle exchange. Healthcare workers giving immunisation should use the opportunity to provide advice on other preventative measures or to arrange referral to appropriate specialist services.

Around 10 to 15% of adults fail to respond to three doses of vaccine or respond poorly. Poor responses are mostly associated with age over 40 years, obesity and smoking (Roome *et al.*, 1993). Lower seroconversion rates have also been reported in alcoholics, particularly those with advanced liver disease (Rosman *et al.*, 1997). Patients who are immunosuppressed or on renal dialysis may respond less well than healthy individuals and may require larger or more frequent doses of vaccine.

Hepatitis B vaccine is highly effective at preventing infection if given shortly after exposure (see below). Ideally, immunisation should commence within 48 hours, although it should still be considered up to a week after exposure.

The vaccine is not effective in patients with acute hepatitis B, and is not necessary for individuals known to have markers of current (HBsAg) or past (anti-HB) infection. However, immunisation should not be delayed while awaiting any test results.

Hepatitis B immunoglobulin

Specific hepatitis B immunoglobulin (HBIG) provides passive immunity and can give immediate but temporary protection after accidental inoculation or contamination with hepatitis B-infected blood. HBIG is given concurrently with hepatitis B vaccine and does not affect the development of active immunity. If infection has already occurred at the time of immunisation, virus multiplication may not be inhibited completely, but severe illness and, most importantly, development of the carrier state may be prevented.

HBIG is used after exposure to give rapid protection until hepatitis B vaccine, which should be given at the same time, becomes effective. The use of HBIG in addition to vaccine is recommended only in high-risk situations or in a known non-responder to vaccine. Whenever immediate protection is required, immunisation with the vaccine should be given. When appropriate, this should be combined with simultaneous administration of HBIG at a different site. Ideally, HBIG should be given within 48 hours, although it should still be considered up to a week after exposure.

HBIG is obtained from the plasma of immunised and screened human donors. Because of a theoretical risk of transmission of vCJD from plasma products, HBIG used in the UK is now prepared from plasma sourced from outside the UK, and supplies are scarce.

All donors are screened for HIV, hepatitis B and hepatitis C, and all plasma pools are tested for the presence of RNA from these viruses. A solvent-detergent inactivation step for envelope viruses is included in the production process. There is no evidence associating the administration of HBIG with acquisition of HIV infection. Not only does the processing of the plasma from which it is prepared render it safe, but the screening of blood donations is routine practice.

Storage

Vaccines should be stored in the original packaging at +2˚C to +8˚C and protected from light. All vaccines are sensitive to some extent to heat and cold. Heat speeds up the decline in potency of most vaccines, thus reducing their shelf life. Effectiveness cannot be guaranteed for vaccines unless they have been stored at the correct temperature. Freezing may cause increased reactogenicity and loss of potency for some vaccines. It can also cause hairline cracks in the container, leading to contamination of the contents.

HBIG should be stored in a refrigerator at +2˚C to +8˚C. These products are tolerant to ambient temperatures for up to one week. They can be distributed in sturdy packaging outside the cold chain if needed.

Presentation

HBIG is a clear, pale yellow fluid or light brown solution dispensed in vials containing 200IU or 500IU in approximately 2ml and 4ml respectively.

Vaccine	Product	Pharmaceutical presentation	Instructions on handling vaccine
Hepatitis B	Engerix B® Fendrix® HBvaxPRO®	Suspension for injection	Shake the vaccine well to obtain a slightly opaque, white suspension
Hepatitis A and B	Twinrix Adult® Twinrix Paediatric®	Suspension for injection	Shake the vaccine well to obtain a slightly opaque, white suspension

Dosage

Currently, licensed vaccines contain different concentrations of antigen per millilitre. The appropriate manufacturer's dosage should be adhered to.

Different hepatitis B vaccine products can be used to complete a primary immunisation course or, where indicated, as a booster dose in individuals who have previously received another hepatitis B vaccine (Bush *et al.*, 1991).

Table 18.1 Dosage of hepatitis B vaccines by age

Vaccine product	Ages and group	Dose	Volume
Engerix B®	0–15 years*	10µg	0.5ml
Engerix B®	16 years or over	20µg	1.0ml
Fendrix®	Patients with renal insufficiency aged 15 years and over	20µg	0.5ml
HBvaxPRO Paediatric®	0–15 years	5µg	0.5ml
HBvaxPRO®	16 years or over	10µg	1.0ml
HBvaxPRO40®	Adult dialysis and pre-dialysis patients	40µg	1.0ml

* 20µg of Engerix B may be given to children 11–15 of years age if using the two-dose schedule (see below)

Table 18.2 Dosage of combined hepatitis A and hepatitis B vaccines by age

Vaccine product	Ages	Dose HAV	Dose HBV	Volume
Twinrix Adult®	16 years or over	720 ELISA units	20µg	1.0ml
Twinrix Paediatric®	1–15 years	360 ELISA units	10µg	0.5ml

Table 18.3 Dosage of HBIG

Age group	Dose
Newborn and children aged 0–4 years	200IU
Children aged 5–9 years	300IU
Adults and children aged 10 years or over	500IU

HBIG is available in 2ml ampoules containing approximately 200IU or 500IU.

Schedule

There are many different immunisation regimes for hepatitis B vaccine (see page 175). Generally the schedule for hepatitis B or combined hepatitis A and hepatitis B vaccine, consists of three doses, with or without a fourth dose. One exception involves the use of adult strength vaccine in children 11–15 years of age, where two doses (given at one and six months) are acceptable.

Administration

Hepatitis B vaccines are routinely given intramuscularly in the upper arm or anterolateral thigh. The buttock must not be used because vaccine efficacy may be reduced.

Hepatitis B-containing vaccines can be given at the same time as other vaccines such as DTaP/IPV/Hib, hepatitis A, MMR, MenC, Td/IPV and other travel vaccines. The vaccines should be given at a separate site, preferably in a different limb. If given in the same limb, they should be given at least 2.5cm apart (American Academy of Pediatrics, 2003). The site at which each vaccine was given should be noted in the individual's records.

For individuals with a bleeding disorder, vaccines should be given by deep subcutaneous injection to reduce the risk of bleeding.

HBIG can be administered in the upper outer quadrant of the buttock or anterolateral thigh (see Chapter 4). If more than 3ml is to be given to young children and infants, or more than 5ml to older children and adults, the immunoglobulin should be divided into smaller amounts and administered to different sites. HBIG may be administered, at a different site, at the same time as hepatitis B vaccine.

Disposal

Equipment used for vaccination, including used vials or ampoules, should be disposed of at the end of a session by sealing in a proper, puncture-resistant 'sharps' box (UN-approved, BS 7320).

Recommendations for the use of the vaccine

Pre-exposure vaccination

The objective of the immunisation programme is to provide a minimum of three doses of hepatitis B vaccine for individuals at high risk of exposure to the virus or complications of the disease.

Pre-exposure immunisation is used for individuals who are at increased risk of hepatitis B because of their lifestyle, occupation or other factors. Immediate post-exposure vaccination is used to prevent infection, especially in babies born to infected mothers or following needlestick injuries (see below).

Where testing for markers of current or past infection is clinically indicated, this should be done at the same time as the administration of the first dose. Vaccination should not be delayed while waiting for results of the tests. Further doses may not be required in those with clear evidence of past exposure. Pre-exposure immunisation is recommended for the following groups.

Injecting drug users

IDUs are a group at particular risk of acquiring hepatitis B infection. Vaccination is recommended for the following:

- all current IDUs, as a high priority
- those who inject intermittently
- those who are likely to 'progress' to injecting, for example those who are currently smoking heroin and/or crack cocaine, and heavily dependent amphetamine users
- non-injecting users who are living with current injectors
- sexual partners of injecting users
- children of injectors.

Individuals who change sexual partners frequently

Those who change sexual partners frequently, particularly MSM and male and female commercial sex workers.

Close family contacts of a case or indivdual with chronic hepatitis B infection

Sexual partners are most at risk, and they and close household contacts should be vaccinated. Blood should be taken at the time of the first dose of vaccine to determine if they have already been infected. Contacts shown to be HBsAg, anti-HBs or anti-HBc positive do not require further immunisation. Advice regarding the appropriate use of condoms should be given; a reasonable level of protection can be assumed following the second dose, provided that completion of the schedule can be assured.

Contacts who have had recent unprotected sex with individuals who have acute hepatitis B or who are HBsAg positive require post-exposure prophylaxis, including HBIG (see below).

Families adopting children from countries with a high or intermediate prevalence of hepatitis B

Members of such families may be at risk, as these children could be chronically infected (Christenson, 1986; Rudin *et al.*, 1990). When the status of the child to be adopted is not known, families adopting children from any high or intermediate-prevalence country should be advised as to the risks and hepatitis B vaccination recommended. In due course, testing such children is advisable because there could be benefits from referring an infected child for further management.

Foster carers

Some children requiring fostering may have been at increased risk of acquiring hepatitis B infection. Emergency placements may be made within a few hours:

foster carers who accept children as emergency placements should be made aware of the risks of undiagnosed infection and how they can minimise the risks of transmission of all blood-borne virus infections. All short-term foster carers who receive emergency placements, and their families, should be offered immunisation against hepatitis B. Permanent foster carers (and their families) who accept a child known to be at high risk of hepatitis B should also be offered immunisation.

Individuals receiving regular blood or blood products and their carers

Those individuals receiving regular blood products, such as people with haemophilia, should be vaccinated. Those receiving regular blood transfusions, for example people with thalassaemia or other chronic anaemia, should be vaccinated against hepatitis B. Carers responsible for the administration of such products should also be vaccinated.

Patients with chronic renal failure

Patients with renal failure may need haemodialysis, at which time they may be at increased risk of hepatitis B. The response to hepatitis B vaccine among patients with renal failure is lower than among healthy adults. Between 45 and 66% of patients with chronic renal failure develop anti-HBs responses and, compared with immunocompetent individuals, levels of anti-HBs decline more rapidly. However, increased response rates have been reported in vaccines formulated for use in patients with chronic renal failure (Tong *et al.*, 2005).

Immunisation against hepatitis B is recommended for patients already on haemodialysis or renal transplantation programmes and for other patients with chronic renal failure as soon as it is anticipated that they may require these interventions. The vaccines formulated for use in patients with chronic renal insufficiency should be used.

Patients with chronic liver disease

Individuals with chronic liver disease may be at increased risk of the consequences of hepatitis B infection. Immunisation against hepatitis B is therefore recommended for patients with severe liver disease, such as cirrhosis, of whatever cause. Vaccine should also be offered to individuals with milder liver disease, particularly those who are chronically infected with hepatitis C virus, who may share risk factors that mean that they are at increased risk of acquiring hepatitis B infection.

Inmates of custodial institutions

Immunisation against hepatitis B is recommended for all sentenced prisoners and all new inmates entering prison in the UK.

Individuals in residential accommodation for those with learning difficulties

A higher prevalence of chronic hepatitis B infection has been found among individuals with learning difficulties in residential accommodation than in the general population. Close, daily living contact and the possibility of behavioural problems may lead to residents being at increased risk of infection. Vaccination is therefore recommended.

Similar considerations may apply to children and adults in day care, schools and centres for those with severe learning disability. Decisions on immunisation should be made on the basis of a local risk assessment. In settings where the individual's behaviour is likely to lead to significant exposure (e.g. biting or being bitten) on a regular basis, immunisation should be offered to individuals even in the absence of documented hepatitis B transmission.

People travelling to or going to reside in areas of high or intermediate prevalence

Travellers to areas of high or intermediate prevalence who place themselves at risk when abroad should be offered immunisation. The behaviours that place them at risk will include sexual activity, injecting drug use, undertaking relief aid work and/or participating in contact sports. Travellers are also at risk of acquiring infection as a result of medical or dental procedures carried out in countries where unsafe therapeutic injections (e.g. the re-use of contaminated needles and syringes without sterilisation) are a risk factor for hepatitis B (Kane *et al.*, 1999; Simonsen *et al.*, 1999). Individuals at high risk of requiring medical or dental procedures in such countries should therefore be immunised, including:

- those who plan to remain in areas of high or intermediate prevalence for lengthy periods
- children and others who may require medical care while travelling to visit families or relatives in high or moderate-endemicity countries
- people with chronic medical conditions who may require hospitalisation while overseas
- those travelling for medical care.

Individuals at occupational risk

Hepatitis B vaccination is recommended for the following groups who are considered at increased risk:

- **healthcare workers in the UK and overseas (including students and trainees):** all healthcare workers who may have direct contact with patients' blood, blood-stained body fluids or tissues, require vaccination. This includes any staff who are at risk of injury from blood-contaminated sharp instruments, or of being deliberately injured or bitten by patients. Advice should be obtained from the appropriate occupational health department.

- **laboratory staff:** any laboratory staff who handle material that may contain the virus require vaccination.

- **staff of residential and other accommodation for those with learning difficulties:** a higher prevalence of hepatitis B carriage has been found among certain groups of patients with learning difficulties in residential accommodation than in the general population. Close contact and the possibility of behavioural problems, including biting and scratching, may lead to staff being at increased risk of infection.

  Similar considerations may apply to staff in day-care settings and special schools for those with severe learning disability. Decisions on immunisation should be made on the basis of a local risk assessment. In settings where the client's behaviour is likely to lead to significant exposures on a regular basis (e.g. biting), it would be prudent to offer immunisation to staff even in the absence of documented hepatitis B transmission.

- **other occupational risk groups:** in some occupational groups, such as morticians and embalmers, there is an established risk of hepatitis B, and immunisation is recommended. Immunisation is also recommended for all prison service staff who are in regular contact with prisoners.

Hepatitis B vaccination may also be considered for other groups such as the police and fire and rescue services. In these workers an assessment of the frequency of likely exposure should be carried out. For those with frequent exposure, pre-exposure immunisation is recommended. For other groups, post-exposure immunisation at the time of an incident may be more appropriate (see below). Such a selection has to be decided locally by the occupational health services or as a result of appropriate medical advice.

Post-exposure immunisation

Post-exposure prophylaxis is recommended for the following groups.

Babies born to mothers who are chronically infected with HBV or to mothers who have had acute hepatitis B during pregnancy

Hepatitis B infection can be transmitted from infected mothers to their babies at or around the time of birth (perinatal transmission). Babies acquiring infection at this time have a high risk of becoming chronically infected with the virus. The development of the carrier state after perinatal transmission can be prevented in over 90% of cases by appropriate vaccination, starting at birth, of all infants born to infected mothers.

UK guidelines (Department of Health, 1998) recommend that all pregnant women should be offered screening for hepatitis B infection during each pregnancy. Confirmatory testing and testing for hepatitis B e-markers of those mothers shown to be infected should follow. Where an unbooked mother presents in labour, an urgent HBsAg test should be performed to ensure that vaccine can be given to babies born to positive mothers within 24 hours of birth.

All babies born to these mothers should receive a complete course of vaccine on time. Arrangements should be in place to ensure that information is shared with appropriate local agencies to facilitate follow up.

Babies born to highly infectious mothers should receive HBIG as well as active immunisation (see Table 18.4). HBIG should preferably be given within 24 hours of delivery, and should be ordered well in advance of the birth. HBIG may be given simultaneously with vaccine but at a different site.

Table 18.4 Vaccination of term babies according to the hepatitis B status of the mother

Hepatitis B status of mother	Baby should receive	
	Hepatitis B vaccine	HBIG
Mother is HBsAg positive and HBeAg positive	Yes	Yes
Mother is HBsAg positive, HBeAg negative and anti-HBe negative	Yes	Yes
Mother is HBsAg positive where e-markers have not been determined	Yes	Yes
Mother had acute hepatitis B during pregnancy	Yes	Yes
Mother is HBsAg positive and anti-HBe positive	Yes	No

Hepatitis B

Vaccination of pre-term babies

There is evidence that the response to hepatitis B vaccine is lower in pre-term, low-birth weight babies (Losonsky *et al.*, 1999). It is, therefore, important that premature infants receive the full paediatric dose of hepatitis B vaccine on schedule. Babies with a birthweight of 1500g or less, born to mothers infected with hepatitis B, should receive HBIG in addition to the vaccine, regardless of the e-antigen status of the mother.

Vaccination schedule and follow-up

For post-exposure prophylaxis in babies born to mothers infected with hepatitis B, the accelerated immunisation schedule is preferred. For these babies this will mean an initial dose of vaccine at birth, with further doses at one and two months of age and a fourth dose at one year of age.

Testing for HBsAg at one year of age will identify any babies for whom this intervention has not been successful and who have become chronically infected with hepatitis B, and will allow them to be referred for assessment and any further management. This testing can be carried out at the same time as the fourth dose is given.

Where immunisation has been delayed beyond the recommended intervals, the vaccine course should be completed, but it is more likely that the child may become infected. In this instance, testing for HBsAg above the age of one year is particularly important.

Other groups potentially exposed to hepatitis B

Any individual potentially exposed to hepatitis B-infected blood or body fluids should be offered protection against hepatitis B, depending on their prior vaccination status and the status of the source. Guidance on post-exposure prophylaxis following exposure to hepatitis B has been issued by the former PHLS Hepatitis Subcommittee (PHLS Hepatitis Subcommittee, 1992). A summary of this guidance is given in Table 18.5.

Sexual partners

Any sexual partner of individuals suffering from acute hepatitis B, and who are seen within one week of last contact, should be offered protection with HBIG and vaccine. Sexual contacts of an individual with newly diagnosed chronic hepatitis B should be offered vaccine; HBIG may be added if unprotected sexual contact occurred in the past week.

Persons who are accidentally inoculated or contaminated

This includes those who contaminate their eyes or mouth, or fresh cuts or abrasions of the skin, with blood from a known HBsAg-positive person. Individuals who sustain such accidents should wash the affected area well with soap and warm water, and seek medical advice. Advice about prophylaxis after such accidents should be obtained by telephone from the nearest public health laboratory or from the local health protection unit (HPU) or virologist on call. Advice following accidental exposure may also be obtained from the occupational health services, hospital control of infection officer.

Primary immunisation

For pre-exposure prophylaxis in groups at high risk and for post-exposure prophylaxis, an accelerated schedule should be used, with vaccine given at zero, one and two months. For those who are at continued risk, a fourth dose is recommended at 12 months. An alternative schedule at zero, one and six months for those 11–15 years of age (see page 167) can be used for pre-exposure prophylaxis where rapid protection is not required and there is a high likelihood of compliance. Where compliance with a more prolonged schedule is difficult to achieve (e.g. in IDUs and genito-urinary medicine clinic attenders), higher completion rates for three doses at zero, one and two months have been reported (Asboe *et al.*, 1996). Improved compliance is likely to offset the slightly reduced immunogenicity when compared with the zero-, one- and six-month schedule, and similar response rates can be achieved by opportunistic use of a fourth dose after 12 months.

Recently, an extension to the product licence for Engerix B® has been granted to allow for a very rapid immunisation schedule of three doses given at 0, 7 and 21 days (Bock *et al.*, 1995). When this schedule is used, a fourth dose is recommended 12 months after the first dose. This schedule is licensed for use in circumstances where adults over 18 years of age are at immediate risk and where a more rapid induction of protection is required. This includes persons travelling to areas of high endemicity, IDUs and prisoners. In teenagers under 18 years of age, response to vaccine is as good or better than in older adults (Plotkin and Orenstein, 2004). Although not licensed for this age group, this schedule can be used in those aged 16 to 18 years where it is important to provide rapid protection and to maximise compliance (e.g. IDUs and those in prison).

Fendrix® is recommended to be given at zero, one, two and six months.

Table 18.5 HBV prophylaxis for reported exposure incidents

	Significant exposure			Non-significant exposure	
HBV status of person exposed	**HBsAg positive source**	**Unknown source**	**HBsAg negative source**	**Continued risk**	**No further risk**
≤ 1 dose HB vaccine pre-exposure	Accelerated course of HB vaccine* HBIG × 1	Accelerated course of HB vaccine*	Initiate course of HB vaccine	Initiate course of HB vaccine	No HBV prophylaxis. Reassure
≥ 2 doses HB vaccine pre-exposure (anti-HBs not known)	One dose of HB vaccine followed by second dose one month later	One dose of HB vaccine	Finish course of HB vaccine	Finish course of HB vaccine	No HBV prophylaxis. Reassure
Known responder to HB vaccine (anti-HBs > 10mIU/ml)	Consider booster dose of HB vaccine	Consider booster dose of HB vaccine	Consider booster dose of HB vaccine	Consider booster dose of HB vaccine	No HBV prophylaxis. Reassure
Known non-responder to HB vaccine (anti-HBs < 10mIU/ml 2–4 months post-immunisation)	HBIG × 1 Consider booster dose of HB vaccine A second dose of HBIG should be given at one month	HBIG × 1 Consider booster dose of HB vaccine A second dose of HBIG should be given at one month	No HBIG Consider booster dose of HB vaccine	No HBIG Consider booster dose of HB vaccine	No prophylaxis. Reassure

*An accelerated course of vaccine consists of doses spaced at zero, one and two months.
A booster dose may be given at 12 months to those at continuing risk of exposure to HBV.
Source: PHLS Hepatitis Subcommittee (1992).

Twinrix® can also be given at 0, 7 and 21 days. This will provide more rapid protection against hepatitis B than other schedules but full protection against hepatitis A will be provided later than with a single dose of single hepatitis A vaccine (see Chapter 17). When this schedule is used, a fourth dose is recommended 12 months after the first dose.

Reinforcing immunisation

The full duration of protection afforded by hepatitis B vaccine has yet to be established (Whittle *et al.*, 2002). Levels of vaccine-induced antibody to hepatitis B decline over time, but there is evidence that immune memory can persist in those successfully immunised (Liao *et al.*, 1999). However, recent evidence suggests that not all individuals may respond in this way (Williams *et al.*, 2003; Boxall *et al.*, 2004). It is, therefore, recommended that individuals at continuing risk of infection should be offered a single booster dose of vaccine, once only, around five years after primary immunisation. Measurement of anti-HBs levels is not required either before or after this dose. Boosters are also recommended after exposure to the virus (as above).

Because of the continued presence of infection in other family members, a single booster dose of hepatitis B vaccine, given with the pre-school booster for other childhood immunisations, is advised for the children born to hepatitis B infected-mothers. This will also provide the opportunity to check whether the child was properly followed up in infancy.

Response to vaccine and the use of additional doses

Except in certain groups (see below), testing for anti-HBs is not recommended.

Those at risk of occupational exposure

In those at risk of occupational exposure, particularly healthcare and laboratory workers, antibody titres should be checked one to four months after the completion of a primary course of vaccine. Under the Control of Substances Hazardous to Health (COSHH) Regulations, individual workers have the right to know whether or not they have been protected. Such information allows appropriate decisions to be made concerning post-exposure prophylaxis following known or suspected exposure to the virus (see above).

Antibody responses to hepatitis B vaccine vary widely between individuals. It is preferable to achieve anti-HBs levels above 100mIU/ml, although levels of 10mIU/ml or more are generally accepted as enough to protect against infection. Some anti-HBs assays are not particularly specific at the lower levels, and anti-HBs levels of 100mIU/ml provide greater confidence that a specific response has been established.

Responders with anti-HBs levels greater than or equal to 100mIU/ml do not require any further primary doses. In immunocompetent individuals, once a response has been established further assessment of antibody levels is not indicated. They should receive the reinforcing dose at five years as recommended above.

Responders with anti-HBs levels of 10 to 100mIU/ml should receive one additional dose of vaccine at that time. In immunocompetent individuals, further assessment of antibody levels is not indicated. They should receive the reinforcing dose at five years as recommended above.

An antibody level below 10mIU/ml is classified as a non-response to vaccine, and testing for markers of current or past infection is good clinical practice. In non-responders, a repeat course of vaccine is recommended, followed by retesting one to four months after the second course. Those who still have anti-HBs levels below 10mIU/ml, and who have no markers of current or past infection, will require HBIG for protection if exposed to the virus (see below).

Patients with renal failure

The role of immunological memory in patients with chronic renal failure on renal dialysis does not appear to have been studied, and protection may persist only as long as anti-HBs levels remain above 10mIU/ml. Antibody levels should, therefore, be monitored annually and if they fall below 10mIU/ml, a booster dose of vaccine should be given to patients who have previously responded to the vaccine.

Booster doses should also be offered to any haemodialysis patients who are intending to visit countries with a high endemicity of hepatitis B and who have previously responded to the vaccine, particularly if they are to receive haemodialysis and have not received a booster in the last 12 months.

Contraindications

There are very few individuals who cannot receive hepatitis B-containing vaccines. When there is doubt, appropriate advice should be sought from a consultant paediatrician, immunisation co-ordinator or local HPU rather than withholding vaccine.

The vaccine should not be given to those who have had:

- a confirmed anaphylactic reaction to a previous dose of a hepatitis B-containing vaccine or
- a confirmed anaphylactic reaction to any component of the vaccine.

Precautions

Minor illnesses without fever or systemic upset are not valid reasons to postpone immunisation. If an individual is acutely unwell, immunisation may be postponed until they have fully recovered. This is to avoid confusing the differential diagnosis of any acute illness by wrongly attributing any signs or symptoms to the adverse effects of the vaccine.

Pregnancy and breast-feeding

Hepatitis B infection in pregnant women may result in severe disease for the mother and chronic infection of the newborn. Immunisation should not be withheld from a pregnant woman if she is in a high-risk category. There is no evidence of risk from vaccinating pregnant women or those who are breast-feeding with inactivated viral or bacterial vaccines or toxoids (Plotkin and Orenstein, 2004). Since hepatitis B is an inactivated vaccine, the risks to the foetus are likely to be negligible, and it should be given where there is a definite risk of infection.

Premature infants

There is evidence that the response to hepatitis B vaccine is lower in pre-term, low-birthweight babies (Losonsky *et al.*, 1999). It is, therefore, important that premature infants receive the full paediatric dose of hepatitis B vaccine on schedule. Babies with a birthweight of 1500g or less, born to mothers infected with hepatitis B, should receive HBIG in addition to the vaccine, regardless of the e-antigen status of the mother.

HIV and immunosuppressed individuals

Hepatitis B vaccine may be given to HIV-infected individuals and should be offered to those at risk, since infection acquired by immunosuppressed, HIV-positive patients can result in higher rates of chronic infection (Bodsworth *et al.*, 1991). Response rates are usually lower depending upon the degree of immunosuppression (Newell and Nelson, 1998; Loke *et al.*, 1990). Increasing the number of doses may improve the anti-HBs response in HIV-infected individuals (Rey *et al.*, 2000).

Further guidance is provided by the Royal College of Paediatrics and Child Health (www.rcpch.ac.uk) the British HIV Association (BHIVA) *immunisation guidelines for HIV-infected adults* (BHIVA, 2006) and the Children's HIV Association of UK and Ireland (CHIVA) immunisation guidelines (www.bhiva.org/chiva).

Precautions for HBIG

When HBIG is being used for prevention of hepatitis B, it must be remembered that it may interfere with the subsequent development of active immunity from live virus vaccines. If immunoglobulin has been administered first, then an interval of three months should be observed before administering a live virus vaccine. If immunoglobulin has been given within three weeks of administering a live vaccine, then the vaccine should be repeated three months later. This does not apply to yellow fever vaccine since HBIG does not contain significant amounts of antibody to this virus.

Adverse reactions

Hepatitis B vaccine is generally well tolerated and the most common adverse reactions are soreness and redness at the injection site. Other reactions that have been reported but may not be causally related include fever, rash, malaise and an influenza-like syndrome, arthritis, arthralgia, myalgia and abnormal liver function tests.

Serious suspected neurological reactions such as Guillain-Barré syndrome and demyelinating disease have been reported, although these have been very rare and a causal relationship with hepatitis B vaccine has not been established (Shaw *et al.*, 1988; McMahon *et al.*, 1992). The results of recent studies indicate no association between hepatitis B immunisation and the development of multiple sclerosis (Ascherio *et al.*, 2001) and that immunisation against hepatitis B does not increase the short-term risk of a relapse in patients with multiple sclerosis (Confavreux *et al.*, 2001).

All suspected reactions in children and severe suspected reactions in adults should be reported to the Commission on Human Medicines using the Yellow Card scheme.

Adverse reactions to HBIG

HBIG is well tolerated. Very rarely, anaphylactoid reactions occur in individuals with hypogammaglobulinaemia who have IgA antibodies, or those who have had an atypical reaction to blood transfusion.

No cases of blood-borne infection acquired through immunoglobulin preparations designed for intramuscular use have been documented in any country.

Supplies

Hepatitis B vaccine

- Engerix B®
- Fendrix®

These vaccines are available from GlaxoSmithKline
(Tel: 0808 100 9997).

- HBvaxPRO®
- HBvaxPRO Paediatric®
- HBvaxPRO® 40

These vaccines are available from Sanofi Pasteur MSD
(Tel: 0800 0855511).

Combined hepatitis A and hepatitis B vaccine

- Twinrix Paediatric®
- Twinrix Adult®

These vaccines are available from GlaxoSmithKline
(Tel: 0808 100 9997).

Hepatitis B immunoglobulin

England and Wales:
Health Protection Agency
Centre for Infections — Tel: 020 8200 6868

Scotland:
HBIG is held by the Blood Transfusion Service:

Aberdeen	Tel: 01224 685685
Dundee	Tel: 01382 645166
Edinburgh	Tel: 0131 5365300
Glasgow	Tel: 0141 357 7700
Inverness	Tel: 01463 704212/3

Northern Ireland:
HBIG is held by the Public Health Laboratory
Belfast City Hospital
Belfast
(Tel: 028 9032 9241 ext 2417)

Note: Supplies of HBIG are limited and demands should be restricted to patients in whom there is a clear indication for its use.

HBIG for use in hepatitis B-infected recipients of liver transplants should be obtained from:

Bioproducts Laboratory
Dagger Lane
Elstree
Herts WD6 3BX
(Tel: 020 8258 2342)

References

American Academy of Pediatrics (2003) Active immunization. In: Pickering LK (ed.) *Red Book: 2003 Report of the Committee on Infectious Diseases*, 26th edition. Elk Grove Village, IL: American Academy of Pediatrics, p 33.

Asboe D, Rice P, de Ruiter A and Bingham JS (1996) Hepatitis B vaccination schedules in genitourinary medicine clinics. *Genitourin Med* **72**(3): 210–12.

Ascherio A, Zhang S, Hernan M *et al.* (2001) Hepatitis B vaccination and the risk of multiple sclerosis. *N Engl J Med* **344**: 327–32.

Aweis D, Brabin BJ, Beeching JN *et al.* (2001) Hepatitis B prevalence and risk factors for HBsAg carriage amongst Somali households in Liverpool. *Commun Dis Public Health* **4**: 247–52.

Bock HL, Löscher T, Scheiermann N *et al.* (1995) Accelerated schedule for hepatitis B immunisation. *J Travel Med* **2**: 213–17.

Bodsworth NJ, Cooper DA and Donovan B (1991) The influence of human immunodeficiency virus type 1 infection on the development of the hepatitis B virus carrier state. *J Infect Dis* **163**: 1138–40.

Boxall E, Skidmore S, Evans C *et al.* (1994) The prevalence of hepatitis B and C in an antenatal population of various ethnic origins. *Epidemiol Infect* **113**: 523–8.

Boxall EH, Sira J, El-Shuhkri N *et al.* (2004) Long term persistence of immunity to hepatitis B after vaccination during infancy in a country where endemicity is low. *J Infect Dis* **190**: 1264–9.

British HIV Association (2006) *Immunisation guidelines for HIV-infected adults:* www.bhiva.org/pdf/2006/Immunisation506.pdf.

Bush LM, Moonsammy GI and Boscia JA (1991) Evaluation of initiating a hepatitis B vaccination schedule with one vaccine and completing it with another. *Vaccine* **9**: 807–9.

Christenson B (1986) Epidemiological aspects of transmission of hepatitis B by HBsAg-positive adopted children. *Scand J Infect Dis* **18**:105–9.

Confavreux C, Suissa S, Saddier P *et al.* for the Vaccines Multiple Sclerosis Study Group (2001) Vaccinations and the risk of relapse in multiple sclerosis. *N Engl J Med* **344**: 319–26.

Department of Health (1998) *Screening of pregnant women for hepatitis B and immunisation of babies at risk.* Health Service Circular HSC 1998/127. Available on the Department of Health website at: www.dh.gov.uk/assetRoot/04/01/18/40/04011840.pdf.

Hutchinson SJ, Wadd S, Taylor A *et al.* (2004) Sudden rise in uptake of hepatitis B vaccination among injecting drug users associated with a universal vaccine programme in prisons. *Vaccine* **23**: 210–14.

Hyams KC (1995) Risks of chronicity following acute hepatitis B virus infection: a review. *Clin Infect Dis* **20**: 992–1000.

Kane A, Lloyd J, Zaffran M *et al.* (1999) Transmission of hepatitis B, hepatitis C and human immunodeficiency viruses through unsafe injections in the developing world: model-based regional estimates. *Bull World Health Org* **77**: 801–7.

Liao SS, Li RC, Li H *et al.* (1999) Long-term efficiency of plasma-derived hepatitis B vaccine: a 15-year follow-up study among Chinese children. *Vaccine* **17**: 2661–6.

Loke RH, Murray-Lyon IM, Coleman JC *et al.* (1990) Diminished response to recombinant hepatitis B vaccine in homosexual men with HIV antibody: an indicator of poor prognosis. *J Med Virol* **31**: 109–11.

Losonsky GA, Wasserman SS, Stephens I *et al.* (1999) Hepatitis B vaccination of premature infants. *Pediatrics* **103** (2): E14.

McMahon BJ, Helminiak C, Wainwright RB *et al.* (1992) Frequency of adverse reactions to hepatitis B in 43,618 persons. *Am J Med* **92**: 254–6.

Newell A and Nelson M (1998) Infectious hepatitis in HIV seropositive patients. *Int J STD AIDS* **9**: 63–9.

PHLS Hepatitis Subcommittee (1992) Exposure to hepatitis B virus: guidance on post exposure prophylaxis. *CDR Review* **2**: R97–R102.

Plotkin SA and Orenstein WA (eds) (2004) *Vaccines*, 4th edition. Phildelphia: WB Saunders Company.

Rey D, Krantz V, Partisani M *et al.* (2000) Increasing the number of hepatitis B injections augments anti-HBs response rate in HIV-infected patients. Effects of HIV-1 viral load. *Vaccine* **18**: 1161–5.

Roome AJ, Walsh SJ, Carter ML *et al.* (1993) Hepatitis B vaccine responsiveness in Connecticut public safety personnel. *JAMA* **270**: 2931–4.

Rosman AS, Basu P, Galvin K *et al.* (1997) Efficacy of high and accelerated dose of hepatitis B vaccine in alcoholic patients: a randomized clinical trial. *Am J Med* **103**: 217–22.

Rudin H, Berger R, Tobler R *et al.* (1990) HIV-1, hepatitis (A, B and C) and measles in Romanian children. *Lancet* **336**: 1592–3.

Shaw FE, Graham DJ, Guess HA *et al.* (1988) Postmarketing surveillance for neurologic adverse events reported after hepatitis B vaccination: experience of the first three years. *Am J Epidemiol* **127**: 337–52.

Simonsen L, Kane A, Lloyd J, *et al.* (1999) Unsafe injections in the developing world and transmission of blood-borne pathogens: a review. *Bull World Health Org* **77**: 789–800.

Tong NK, Beran J, Kee SA *et al.* (2005) Immunogenicity and safety of an adjuvanted hepatitis B vaccine in pre-hemodialysis and hemodialysis patients. *Kidney Int* **68**(5): 2298–303.

Whittle H, Jaffar S, Wansbrough M *et al.* (2002) Observational study of vaccine efficacy 14 years after trial of hepatitis B vaccination in Gambian children. *BMJ* **325**: 569–73.

Williams IT, Goldstein ST, Tufa J *et al.* (2003) Long-term antibody response to hepatitis B vaccination beginning at birth and to subsequent booster vaccination. *Paediatr Infect Dis J.* **22**: 157–63.

19

Influenza

The disease

Influenza is an acute viral infection of the respiratory tract. There are three types of influenza virus: A, B and C. Influenza A and influenza B are responsible for most clinical illness. Influenza is highly infectious with an incubation period of one to three days.

The disease is characterised by the sudden onset of fever, chills, headache, myalgia and extreme fatigue. Other common symptoms include a dry cough, sore throat and stuffy nose. For otherwise healthy individuals, influenza is an unpleasant but usually self-limiting disease with recovery in two to seven days. The illness may be complicated by (and may present as) bronchitis, secondary bacterial pneumonia or (in children) otitis media. Severe influenza can be complicated by meningitis, encephalitis or meningoencephalitis. Serious illness and mortality from influenza are highest among neonates, older people and those with underlying disease, particularly chronic respiratory and cardiac disease, or those who are immunosuppressed. Primary influenzal pneumonia is a rare complication that may occur at any age and carries a high case fatality rate (Barker and Mullooly, 1982). Serological studies in healthcare professionals show that approximately 30 to 50% of influenza infections are asymptomatic (Wilde *et al.*, 1999).

Transmission is by aerosol, droplets or direct contact with respiratory secretions of someone with the infection. Influenza spreads rapidly, especially in closed communities. Most cases in the UK tend to occur during a six to eight-week period during the winter. The timing, extent and severity of this 'seasonal' influenza can all vary. Influenza A viruses cause outbreaks most years and these viruses are the usual cause of epidemics. Large epidemics occur intermittently. Influenza B tends to cause less severe disease and smaller outbreaks, although in children the severity of illness may be similar to that associated with influenza A.

Changes in the principal surface antigens of influenza A – haemagglutinin and neuraminidase – make these viruses antigenically labile. Minor changes (antigenic drift) occur progressively from season to season. Major changes (antigenic shift) occur periodically, resulting in the emergence of a new

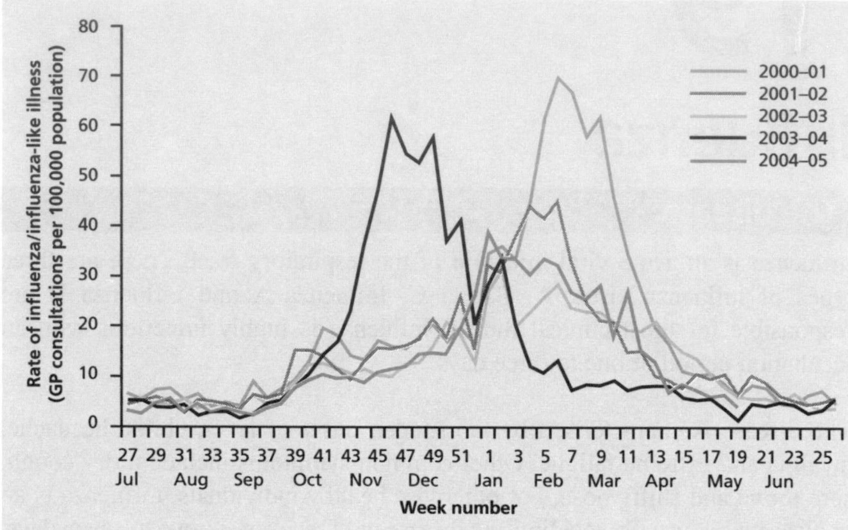

Figure 19.1 Rate of influenza/influenza-like illness episodes in England (weekly returns to Royal College of General Practitioners), 2000–01 to 2004–05

subtype with a different haemagglutinin protein. A new subtype can cause widespread epidemics or even a pandemic if populations have little or no immunity. Three influenza pandemics occurred in the last century (in 1918, 1957 and 1968) and the conditions continue to exist for the emergence of future strains with pandemic potential. Influenza B viruses are subject to antigenic drift but with less frequent changes.

History and epidemiology of the disease

Influenza activity is monitored in the UK through reports of new consultations for influenza-like illness from sentinel GP practices, combined with virological surveillance. Activity was modest during the five influenza seasons from 2000–01 to 2004–05 compared with 1996–97, 1998–99 and 1999–2000 (Goddard *et al.*, 2003). Severe epidemics were recorded in 1975–76 and 1989–90, resulting in an estimated 29,646 and 23,046 deaths respectively in England and Wales (Nicholson, 1996). Even in winters when the incidence is low, 3000–4000 deaths have been attributed to influenza (Watson *et al.*, 2001).

Figure 19.1 shows the number of GP consultations for influenza-like illness per 100,000 population in England from 2000–2005. In this period, the GP consultation rate reached its highest (70 per 100,000 per week) in 2000–01. However, this compares with a peak rate of 583 per 100,000 per week in the epidemic of 1989–90. In Scotland, the same pattern was seen where consultation rates peaked in calendar week 1 of 1999–2000 at 839 per 100,000 compared with a peak rate of 1184 per 100,000 during 1989–90.

Influenza immunisation has been recommended in the UK since the late 1960s, with the aim of directly protecting those at a higher risk of serious morbidity and mortality. In 2000, the policy was extended to include all people aged 65 years or over. Uptake of vaccination in those aged 65 years or over in the UK is shown in Table 19.1.

Table 19.1 Vaccine uptake in the UK since the start of the influenza immunisation programme for people aged 65 years or over

Year	England %	Scotland %	Wales %	Northern Ireland %
2000–01	65.4	65	39	68
2001–02	67.5	65	59	72
2002–03	68.6	69	54*	72.1
2003–04	71.0	72.5	63	73.4
2004–05	71.5	71.7	63	72.7
2005–06	75.3	77.8	68	80.9

*Some GP practices experienced problems in collating and reporting data

The influenza vaccination

Because of their changing nature, the World Health Organization (WHO) monitors influenza viruses throughout the world. Each year the WHO makes recommendations about the strains to be included in vaccines for the forthcoming winter (www.who.int/csr/disease/influenza). To provide continuing protection, annual immunisation with vaccine against the currently prevalent strains is necessary.

Influenza vaccines are prepared using virus strains in line with the WHO recommendations. Current vaccines are trivalent, containing two subtypes of influenza A and one type B virus; in recent years these have closely matched viruses circulating subsequently. Should a new influenza A subtype emerge with epidemic or pandemic potential, a monovalent vaccine against that strain would be considered.

The viruses are grown in embryonated hens' eggs, chemically inactivated and then further treated and purified. Three types of influenza vaccine are currently available:

- 'split virion, inactivated' or 'disrupted virus' vaccines containing virus components prepared by treating whole viruses with organic solvents or detergents
- 'surface antigen, inactivated' vaccines containing highly purified haemagglutinin and neuraminidase antigens prepared from disrupted virus particles and
- 'surface antigen, inactivated, virosome' vaccines containing highly purified haemagglutinin and neuraminidase antigens prepared from disrupted virus particles reconstituted into virosomes with phospholipids.

The vaccines are equivalent in efficacy and adverse reactions. The vaccines are inactivated, do not contain live organisms and cannot cause the diseases against which they protect.

Some influenza vaccines currently contain thiomersal. Other influenza vaccines are thiomersal-free. They have equivalent efficacy and safety. If a thiomersal-free influenza vaccine is not available, then a thiomersal-containing vaccine should be given.

The currently available influenza vaccines give 70 to 80% protection against infection with influenza virus strains well matched with those in the vaccine (Fleming *et al.*, 1995). Protection afforded by the vaccine lasts for about one year. In the elderly, protection against infection may be less, but immunisation has been shown to reduce the incidence of bronchopneumonia, hospital admissions and mortality (Wright *et al.*, 1977).

After immunisation, antibody levels may take up to 10 to 14 days to reach protective levels. While influenza activity is not usually significant before the middle of November, the influenza season can start early (as it did in 2003–04), and therefore the ideal time for immunisation is between September and early November.

Manufacture of influenza vaccines is complex and conducted to a tight schedule, constrained by the length of time available between the WHO recommendations and the opportunity to vaccinate before the influenza season. Manufacturers may not be able to respond to unexpected demands for vaccine at short notice.

Other influenza vaccines are being developed, such as an intranasal vaccine and an attenuated live vaccine, but these are not currently available in the UK.

Storage

Vaccines should be stored in the original packaging at +2˚C to +8˚C and protected from light. All vaccines are sensitive to some extent to heat and cold. Heat speeds up the decline in potency of most vaccines, thus reducing their shelf life. Effectiveness cannot be guaranteed for vaccines unless they have been stored at the correct temperature. Freezing may cause increased reactogenicity and loss of potency for some vaccines. It can also cause hairline cracks in the container, leading to contamination of the contents.

Presentation

Influenza vaccines are all supplied as suspensions of inactivated vaccines in pre-filled syringes. They should be shaken well before they are given.

Dosage and schedule

Age	Dose
Children aged 6–35 months	0.25ml or 0.5ml (depending on manufacturer's Summary of Product Characteristics (SPC)), repeated 4–6 weeks later if receiving influenza vaccine for the first time
Children aged 3–12 years	0.5ml, repeated after 4–6 weeks if receiving influenza vaccine for the first time
Adults and children over 13 years	A single injection of 0.5ml

Children and pregnant women should preferably receive a thiomersal-free influenza vaccine. If a thiomersal-free vaccine is not available then a thiomersal-containing vaccine should be given. The benefits of vaccination outweigh the risks, if any, of exposure to thiomersal-containing vaccines.

Administration

The vaccine is given by intramuscular injection, preferably into the upper arm or anterolateral thigh. However, individuals with a bleeding disorder should be given the vaccine by deep subcutaneous injection to reduce the risk of bleeding.

Influenza vaccine can be given at the same time as other vaccines. The vaccines should be given at separate sites, preferably in a different limb. If given in the same limb, they should be given at least 2.5cm apart (American Academy of Pediatrics, 2003). The site at which each vaccine is given and the batch numbers of the vaccines should be recorded in the individual's records.

Where the vaccine is given for occupational reasons, it is recommended that the employer keeps a vaccination record.

Disposal

Equipment used for vaccination, including used vials or ampoules, should be disposed of at the end of a session by sealing in a proper, puncture-resistant 'sharps' box (UN-approved, BS 7320).

Recommendations for the use of the vaccine

The objective of the influenza immunisation programme is to protect those who are most at risk of serious illness or death should they develop influenza. To facilitate this, general practitioners are required to compile a register of those patients for whom influenza immunisation is recommended. Sufficient vaccine can then be ordered in advance and patients can be invited to planned immunisation sessions or appointments.

Patients should be advised that many other organisms cause respiratory infections similar to influenza during the influenza season, e.g. the common cold and respiratory syncytial virus (RSV). Influenza vaccine will not protect against these diseases.

Influenza vaccine is offered annually between September and early November to:

- all those aged 65 years or over;
- all those aged six months or over in the clinical risk groups shown in Table 19.2.

The medical practitioner should take into account the risk of influenza infection exacerbating any underlying disease that the patient may have, as well as the risk of serious illness from influenza itself.

Table 19.2 Clinical risk groups who should receive the influenza immunisation

Clinical risk category	Some examples
Chronic respiratory disease, including asthma	Chronic obstructive pulmonary disease (COPD), including chronic bronchitis and emphysema, and such conditions as bronchiectasis, cystic fibrosis, interstitial lung fibrosis, pneumoconiosis and bronchopulmonary dysplasia (BPD). Asthma requiring continuous or repeated use of inhaled or systemic steroids or with previous exacerbations requiring hospital admission. Children who have previously been admitted to hospital for lower respiratory tract disease.
Chronic heart disease	Congenital heart disease hypertension, with cardiac complications,chronic heart failure and individuals requiring regular medication and/or follow-up for ischaemic heart disease.
Chronic renal disease	Nephrotic syndrome, chronic renal failure and renal transplantation.
Chronic liver disease	Cirrhosis, biliary atresia and chronic hepatitis.
Diabetes requiring insulin or oral hypoglycaemic drugs	Type 1 diabetes, and type 2 diabetes requiring oral hypoglycaemic drugs.
Immunosuppression	Due to disease or treatment. Asplenia or splenic dysfunction and human immunodeficiency virus (HIV) infection at all stages. Patients undergoing chemotherapy leading to immunosuppression. Individuals on or likely to be on systemic steroids for more than a month at a dose equivalent to prednisolone at 20mg or more per day (any age) or for children under 20kg a dose of 1mg or more per kg per day. *However, some immunocompromised patients may have a suboptimal immunological response to the vaccine.*

In addition to the above, immunisation is provided to reduce the transmission of influenza within health and social-care premises, to contribute to the protection of individuals who may have a suboptimal response to their own immunisations, or to avoid disruption to services that provide their care. Annual immunisation is recommended for:

- health and social care staff directly involved in patient care
- those living in long-stay residential care homes or other long-stay care facilities where rapid spread is likely to follow introduction of infection and cause high morbidity and mortality (this does not include prisons, young offender institutions, university halls of residence etc.) and
- those who are the main carer for an elderly or disabled person whose welfare may be at risk if their carer falls ill. Vaccination should be given at the GP's discretion.

Consideration should also be given to the vaccination of household contacts of immunocompromised individuals.

At-risk children

Children who have medical conditions that increase the risk of complications from influenza should be vaccinated before the influenza season.

Studies have shown that two doses of inactivated vaccine are required to achieve adequate antibody levels in children under 13 years of age as they may never have been exposed to influenza or been vaccinated (Wright *et al.*, 1977). The vaccines are interchangeable; the second dose should be given four to six weeks after the first dose in accordance with the manufacturer's SPC for that vaccine.

Contraindications

There are very few individuals who cannot receive influenza vaccine. When there is doubt, appropriate advice should be sought from an immunisation co-ordinator, consultant in communicable disease control or consultant paediatrician, so that the period the individual is left unvaccinated is minimised.

The vaccines should not be given to those who have had:

- a confirmed anaphylactic reaction to a previous dose of the vaccine, or
- a confirmed anaphylactic reaction to any component of the vaccine, or
- a confirmed anaphylactic hypersensitivity to egg products as the vaccines are prepared in hens' eggs.

Confirmed anaphylaxis is rare. Other allergic conditions such as rashes may occur more commonly and are not contraindications to further immunisation. A careful history of the event will often distinguish between true anaphylaxis and other events that are either not due to the vaccine or are not life threatening. In the latter circumstance, it may be possible to continue the immunisation course. Specialist advice must be sought on the vaccines and the circumstances in which they could be given. The risk to the individual of not being immunised must be taken into account.

Precautions

Minor illnesses without fever or systemic upset are not valid reasons to postpone immunisation. If an individual is acutely unwell, immunisation may be postponed until they have fully recovered. This is to avoid confusing the differential diagnosis of any acute illness by wrongly attributing any signs or symptoms to the adverse effects of the vaccine.

Pregnancy and breast-feeding

Pregnant women in the risk groups listed in Table 19.2 above should be vaccinated before the influenza season, regardless of the stage of pregnancy. A study of over 2000 pregnant women who received influenza vaccine demonstrated no associated adverse fetal effects (Heinonen *et al.*, 1973). There is no evidence of risk from vaccinating pregnant women, or those who are breast-feeding, with inactivated viral or bacterial vaccines or toxoids (Plotkin and Orenstein, 2004).

Where possible, pregnant women should receive a thiomersal-free influenza vaccine. If a thiomersal-free influenza vaccine is unavailable then a thiomersal-containing vaccine should be given. The benefits of vaccination outweigh the risks, if any, of exposure to thiomersal-containing vaccines.

Premature infants

It is important that premature infants who have risk factors have their immunisations at the appropriate chronological age. Influenza immunisation should be considered after the child has reached six months of age.

Where possible, infants should receive a thiomersal-free influenza vaccine. If a thiomersal-free influenza vaccine is unavailable then a thiomersal-containing vaccine should be given. The benefits of vaccination outweigh the risks, if any, of exposure to thiomersal-containing vaccines.

Immunosuppression and HIV infection

Individuals with immunosuppression and HIV infection (regardless of CD4 count) should be given influenza vaccine in accordance with the recommendations above. These individuals may not make a full antibody response.

Further guidance is provided by the Royal College of Paediatrics and Child Health (www.rcpch.ac.uk), the British HIV Association (BHIVA) *Immunisation guidelines for HIV-infected adults* (BHIVA, 2006) and the Children's HIV Association of UK and Ireland (CHIVA) immunisation guidelines (www.bhiva.org/chiva).

Adverse reactions

Pain, swelling or redness at the injection site, low grade fever, malaise, shivering, fatigue, headache, myalgia and arthralgia are among the commonly reported symptoms of vaccination. A small painless nodule (induration) may also form at the injection site. These reactions usually disappear within one to two days without treatment.

Immediate reactions such as urticaria, angio-oedema, bronchospasm and anaphylaxis can occur, most likely due to hypersensitivity to residual egg protein.

Neuralgia, paraesthesiae, convulsions and transient thrombocytopenia have been reported rarely.

Guillain-Barré syndrome has been reported very rarely after immunisation with influenza vaccine (one case per million people vaccinated in one US study (Lasky *et al.*, 1998). However, a causal relationship has not been established.

Vasculitis with transient renal involvement and neurological disorders such as encephalomyelitis and neuritis occur very rarely.

All suspected reactions in children and severe suspected reactions in adults should be reported to the Commission on Human Medicines using the Yellow Card scheme.

Management of suspected cases, contacts and outbreaks

There are antiviral drugs available which can be used under certain circumstances to either prevent influenza or to treat it.

Guidance on the treatment and prevention of influenza with antiviral drugs applicable in England, Wales and Northern Ireland was issued by the National Institute for Health and Clinical Excellence (NICE) in February 2003 and September 2003 respectively (www.nice.org.uk). These drugs are not a substitute for influenza immunisation.

Similar treatment guidance endorsing the recommendations of NICE was issued by Quality Improvement Scotland (QIS) in February 2003 (www.nhshealthquality.org/nhsqis/qis_display_findings.jsp?pContentID=1096&p_applic=CCC&p_service=Content.show&).

This guidance applies when influenza A or B is known to be circulating in the community. The Department of Health posts this information on its website (www.dh.gov.uk/PolicyAndGuidance/HealthAndSocialCareTopics/Flu/FluGeneralInformation/fs/en) and this should be checked regularly during the influenza season.

Antivirals in the prevention and treatment of influenza

Antiviral drugs can be used for either the prevention or treatment of influenza.

Oseltamivir and amantadine are licensed for the prevention of influenza. Zanamivir, oseltamivir and amantadine are licensed for the treatment of influenza. Zanamivir and oseltamivir are neuraminidase inhibitors, active against influenza A and B; amantadine is an M2 inhibitor, active against influenza A only.

Zanamivir is taken using a special inhaler (Diskhaler®) and is licensed for individuals aged 12 years or over; oseltamivir is taken orally and is licensed for individuals aged one year or over; amantadine is taken orally and licensed for individuals aged ten years or over.

NICE guidance on the use of antiviral drugs for the *prevention* of influenza

When influenza A or B virus is circulating in the community, as defined on the Department of Health website, oseltamivir should be prescribed for the prevention of influenza in individuals aged 13 years or over, who:

- belong to an 'at-risk' group **and**
- have not had an influenza immunisation this season, or who have had one within the last two weeks, or have had an influenza immunisation but the vaccine did not match the virus circulating in the community **and**
- have been in close contact with someone with influenza-like symptoms **and**
- can start taking oseltamivir within 48 hours of being in contact with the person with influenza-like symptoms.

Oseltamivir has recently been licensed for prophylactic use in children aged one year and over (31 January 2006). In the interim, until NICE formally reviews its recommendation, it would therefore be appropriate to use oseltamivir for prophylaxis in persons aged one year and over according to the other conditions laid out by NICE as summarised above.

Prescribers should also note a concomitant change to the licensed duration of post-exposure prophylaxis in children and adults, now ten days (as opposed to the previous seven).

Oseltamivir should **not** be used for the prevention of influenza in otherwise healthy people under 65 years of age, even if they have been in contact with people with influenza-like symptoms.

Amantadine should **not** be used for the prevention of influenza in either group.

Dosage for the prevention of influenza

Individuals aged 13 years or over

Therapy should begin within 48 hours of exposure. A daily dose of oseltamivir 75mg should be given for seven days. It can be given for up to six weeks during a community outbreak.

Contraindications for prevention

Oseltamivir should not be used in children under one year of age.

Precautions for prevention

There are no adequate data for the use of oseltamivir in pregnant or breast-feeding women. Oseltamivir should not be used during pregnancy or in breast-feeding women unless the potential benefit to the woman overrides the potential risk for the fetus or infant.

The dose of oseltamivir should be reduced for people with moderate to severe renal impairment.

Adverse reactions

Oseltamivir

Nausea, vomiting, diarrhoea, abdominal pains and headache have been reported.

NICE guidance on the use of antiviral drugs for the *treatment* of influenza

Zanamivir and oseltamivir are recommended for the treatment of influenza in at-risk children or adults who present with influenza-like illness and who can start treatment within 48 hours of the onset of symptoms.

NICE does not recommend amantadine for the treatment of influenza.

Dosage for the treatment of influenza

Individuals aged over one year and under 13 years of age

Treatment should start within 48 hours of the onset of symptoms. Oseltamivir is licensed for the **treatment** of children over one year of age. The dosage depends on body weight.

Body weight	Dosage
15kg or under	30mg every 12 hours
16–23kg	45mg every 12 hours
24–40kg	60mg every 12 hours
Over 40kg	75mg every 12 hours

Zanamivir is not used in this age group.

Individuals aged 12 years or over

Treatment should start within 48 hours of the onset of symptoms. For zanamivir, the dose is 10mg, by inhalation, twice a day for five days. For oseltamivir, the dose is 75mg every 12 hours for five days.

Contraindications for treatment

Oseltamivir is contraindicated in children under one year; zanamivir should not be used in children under 13 years of age.

Zanamivir is not recommended in women who are breast-feeding.

Precautions for treatment

There are no adequate data for the use of oseltamivir in pregnant or breast-feeding women. It should not be used during pregnancy or in breast-feeding women unless the potential benefit to the mother overrides the potential risk for the fetus or infant.

Zanamivir should be used with caution in individuals with asthma or chronic pulmonary disease because of the risk of bronchospasm. It should not be used during pregnancy unless the potential benefit to the mother overrides the potential risk for the fetus.

The dose of oseltamivir should be reduced for people with moderate to severe renal impairment.

Adverse reactions

Oseltamivir

Nausea, vomiting, diarrhoea, abdominal pains and headache have been reported.

Zanamivir

Headache and gastro-intestinal disturbances have been reported rarely.

Supplies

Vaccines

Demand for influenza vaccine sometimes increases unpredictably in response to speculation about influenza illness in the community. It is, therefore, recommended that practices order sufficient vaccine for their needs, based on their 'At risk' registers, well in advance of the immunisation season.

Information on current vaccines is given in the latest Chief Medical Officer's letter from the Department of Health. At the time of publication, vaccines are available as follows:

Manufacturer	Name of product	Vaccine type	Contact details
Sanofi Pasteur MSD	Inactivated influenza vaccine	Split virion	0800 085 5511
	Inactivated influenza vaccine for paediatric use	Split virion	
	Inflexal V®	Surface antigen	
Novartis Vaccines	Enzira®	Split virion	08457 451 500
	Generic brand	Split virion	
GlaxoSmithKline	Fluarix®*	Split virion	0808 100 9997
MASTA	MASTAFLU®	Surface antigen	0113 238 7500
Solvay Healthcare	Influvac®	Surface antigen, inactivated, subunit	0800 358 7468
	Invivac®	Surface antigen, inactivated, virosome	
Wyeth Vaccines	Begrivac®	Split virion	01628 685 437

* Contains thiomersal. The Commission on Human Medicines' statement on the safety of vaccines containing thiomersal can be found at www.mhra.gov.uk and typing 'thiomersal' in the search box.

Antiviral drugs

Oseltamivir is supplied by Roche (Tel: 0800 731 5711).
Zanamivir is supplied by GlaxoSmithKline (Tel: 0808 100 9997).

References

American Academy of Pediatrics (2003) Active immunization. In: Pickering LK (ed.) *Red Book: 2003 Report of the Committee on Infectious Diseases,* 26th edition. Elk Grove Village, IL: American Academy of Pediatrics, p. 33.

Barker WH and Mullooly JP (1982) Pneumonia and influenza deaths during epidemics. *Arch Int Med* **142**: 85–9.

British HIV Association (2006) *Immunisation guidelines for HIV-infected adults:* www.bhiva.org/pdf/2006/Immunisation506.pdf.

Fleming DM, Watson JM, Nicholas S *et al.* (1995) Study of the effectiveness of influenza vaccination in the elderly in the epidemic of 1989/90 using a general practice database. *Epidemiol Infect* **115**: 581–9.

Goddard NL, Kyncl J and Watson JM (2003) Appropriateness of thresholds currently used to describe influenza activity in England. *Common Dis Public Health* **6**: 238–45.

Heinonen OP, Shapiro S, Monson RR *et al.* (1973) Immunization during pregnancy against poliomyelitis and influenza in relation to childhood malignancy. *Int J Epidemiol* **2**: 229–35.

Lasky T, Terracciano GJ, Magder L *et al.* (1998) The Guillain-Barré syndrome and the 1992–1993 and 1993–1994 influenza vaccines. *N Engl J Med* **339**: 1797–1802.

Nicholson KG (1996) Impact of influenza and respiratory syncytial virus on mortality in England and Wales from January 1975 to December 1990. *Epidemiol Infect* **116**: 51–63.

Plotkin SA and Orenstein WA (eds) (2004) *Vaccines,* 4th edition. Philadelphia: WB Saunders Company, Chapter 8.

Watson JM, Goddard N, Joseph C and Zambon MC (2001) Influenza: the impact of the 1999/2000 epidemic on morbidity and mortality in the UK. In: Osterhaus ADME (ed.) *Options for the control of influenza*. Elsevier, pp 21–3.

Wilde JA, McMillan JA, Serwint J *et al.* (1999) Effectiveness of influenza vaccine in health care professionals: a randomised trial. *JAMA* **281**: 908–13.

Wright PF, Thompson J, Vaughn WK *et al.* (1977) Trials of influenza A/New Jersey/76 virus vaccine in normal children: an overview of age-related antigenicity and reactogenicity. *J Infect Dis* **136** (suppl): S731–41.

20

Japanese encephalitis

The disease

Japanese encephalitis (JE) is a mosquito-borne viral encephalitis caused by a flavivirus. It is the leading cause of childhood encephalitis in Asia, with 20,000 to 50,000 cases per annum (Plotkin and Orenstein, 2004; World Health Organization, 1998).

It is endemic in rural areas, especially where rice growing and pig farming coexist, and epidemics occur in rural and occasionally in urban areas. Highest transmission rates occur during and just after wet seasons, when mosquitoes are most active, but seasonal patterns vary both within individual countries and from year to year. This disease is not transmitted from person to person.

The incubation period is from five to 15 days. Illness ranges from asymptomatic infection (about one in 250 infections is estimated to become clinically apparent) to severe encephalitis with a high mortality and a high rate of permanent neurological sequelae (approximately 30%) in survivors (Plotkin and Orenstein, 2004).

History and epidemiology of the disease

Outbreaks were recorded in Japan as early as 1871; the first major epidemic in Japan was described in 1924 and involved 6000 cases. JE spread throughout Asia but national immunisation campaigns and urban development in the 1960s led to the near-elimination of JE in Japan, Korea, Singapore and Taiwan. However, JE remains endemic in much of the rest of Asia. The virus was isolated in the 1930s, and inactivated mouse-brain derived vaccines were produced in the same decade.

The Japanese encephalitis vaccination

There are two vaccines available for use in the UK – JE-VAX and 'Green Cross'. Both are currently unlicensed in the UK, and have similar schedules for rapid and normal vaccination.

The vaccines contain formalin-inactivated Nakayama strain viruses derived from mouse brains. They contain small amounts of thiomersal. They are inactivated, do not contain live organisms and cannot cause the disease against which they protect.

Storage

Vaccines should be stored in the original packaging at +2˚C to +8˚C and protected from light. All vaccines are sensitive to some extent to heat and cold. Heat speeds up the decline in potency of most vaccines, thus reducing their shelf life. Effectiveness cannot be guaranteed for vaccines unless they have been stored at the correct temperature. Freezing may cause increased reactogenicity and loss of potency for some vaccines. It can also cause hairline cracks in the container, leading to contamination of the contents.

Presentation

JE-VAX is lyophilised; each vial contains a single-dose of vaccine which should be reconstituted with 1.3ml of sterile water for injection to provide a 1.0ml dose. The reconstituted vaccine should be used within eight hours and not stored.

Green Cross vaccine is available in 1ml single-dose, rubber-capped vials as a solution.

Dosage and schedule

- First dose of 1ml (0.5ml under 36 months of age) at day 0.
- Second dose of 1ml (0.5ml under 36 months of age) at days 7–14.
- Third dose of 1ml (0.5ml under 36 months of age) at days 28–30.

Administration

Vaccines should be given by deep subcutaneous injection only. The vaccines should be shaken before administration.

JE vaccines can be given at the same time as other travel or routine vaccines. The vaccines should be given at a separate site, preferably in a different limb. If given in the same limb, they should be given at least 2.5cm apart (American Academy of Pediatrics, 2003).

Disposal

Equipment used for vaccination, including empty vials or ampoules, should be put into a 'sharps' bin. Discarded doses of vaccine should be disposed of by incineration at a suitably authorised facility.

Recommendations for the use of the vaccine

The objective of JE vaccination is to protect individuals at high risk of exposure through travel or in the course of their occupation. Guidance on the employer's responsibility under Control of Substances Hazardous to Health (COSHH) Regulations is described in Chapter 12.

Primary immunisation

Infants, and children under 36 months of age

The recommended vaccine schedule is three doses of 0.5ml on days 0, 7–14 and 28–30. Full immunity takes up to a month to develop.

There are no safety or efficacy data in children under one year of age. As the immune response under one year of age is unpredictable, the vaccine is not usually recommended in children under one year of age in the UK.

Children aged three years or over, and adults

The recommended vaccine schedule is three doses of 1ml in those three years of age or older, on days 0, 7–14 and 28–30. Full immunity takes up to a month to develop.

Under exceptional circumstances, when time constraints preclude giving three doses over one month, a two-dose schedule at 0 and 7–14 days, or three doses at 0, 7 and 14 days, can be given. These abbreviated courses may result in lower antibody titres and a shorter duration of persistence of antibody (Poland *et al.*, 1990; Henderson, 1984; Centers for Disease Control and Prevention, 1993).

Reinforcing immunisation

The duration of protection is not known, but neutralising antibody persists for at least two years after a three-dose primary course of JE-VAX (Gambel *et al.*, 1995; Kurane and Takashi, 2000).

For JE-VAX, boosters are given at two-year intervals.

For the Green Cross vaccine, a booster dose is given one year after completion of the primary course and then at three-year intervals.

Travellers and those going to reside abroad

There is geographical variation in transmission periods – from all year round to seasonal. In temperate regions of Asia, transmission is generally from May to September. It extends from March through to October in areas further south, and may be year round in tropical areas.

All travellers should undergo a careful risk assessment that takes into consideration their itinerary, season of travel, duration of stay and planned activities. The risk of JE should then be balanced against the risk of adverse events from vaccination. JE vaccine is recommended for those who are going to reside in an area where JE is endemic or epidemic. Travellers to South-East Asia and the Far East should be immunised if staying for a month or longer in endemic areas during the transmission season, especially if travel will include rural areas. Other travellers with shorter exposure periods should be immunised if the risk is considered sufficient. For example, those spending a short period of time in rice fields (where the mosquito vector breeds) or close to pig farming (a reservoir host for the virus) should be considered for vaccination. Country-specific recommendations and information on the global epidemiology of JE can be found in the Yellow Book, *Health information for overseas travel* (Department of Health, 2001; www.nathnac.org).

Laboratory workers

Immunisation is recommended for all research laboratory staff who have potential exposure to the virus. Worldwide there have been more than 20 cases of laboratory-acquired JE virus infection (Plotkin and Orenstein, 2004).

Contraindications

There are very few individuals who cannot receive JE vaccine. When there is doubt, appropriate advice should be sought from a travel health specialist.

The vaccine should not be given to those who have had:

- a confirmed anaphylactic or serious systemic reaction to a previous dose of JE vaccine, or
- a confirmed anaphylactic reaction to any component of the vaccine.

Precautions

Individuals with pre-existing allergies

Hypersensitivity reactions to mouse-brain derived JE vaccine are more common among those with allergic conditions such as asthma, allergic rhinitis, and drug, food, gelatin or bee-sting allergy. Such patients should be advised about the risk of vaccine-related angioedema and generalised urticaria. A risk assessment needs to take into account the likelihood of exposure to JE and the possible adverse effects of the vaccine.

Neurological conditions

Individuals with unstable neurological conditions, including convulsions in the past year, may be at higher risk of adverse events following JE vaccination. The risk of JE infection should always be balanced against the risk of adverse events from vaccination, and specialist advice may need to be obtained. When high-risk travel is essential in this group of travellers, the JE-VAX is recommended in preference to the Green Cross vaccine, owing to the differences in contraindications listed in the Summary of Product Characteristics.

Anecdotal reports suggest that JE vaccine should not be used in individuals who have recovered from acute disseminated encephalomyelitis or Guillain-Barré syndrome or who have multiple sclerosis or other demyelinating disorders (Plotkin and Orenstein, 2004).

Pregnancy and breast-feeding

There is no evidence of risk from vaccinating pregnant women or those who are breast-feeding with inactivated viral or bacterial vaccines or toxoids (Plotkin and Orenstein, 2004). Specifically, JE vaccines have not been associated with adverse outcomes of pregnancy. However, travellers and their medical advisers must make a risk assessment of the theoretical risks of JE vaccine in pregnancy against the potential risk of acquiring JE. Miscarriage has been associated with JE virus infection when acquired in the first two trimesters of pregnancy (Canadian Medical Association, 2002).

Systemic and local reactions following a previous immunisation

Local reaction at the injection site (10–20%) and non-specific reactions may occur as for all vaccines. About 10–30% experience systemic reactions such as fever, headache, malaise, chills, dizziness, aching muscles, nausea and/or vomiting (Plotkin and Orenstein, 2004).

Hypersensitivity reactions such as urticaria and angioedema have occurred. They are much more likely to occur in those with a history of allergic conditions, as outlined above. Such reactions can happen following any dose and, although most will occur in the first 24 to 48 hours after immunisation, they may develop after up to ten days or more. Ideally travel should be delayed until ten days after receiving the last dose of the vaccine or travellers should remain in an area with ready access to hospital care.

Neurological adverse events may rarely occur. In Japan, these have been noted to occur in less than one in a million doses given (Ohtaki *et al.*, 1993). A Danish study found a higher level of risk of one in 50,000 to 75,000 vaccinees (Plesner *et al.*, 1996). No specific UK data are available.

Management of cases

No specific therapy is available for JE. Supportive treatment can significantly reduce morbidity and mortality. Diagnostic testing is available through the Health Protection Agency (HPA).

Supplies

- Japanese encephalitis (JE) Vaccine (Green Cross Corporation) is manufactured by Berna Biotech and supplied by MASTA (Tel: 0113 238 7555).

- JE-VAX® is manufactured by the Research Foundation for Microbial Diseases of Osaka, Japan, and is supplied by Sanofi Pasteur MSD (Tel: 0800 0855511).

References

American Academy of Pediatrics (2003) Active immunization. In: Pickering LK (ed.) *Red Book: 2003 Report of the Committee on Infectious Diseases* 26th edition. Elk Grove Village, IL: American Academy of Pediatrics, p 33.

Canadian Medical Association (2002) General considerations. In: *Canadian Immunization Guide,* 6th edition. Canadian Medical Association, p 14.

Centers for Disease Control and Prevention (1993) Inactivated Japanese encephalitis virus vaccine. Recommendations of the advisory committee on immunization practices (ACIP). *MMWR* **42** (No. RR-1): 1–15.

Department of Health (2001) *Health information for overseas travel*, 2nd edition. London: TSO.

Gambel JM, DeFraites R, Hoke C *et al.* (1995) Japanese encephalitis vaccine: persistence of antibody up to 3 years after a three-dose primary series (letter). *J Infect Dis* **171**: 1074.

Henderson A (1984) Immunization against Japanese encephalitis in Nepal: experience of 1152 subjects. *J R Army Med Corps* **130**: 188–91.

Kurane I and Takashi T (2000) Immunogenicity and protective efficacy of the current inactivated Japanese encephalitis vaccine against different Japanese encephalitis virus strains. *Vaccine* **18** (suppl 2): 33–5.

Ohtaki T, Masuda Y, Ishibashi Y *et al* (1993) Purification and characterization of the receptor for pituitary adenylate cyclase–activating polypeptide. *J Biol Chem* **268** (35): 26650–7.

Plesner AM, Soborg PA and Herning M (1996) Neurological complications and Japanese encephalitis vaccination. *Lancet* **348**: 202–3.

Plotkin SA and Orenstein WA (eds) (2004) *Vaccines*, 4th edition. Philadelphia: WB Saunders Company, 672–710.

Poland JD, Cropp CB, Craven RB and Monath TP (1990) Evaluation of the potency and safety of inactivated Japanese encephalitis vaccine in US inhabitants. *J Infect Dis* **161**: 878–82.

World Health Organization (1998) Japanese encephalitis vaccines. WHO position paper. www.who.int/docstore/wer/pdf/1998/wer7344.pdf.

21

Measles

NOTIFIABLE

The disease

Measles is an acute viral illness caused by a morbillivirus of the paramyxovirus family. The prodromal stage is characterised by the onset of fever, malaise, coryza, conjunctivitis and cough. The rash is erythematous and maculopapular, starting at the head and spreading to the trunk and limbs over three to four days. Koplik spots (small red spots with bluish-white centres) may appear on the mucous membranes of the mouth one to two days before the rash appears and may be seen for a further one to two days afterwards.

Measles is spread by airborne or droplet transmission. Individuals are infectious from the beginning of the prodromal period (when the first symptom appears) to four days after the appearance of the rash. It is one of the most highly communicable infectious diseases. The incubation period is about ten days (ranging between seven and 18 days) with a further two to four days before the rash appears (Chin, 2000).

The following features are strongly suggestive of measles:

- rash for at least three days
- fever for at least one day, and
- at least one of the following – cough, coryza or conjunctivitis.

Laboratory confirmation of suspected cases is required (see section below on diagnosis).

The most common complications of measles infection are otitis media (7 to 9% of cases), pneumonia (1 to 6%), diarrhoea (8%) and convulsions (one in 200). Other, more rare complications include encephalitis (overall rate of one per 1000 cases of measles) and sub-acute sclerosing pan-encephalitis (SSPE) (see below) (Plotkin and Orenstein, 2004; Norrby and Oxman, 1990; Perry and Halsey, 2004; McLean and Carter, 1990; Miller, 1978). Death occurs in one in 5000 cases in the UK (Miller, 1985). The case–fatality ratio for measles is age-related and is high in children under one year of age, lower in children aged one to nine years and rises again in teenagers and adults (Plotkin and Orenstein, 2004, Chapter 19). Complications are more common and more severe in poorly nourished and/or chronically ill children, including those who are immunosuppressed.

Measles encephalitis

There are different forms of measles encephalitis which occur at different times in relation to the onset of rash:

- post-infectious encephalomyelitis occurs at around one week after onset of the rash. Infectious virus is rarely found in the brain. The condition is associated with demyelination and is thought to have an auto-immune basis (Perry and Halsey, 2004).
- acute measles encephalitis of the delayed type (Barthez Carpentier *et al.*, 1992) occurs in immunocompromised patients. It may occur without a preceding measles-like illness (Kidd *et al.*, 2003) although there may be a history of exposure to measles several weeks or months previously (Alcardi *et al.*, 1997). It is characterised by acute neurological compromise and deterioration of consciousness, seizures and progressive neurological damage.
- SSPE is a rare, fatal, late complication of measles infection. One case of SSPE occurs in every 25,000 measles infections (Miller *et al.*, 2004). In children infected under the age of two, the rate is one in 8000 infections (Miller *et al.*, 2004; Miller *et al.*, 1992). Developing measles under one year of age carries a risk of SSPE 16 times greater than in those infected over five years of age (Miller *et al.*, 1992). The median interval from measles infection to onset of symptoms is around seven years but may be as long as two to three decades. SSPE may follow an unrecognised measles infection. Wild measles virus has been found in the brain of people with SSPE including those with no history of measles disease (Miller *et al.*, 2004).

History and epidemiology of the disease

Notification of measles began in England and Wales in 1940. Before the introduction of measles vaccine in 1968, annual notifications varied between 160,000 and 800,000, with peaks every two years (see Figure 21.1), and around 100 deaths from acute measles occurred each year.

From the introduction of measles vaccination in 1968 until the late 1980s coverage was low (Figure 21.1) and was insufficient to interrupt measles transmission. Therefore, annual notifications only fell to between 50,000 and 100,000 and measles remained a major cause of morbidity and mortality. Between 1970 and 1988, there continued to be an average of 13 acute measles

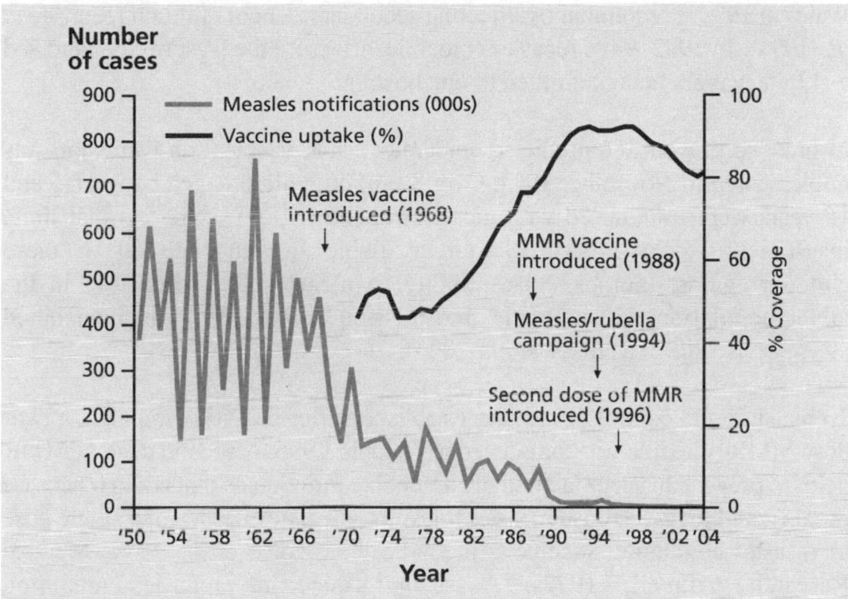

Figure 21.1 Coverage of measles vaccination and measles notifications from 1950 to 2004.

deaths each year. Measles remained a major cause of mortality in children who could not be immunised because they were receiving immunosuppressive treatment. Between 1974 and 1984, of 51 children who died when in first remission from acute lymphatic leukaemia, 15 of the deaths were due to measles or its complications (Gray *et al.*, 1987). Between 1970 and 1983, however, more than half the acute measles deaths that occurred were in previously healthy children who had not been immunised (Miller, 1985).

Following the introduction of measles, mumps and rubella (MMR) vaccine in October 1988 and the achievement of coverage levels in excess of 90%, measles transmission was substantially reduced and notifications of measles fell progressively to very low levels.

Because of the substantial reduction in measles transmission in the UK, children were no longer exposed to measles infection and, if they had not been immunised, they remained susceptible to an older age. Seroprevalence studies confirmed that a higher proportion of school-age children were susceptible to measles in 1991 than in 1986/7 (Gay *et al.*, 1995). A major resurgence of measles was predicted, mainly affecting the school-age population (Gay *et al.*, 1995; Babad *et al.*, 1995). Small outbreaks of measles occurred in England and

Wales in 1993, predominantly affecting secondary school children (Ramsay *et al.*, 1994). In 1993–94, a measles epidemic, affecting the west of Scotland, led to 138 teenagers being admitted to one hospital.

In order to prevent the predicted epidemic, a UK vaccination campaign was implemented in November 1994. Over 8 million children aged between 5 and 16 years were immunised with measles-rubella (MR) vaccine. At that time, insufficient stocks of MMR were available to vaccinate all of these children against mumps. Susceptibility to measles fell seven-fold in the target population and endemic transmission of measles was interrupted (Vyse *et al.*, 2002; Ramsay *et al.*, 2003).

To maintain the control of measles established after the MR campaign, a two-dose MMR schedule was introduced in October 1996. A second dose of MMR helps to prevent an accumulation of susceptible individuals that could otherwise be sufficient to re-establish measles transmission. The efficacy of a single dose of measles-containing vaccine is around 90% (Morse *et al.*, 1994; Medical Research Council, 1977). A second dose of measles-containing vaccine protects those who do not respond to the first dose. In order to eliminate measles, the World Health Organization (WHO) recommends two doses of a measles-containing vaccine (see www.who.int/mediacentre/factsheets/fs286/en/).

In Finland, a two-dose MMR schedule was introduced in 1982; high coverage of each dose has been achieved consistently. Indigenous measles, mumps and rubella have been eliminated since 1994 (Peltola *et al.*, 1994). The United States introduced its two-dose schedule in 1989, and in 2000 it announced that it had interrupted endemic transmission (Plotkin and Orenstein, 2004). MMR is now routinely given in over 100 countries, including those in the European Union, North America and Australasia.

Until 2006, the last confirmed death due to acute measles in the UK had been in 1992. In 2006, an unimmunised 13-year-old boy who was immunocompromised died from acute measles. Since the MR campaign, between 1995 and 2003 there have been 13 deaths recorded to measles in England and Wales. All except one of these were due to late effects of measles acquired before 1995 (www.hpa.org.uk/infections/topics_az/measles/data_death_age.htm). In the remaining case, measles infection was subsequently excluded by laboratory testing.

The reduced incidence of measles, brought about by vaccination, has caused the almost total disappearance of SSPE in England and Wales. In the early

1970s, when the SSPE Register was put in place, around 20 cases were reported each year. By the early 1990s, the annual total had fallen to around six cases and this has fallen further to between one and two in recent years (Miller *et al.*, 2004). In a UK study of 11 cases of SSPE, sequencing of the measles virus strains identified wild-type (and not vaccine-type) virus in all individuals, including five with a history of measles-containing vaccine (Jin *et al.*, 2002). The presence of wild and not vaccine strains of measles virus has been confirmed by studies of SSPE cases in other countries (Miki *et al.*, 2002).

The MMR vaccination

MMR vaccines are freeze-dried preparations containing live, attenuated strains of measles, mumps and rubella viruses. The three attenuated virus strains are cultured separately in appropriate media and mixed before being lyophilised. These vaccines contain the following:

Priorix®

Each 0.5ml dose of reconstituted vaccine contains:

not less than $10^{3.0}$ cell culture infective $dose_{50}$ ($CCID_{50}$) of the Schwarz measles virus
not less than $10^{3.7}$ $CCID_{50}$ of the RIT 4385 mumps virus
not less than $10^{3.0}$ $CCID_{50}$ of the Wistar RA 27/3 rubella virus strains.

M-M-R™II

Each 0.5ml dose when reconstituted contains not less than the equivalent of:

1000 tissue culture infective $dose_{50}$ ($TCID_{50}$) of the more attenuated Enders line of the Edmonston strain of measles virus
20,000 $TCID_{50}$ of mumps virus (Jeryl Lynn® Level B strain)
1000 $TCID_{50}$ of rubella virus (Wistar RA 27/3 strain).

MMR vaccine does not contain thiomersal or any other preservatives. The vaccine contains live organisms that have been attenuated (modified). MMR is recommended when protection against measles, mumps and/or rubella is required.

Human normal immunoglobulin (HNIG)

Human normal immunoglobulin (HNIG) is prepared from pooled plasma derived from blood donations and contains antibody to measles and other viruses prevalent in the population. There is no currently accepted minimum level of measles antibody required in HNIG.

Because of a theoretical risk of transmission of vCJD from plasma products, HNIG used in the UK is now prepared from plasma sourced from outside the UK, and supplies are scarce.* All donors are screened for HIV and hepatitis B and C, and all plasma pools are tested for the presence of RNA from these viruses. A solvent detergent inactivation step for envelope viruses is included in the production process.

Storage

The unreconstituted MMR vaccine and its diluent should be stored in the original packaging at +2˚C to +8˚C and protected from light. All vaccines are sensitive to some extent to heat and cold. Heat speeds up the decline in potency of most vaccines, thus reducing their shelf life. Effectiveness cannot be guaranteed for vaccines unless they have been stored at the correct temperature. Freezing may cause increased reactogenicity and loss of potency for some vaccines. It can also cause hairline cracks in the container, leading to contamination of the contents.

The vaccines should be reconstituted with the diluent supplied by the manufacturer and either used within one hour or discarded.

HNIG should be stored in the original packaging in a refrigerator at +2˚C to +8˚C. These products are tolerant to ambient temperatures for up to one week. They can be distributed in sturdy packaging outside the cold chain if needed.

Presentation

Measles vaccine is only available as part of a combined product (MMR).

Priorix is supplied as a whitish to slightly pink pellet of lyophilised vaccine for reconstitution with the diluent supplied. The reconstituted vaccine must be shaken well until the pellet is completely dissolved in the diluent.

M-M-R II is supplied as a lyophilised powder for reconstitution with the diluent supplied. The reconstituted vaccine must be shaken gently to ensure thorough mixing. The reconstituted vaccine is yellow in colour and should only be used if clear and free from particulate matter.

Dosage and schedule

Two doses of 0.5ml at the recommended interval (see below).

---

* Normal immunoglobulin for measles prophylaxis is in short supply and from time to time alternative products and doses may need to be used. For latest advice please check with the Health Protection Agency (www.hpa.org.uk) or Health Protection Scotland (www.hps.scot.nhs.uk).

Administration

Vaccines are routinely given intramuscularly into the upper arm or anterolateral thigh. However, for individuals with a bleeding disorder, vaccines should be given by deep subcutaneous injection to reduce the risk of bleeding.

MMR vaccine can be given at the same time as other vaccines such as DTaP/IPV, MenC, PCV and hepatitis B. The vaccine should be given at a separate site, preferably in a different limb. If given in the same limb, they should be given at least 2.5cm apart (American Academy of Pediatrics, 2003). If MMR cannot be given at the same time as an inactivated vaccine, it can be given at any interval before or after.

MMR should ideally be given at the same time as other live vaccines, such as BCG. If live vaccines are given simultaneously, then each vaccine virus will begin to replicate and an appropriate immune response is made to each vaccine. After a live vaccine is given, natural interferon is produced in response to that vaccine. If a second live vaccine is given during this response, the interferon may prevent replication of the second vaccine virus. This may attenuate the response to the second vaccine. Based on evidence that MMR vaccine can lead to an attenuation of the varicella vaccine response (Mullooly and Black, 2001), the recommended interval between live vaccines is currently four weeks. For this reason, if live vaccines cannot be administered simultaneously, a four-week interval is recommended.

Four weeks should be left between giving MMR vaccine and carrying out tuberculin testing. The measles vaccine component of MMR can reduce the delayed-type hypersensitivity response. As this is the basis of a positive tuberculin test, this could give a false negative response.

When MMR is given within three months of receiving blood products, such as immunoglobulin, the response to the measles component may be reduced. This is because such blood products may contain significant levels of measles-specific antibody, which could then prevent vaccine virus replication. Where possible, MMR should be deferred until three months after receipt of such products. If immediate measles protection is required in someone who has recently received a blood product, MMR vaccine should still be given. To confer longer-term protection, MMR should be repeated after three months.

HNIG can be administered in the upper outer quadrant of the buttock or anterolateral thigh (see Chapter 4). If more than 3ml is to be given to young children and infants, or more than 5ml to older children and adults, the immunoglobulin should be divided into smaller amounts and given into different sites.

Disposal

Equipment used for vaccination, including used vials or ampoules, should be disposed of at the end of a session by sealing in a proper, puncture-resistant 'sharps' box (UN-approved, BS 7320).

Recommendations for the use of the vaccine

The objective of the immunisation programme is to provide two doses of MMR vaccine at appropriate intervals for all eligible individuals.

Over 90% of individuals will seroconvert to measles, mumps and rubella antibodies after the first dose of the MMR vaccines currently used in the UK (Tischer and Gerike, 2000). Antibody responses from pre-licence studies may be higher, however, than clinical protection under routine use. Evidence shows that a single dose of measles-containing vaccine confers protection in around 90% of individuals for measles (Morse *et al.*, 1994; Medical Research Council, 1977). A single dose of a rubella-containing vaccine confers around 95 to 100% protection (Plotkin and Orenstein, 2004). A single dose of a mumps-containing vaccine used in the UK confers between 61 and 91% protection against mumps (Plotkin and Orenstein, 2004, Chapter 20). A more recent study in the UK suggested that a single dose of MMR is around 64% effective against mumps (Harling *et al.*, 2005). Therefore, two doses of MMR are required to produce satisfactory protection against measles, mumps and rubella.

MMR is recommended when protection against measles, mumps and/or rubella is required. MMR vaccine can be given irrespective of a history of measles, mumps or rubella infection or vaccination. There are no ill effects from immunising such individuals because they have pre-existing immunity that inhibits replication of the vaccine viruses.

Children under ten years of age

The first dose of MMR should be given at any time after the first birthday, ideally at 13 months of age. Immunisation before 13 months of age provides earlier protection in localities where the risk of measles is higher, but residual maternal antibodies may reduce the response rate to the vaccine. The optimal age chosen for scheduling children is therefore a compromise between risk of disease and level of protection.

If a dose of MMR is given before the first birthday, either because of travel to an endemic country, or because of a local outbreak, then this dose should be ignored, and two further doses given at the recommended times after the first birthday and pre-school.

A second dose is normally given before school entry but can be given routinely at any time from three months after the first dose. Allowing three months between doses is likely to maximise the response rate, particularly in young children under the age of 18 months where maternal antibodies may reduce the response to vaccination (Orenstein *et al.*, 1986; Redd *et al.*, 2004; De Serres *et al.*, 1995). Where protection against measles is urgently required, the second dose can be given one month after the first (Anon., 1998). If the child is given the second dose less than three months after the first dose and at less than 18 months of age, then the routine pre-school dose (a third dose) should be given in order to ensure full protection.

Children with chronic conditions such as cystic fibrosis, congenital heart or kidney disease, failure to thrive or Down's syndrome are at particular risk from measles infection and should be immunised with MMR vaccine.

Children aged ten years or over and adults

All children should have received two doses of MMR vaccine before they leave school. The teenage (school-leaving) booster session or appointment is an opportunity to ensure that unimmunised or partially immunised children are given MMR. If two doses of MMR are required, then the second dose should be given one month after the first.

MMR vaccine can be given to individuals of any age. Entry into college, university or other higher education institutions, prison or military service provides an opportunity to check an individual's immunisation history. Those who have not received MMR should be offered appropriate MMR immunisation.

The decision on when to vaccinate adults needs to take into consideration the past vaccination history, the likelihood of an individual remaining susceptible and the future risk of exposure and disease:

- individuals who were born between 1980 and 1990 may not be protected against mumps but are likely to be vaccinated against measles and rubella. They may never have received a mumps-containing vaccine or had only one dose of MMR, and had limited opportunity for exposure to natural mumps. They should be recalled and given MMR vaccine. If this is their first dose, a further dose of MMR should be given from one month later

- individuals born between 1970 and 1979 may have been vaccinated against measles and many will have been exposed to mumps and rubella during childhood. However, this age group should be offered MMR wherever feasible, particularly if they are considered to be at high risk of exposure. Where such adults are being vaccinated because they have been demonstrated to be susceptible to at least one of the vaccine components, then either two doses should be given, or there should be evidence of seroconversion to the relevant antigen
- individuals born before 1970 are likely to have had all three natural infections and are less likely to be susceptible. MMR vaccine should be offered to such individuals on request or if they are considered to be at high risk of exposure. Where such adults are being vaccinated because they have been demonstrated to be susceptible to at least one of the vaccine components, then either two doses should be given or there should be evidence of seroconversion to the relevant antigen.

Individuals with unknown or incomplete vaccination histories

Children coming from developing countries will probably have received a measles-containing vaccine in their country of origin but may not have received mumps or rubella vaccines (www.who.int/immunization_monitoring/en/globalsummary/countryprofileselect.cfm). Unless there is a reliable history of appropriate immunisation, individuals should be assumed to be unimmunised and the recommendations above should be followed. Individuals aged 18 months and over who have not received MMR should receive two doses at least one month apart. An individual who has already received one dose of MMR should receive a second dose to ensure that they are protected.

Healthcare workers

Protection of healthcare workers is especially important in the context of their ability to transmit measles, mumps or rubella infections to vulnerable groups. While they may need MMR vaccination for their own benefit, on the grounds outlined above, they also should be immune to measles, mumps and rubella for the protection of their patients.

Satisfactory evidence of protection would include documentation of:

- having received two doses of MMR, or
- positive antibody tests for measles and rubella.

Individuals who are travelling or going to reside abroad

All travellers to epidemic or endemic areas should ensure that they are fully immunised according to the UK schedule (see above). Infants from six months of age travelling to measles endemic areas or to an area where there is a current outbreak should receive MMR. As the response to MMR in infants is sub-optimal where the vaccine has been given before one year of age, immunisation with two further doses of MMR should be given at the recommended ages. Children who are travelling who have received one dose of MMR at the routine age should have the second dose brought forward to at least one month after the first. If the child is under 18 months of age and the second dose is given within three months of the first dose, then the routine pre-school dose (a third dose) should be given in order to ensure full protection.

Contraindications

There are very few individuals who cannot receive MMR vaccine. When there is doubt, appropriate advice should be sought from a consultant paediatrician, immunisation co-ordinator or consultant in communicable disease control rather than withholding the vaccine.

The vaccine should not be given to:

- those who are immunosuppressed (see chapter 6 for more detail)
- those who have had a confirmed anaphylactic reaction to a previous dose of a measles-, mumps- or rubella-containing vaccine
- those who have had a confirmed anaphylactic reaction to neomycin or gelatin
- pregnant women.

Anaphylaxis after MMR is extremely rare (3.5 to 14.4 per million doses) (Bohlke *et al.*, 2003; Patja *et al.*, 2000; Pool *et al.*, 2002; D'Souza *et al.*, 2000). Minor allergic conditions may occur and are not contraindications to further immunisation with MMR or other vaccines. A careful history of that event will often distinguish between anaphylaxis and other events that are either not due to the vaccine or are not life-threatening. In the latter circumstances, it may be possible to continue the immunisation course. Specialist advice must be sought on the vaccines and circumstances in which they could be given. The lifelong risk to the individual of not being immunised must be taken into account.

Precautions

Minor illnesses without fever or systemic upset are not valid reasons to postpone immunisation. If an individual is acutely unwell, immunisation should be postponed until they have fully recovered. This is to avoid confusing the differential diagnosis of any acute illness by wrongly attributing any signs or symptoms to the adverse effects of the vaccine.

Idiopathic thrombocytopaenic purpura

Idiopathic thrombocytopaenic purpura (ITP) has occurred rarely following MMR vaccination, usually within six weeks of the first dose. The risk of developing ITP after MMR vaccine is much less than the risk of developing it after infection with wild measles or rubella virus.

If ITP has occurred within six weeks of the first dose of MMR, then blood should be taken and tested for measles, mumps and rubella antibodies before a second dose is given. Serum should be sent to the Health Protection Agency (HPA) Virus Reference Laboratory (Colindale), which offers free, specialised serological testing for such children. If the results suggest incomplete immunity against measles, mumps or rubella, then a second dose of MMR is recommended.

Allergy to egg

Children with egg allergy should have MMR vaccine. Recent data suggest that anaphylactic reactions to MMR vaccine are not associated with hypersensitivity to egg antigens but to other components of the vaccine (such as gelatin) (Fox and Lack, 2003). In three large studies with a combined total of over 1000 patients with egg allergy, no severe cardiorespiratory reactions were reported after MMR vaccination (Fasano *et al.*, 1992; Freigang *et al.*, 1994; Aickin *et al.*, 1994; Khakoo and Lack, 2000).

If there is a history of confirmed anaphylactic reaction to egg-containing food, paediatric advice should be sought with a view to immunisation under controlled conditions such as admission to hospital as a day case.

Pregnancy and breast-feeding

There is no evidence that rubella-containing vaccines are teratogenic. In the USA, UK and Germany, 661 women were followed through active surveillance, including 293 who were vaccinated (mainly with single rubella vaccine) in the high-risk period (i.e. the six weeks after the last menstrual period). Only 16 infants had evidence of infection and none had permanent abnormalities compatible with congenital rubella syndrome (Best *et al.*, 2004). However, as a precaution, MMR vaccine should not be given to women known to be pregnant. If MMR vaccine is given to adult women, they should be advised to guard against pregnancy for one month.

Termination of pregnancy following inadvertent immunisation should not be recommended (Tookey *et al.*, 1991). The potential parents should be given information on the evidence of lack of risk from vaccination in pregnancy. Surveillance of inadvertent MMR administration in pregnancy is being conducted by the HPA Immunisation Department, to whom such cases should be reported (Tel: 020 8200 4400).

Breast-feeding is not a contraindication to MMR immunisation, and MMR vaccine can be given to breast-feeding mothers without any risk to their baby. Very occasionally, rubella vaccine virus has been found in breast milk, but this has not caused any symptoms in the baby (Buimovici-Klein *et al.*, 1997; Landes *et al.*, 1980; Losonsky *et al.*, 1982). The vaccine does not work when taken orally. There is no evidence of mumps and measles vaccine viruses being found in breast milk.

Premature infants

It is important that premature infants have their immunisations at the appropriate chronological age, according to the schedule (see Chapter 11).

Immunosuppression and HIV

MMR vaccine is not recommended for patients with severe immunosuppression (see Chapter 6) (Angel *et al.*, 1996). MMR vaccine can be given to HIV-positive patients without or with moderate immunosuppression (as defined in Table 21.1).

Table 21.1 CD4 count/μl (% of total lymphocytes)

Age	<12 months	1–5 years	6–12 years	>12 years
No suppression	≥1500 (≥25%)	≥1000 (15–24%)	≥500 (≥25%)	≥500 (≥25%)
Moderate suppression	750–1499 (15–24%)	500–999 (15–24%)	200–499 (15–24%)	200–499 (15–24%)
Severe suppression	<750 (<15%)	<500 (<15%)	<200 (<15%)	<200 (<15%)

Further guidance is provided by the Royal College of Paediatrics and Child Health (www.rcpch.ac.uk), the British HIV Association (BHIVA) *Immunisation guidelines for HIV-infected adults* (BHIVA, 2006) and the Children's HIV Association of UK and Ireland (CHIVA) immunisation guidelines (www.bhiva.org/chiva).

Neurological conditions

The presence of a neurological condition is not a contraindication to immunisation. If there is evidence of current neurological deterioration, including poorly controlled epilepsy, immunisation should be deferred until the condition has stabilised. Children with a personal or close family history of seizures should be given MMR vaccine. Advice about likely timing of any fever and management of a fever should be given. Doctors and nurses should seek specialist paediatric advice rather than refuse immunisation.

Adverse reactions

Adverse reactions following the MMR vaccine (except allergic reactions) are due to effective replication of the vaccine viruses with subsequent mild illness. Such events are to be expected in some individuals. Events due to the measles component occur six to 11 days after vaccination. Events due to the mumps and rubella components usually occur two to three weeks after vaccination but may occur up to six weeks after vaccination. These events only occur in individuals who are susceptible to that component, and are therefore less common after second and subsequent doses. Individuals with vaccine-associated symptoms are not infectious to others.

Common events

Following the first dose of MMR vaccine, malaise, fever and/or a rash may occur, most commonly about a week after immunisation, and last about two to three days. In a study of over 6000 children aged one to two years, the symptoms reported were similar in nature, frequency, time of onset and duration to those commonly reported after measles vaccine alone (Miller *et al.*, 1989). Parotid swelling occurred in about 1% of children of all ages up to four years, usually in the third week.

Adverse reactions are considerably less common after a second dose of MMR vaccine than after the first dose. One study showed no increase in fever or rash after re-immunisation of college students compared with unimmunised controls (Chen *et al.*, 1991). An analysis of allergic reactions reported through the US Vaccine Adverse Events Reporting System in 1991–93 showed fewer reactions among children aged six to 19 years, considered to be second-dose recipients, than among those aged one to four years, considered to be first-dose recipients (Chen *et al.*, 1991). In a study of over 8000 children, there was no increased risk of convulsions, rash or joint pain in the months after the second dose of the MMR vaccination given between four and six years of age (Davis *et al.*, 1997).

Rare and more serious events

Febrile seizures are the most commonly reported neurological event following measles immunisation. Seizures occur during the sixth to eleventh day in one in 1000 children vaccinated with MMR– a rate similar to that reported in the same period after measles vaccine. The rate of febrile seizures following MMR is lower than that following infection with measles disease (Plotkin and Orenstein, 2004). There is good evidence that febrile seizures following MMR immunisation do not increase the risk of subsequent epilepsy compared with febrile seizures due to other causes (Vestergaard *et al.*, 2004).

One strain of mumps virus (Urabe) in an MMR vaccine previously used in the UK was associated with an increased risk of aseptic meningitis (Miller *et al.*, 1993). This vaccine was replaced in 1992 (Department of Health, 1992) and is no longer licensed in the UK. A study in Finland using MMR containing a different mumps strain (Jeryl Lynn), similar to those used currently in MMR in the UK, did not identify any association between MMR and aseptic meningitis (Makela *et al.*, 2002).

Because MMR vaccine contains live, attenuated viruses, it is biologically plausible that it may cause encephalitis. A recent large record-linkage study in Finland, looking at over half a million children aged between one and seven years, did not identify any association between MMR and encephalitis. (Makela *et al.*, 2002)

ITP is a condition that may occur following MMR and is most likely due to the rubella component. This usually occurs within six weeks and resolves spontaneously. One case of ITP attributable to vaccine, occurs for every 32,000 doses administered (Miller *et al.*, 2001). If ITP has occurred within six weeks of the first dose of MMR, then blood should be taken and tested for measles, mumps and rubella antibodies before a second dose is given (see above).

Arthropathy (arthralgia or arthritis) has also been reported to occur rarely after MMR immunisation, probably due to the rubella component. If it is caused by the vaccine, it should occur between 14 and 21 days after immunisation. Where it occurs at other times, it is highly unlikely to have been caused by vaccination. Several controlled epidemiological studies have shown no excess risk of chronic arthritis in women (Slater, 1997).

All suspected adverse reactions to vaccines occurring in children, or in individuals of any age after vaccines labelled with a black triangle (▼), should be reported to the Commission on Human Medicines using the Yellow Card scheme. Serious, suspected adverse reactions to vaccines in adults should be reported through the Yellow Card scheme.

Other conditions reported after vaccines containing measles, mumps and rubella

Following the November 1994 MR immunisation campaign, only three cases of Guillain-Barré syndrome (GBS) were reported. From the background rate, between one and eight cases would have been expected in this population over this period. Therefore, it is likely that these three cases were coincidental and not caused by the vaccine. Analysis of reporting rates of GBS from acute flaccid paralysis surveillance undertaken in the WHO Region of the Americas has shown no increase in rates of GBS following measles immunisation campaigns when 80 million children were immunised (da Silveira *et al.*, 1997). In a population that received 900,000 doses of MMR, there was no increased risk of GBS at any time after the vaccinations were administered (Patja *et al.*, 2001). This evidence refutes the suggestion that MMR causes GBS.

Although gait disturbance has been reported after MMR, a recent epidemiological study showed no evidence of a causal association between MMR and gait disturbance (Miller *et al.*, 2005).

In recent years, the postulated link between measles vaccine and bowel disease has been investigated. There was no increase in the incidence of inflammatory bowel disorders in those vaccinated with measles-containing vaccines when compared with controls (Gilat *et al.*, 1987; Feeney *et al.*, 1997). No increase in the incidence of inflammatory bowel disease has been observed since the introduction of MMR vaccination in Finland (Pebody *et al.*,1998) or in the UK (Seagroatt, 2005).

There is now overwhelming evidence that MMR does not cause autism (www.iom.edu/report.asp?id=20155). Over the past seven years, a large number of studies have been published looking at this issue. Such studies have shown:

- no increased risk of autism in children vaccinated with MMR compared with unvaccinated children (Farrington *et al.*, 2001; Madsen and Vertergaard, 2004)
- no clustering of the onset of symptoms of autism in the period following MMR vaccination (Taylor *et al.*, 1999; De Wilde *et al.*, 2001; Makela *et al.*, 2002)
- that the increase in the reported incidence of autism preceded the use of MMR in the UK (Taylor *et al.*, 1999)
- that the incidence of autism continued to rise after 1993 in Japan despite withdrawal of MMR (Honda *et al.*, 2005)
- that there is no correlation between the rate of autism and MMR vaccine coverage in either the UK or the USA (Kaye *et al.*, 2001; Dales *et al.*, 2001)
- no difference between the proportion of children developing autism after MMR who have a regressive form compared with those who develop autism without vaccination (Fombonne, 2001; Taylor *et al.*, 2002; Gillberg and Heijbel, 1998)
- no difference between the proportion of children developing autism after MMR who have associated bowel symptoms compared with those who develop autism without vaccination (Fombonne, 1998, Fombonne, 2001; Taylor *et al.*, 2002)
- that no vaccine virus can be detected in children with autism using the most sensitive methods available (Afzal *et al.*, 2006; D'Souza *et al.*, 2006).

For the latest evidence, see the Department of Health's website: www.mmrthe facts.nhs.uk.

It has been suggested that combined MMR vaccine could potentially overload the immune system. From the moment of birth, humans are exposed to countless numbers of foreign antigens and infectious agents in their everyday environment. Responding to the three viruses in MMR would use only a tiny proportion of the total capacity of an infant's immune system (Offit *et al.*, 2002). The three viruses in MMR replicate at different rates from each other and would be expected to reach high levels at different times.

A study examining the issue of immunological overload found a lower rate of admission for serious bacterial infection in the period shortly after MMR vaccination compared with other time periods. This suggests that MMR does not cause any general suppression of the immune system (Miller *et al.*, 2003).

Management of cases, contacts and outbreaks

Diagnosis

Prompt notification of measles, mumps and rubella to the local health protection unit (HPU) is required to ensure that public health action can be taken promptly. Notification should be based on clinical suspicion and should not await laboratory confirmation. Since 1994, few clinically diagnosed cases have been subsequently confirmed to be true measles, mumps or rubella. Confirmation rates do increase, however, during outbreaks and epidemics.

The diagnosis of measles, mumps and rubella can be confirmed through non-invasive means. Detection of specific IgM in oral fluid (saliva) samples, ideally between one and six weeks after the onset of rash or parotid swelling, has been shown to be highly sensitive and specific for confirmation of these infections (Brown *et al.*, 1994; Ramsay *et al.*, 1991; Ramsay *et al.*, 1998). It is recommended that oral fluid samples should be obtained from all notified cases, other than during a large epidemic. Advice on this procedure can be obtained from the local HPU.

Protection of contacts with MMR

As vaccine-induced measles antibody develops more rapidly than that following natural infection, MMR vaccine should be used to protect susceptible contacts from suspected measles. To be effective against this exposure, vaccine must be administered very promptly, ideally within three days. Even where it is too late to provide effective post-exposure prophylaxis with MMR, the vaccine can provide protection against future exposure to all three infections. Therefore, contact with suspected measles, mumps or rubella provides a good opportunity to offer MMR vaccine to previously unvaccinated individuals. If the individual is already incubating measles, mumps or rubella, MMR vaccination will not exacerbate the symptoms. In these circumstances, individuals should be advised that a measles-like illness occurring shortly after vaccination is likely to be due to natural infection. If there is doubt about an individual's vaccination status, MMR should still be given as there are no ill effects from vaccinating those who are already immune.

Immunoglobulin is available for post-exposure prophylaxis in individuals for whom vaccine is contraindicated (see above). Antibody responses to the rubella and mumps components of MMR vaccine do not develop soon enough to provide effective prophylaxis after exposure to these infections.

Where immediate protection against measles is required, for example following exposure, MMR may be given from six months of age. As response to MMR in infants is sub-optimal, where the vaccine has been given before 12 months of age, immunisation with two further doses of MMR should be given at the normal ages. Where children who have received the first dose of MMR require immediate protection against measles, the interval between the first and second doses may be reduced to one month. If the child is under 18 months of age when the second dose is given, then the routine pre-school dose (a third dose) should be given in order to ensure full protection.

Protection of contacts with immunoglobulin

Children and adults with compromised immune systems who come into contact with measles should be considered for treatment with human normal immunoglobulin (HNIG) as soon as possible after exposure – at least within six days. Such protection should not await confirmation in the index case, but will require a detailed epidemiological and clinical risk assessment of the likelihood of true measles.

This should be conducted in collaboration with the local HPU or microbiologist. Testing of the index case, however, may inform the future management of contacts and so should be undertaken as soon as possible. Testing the immunocompromised individual for measles IgG antibody may delay the administration of HNIG, and neither previous vaccination nor a low level of antibody will guarantee protection against measles in the profoundly immunosuppressed. The benefit of HNIG, however, is likely to be limited in individuals with detectable antibody and so, where an individual is known or likely to have pre-existing measles antibody, HNIG may not be required, particularly where the degree of immunosuppression is less severe.

Children under nine months in whom there is a particular reason to avoid measles (such as recent severe illness) can also be given immunoglobulin; MMR vaccine should then be given after an interval of at least three months, at around the usual age.

Measles infection in pregnancy can lead to intra-uterine death and pre-term delivery, but is not associated with congenital infection or damage. Pregnant women who are exposed to measles may be considered for HNIG. A very high proportion of such women will be immune and therefore, wherever possible, measles IgG testing should be undertaken. Where the diagnosis in the index case is uncertain, this assessment should be done as part of the investigation of exposure to rash in pregnancy (www.hpa.org.uk/infections/topics_az/rubella/rash.pdf)

To prevent or attenuate an attack*:

Age	Dose
Under 1 year	250mg
1–2 years	500mg
3 and over	750mg

An interval of at least three months must be allowed before subsequent MMR immunisation.

Supplies

MMR vaccine

- M-M-R II – manufactured by Sanofi Pasteur MSD.
- Priorix – manufactured by GlaxoSmithKline.

These vaccines are supplied by Healthcare Logistics (Tel: 0870 8711890) as part of the national childhood immunisation programme.

In Scotland, supplies should be obtained from local childhood vaccine-holding centres. Details of these are available from Scottish Healthcare Supplies (Tel: 0131 275 6154).

In Northern Ireland, supplies should be obtained from local childhood vaccineholding centres. Details of these are available from the regional pharmaceutical procurement service
(Tel: 02890 552368).

Human normal immunoglobulin

England and Wales:
Health Protection Agency, Centre for Infections
(Tel: 0208 200 6868)

Scotland:
Blood Transfusion Service
(Tel: 0141 3577700)

* Normal immunoglobulin for measles prophylaxis is in short supply and from time to time alternative products and doses may need to be used. For latest advice please check with the Health Protection Agency (www.hpa.org.uk) or Health Protection Scotland (www.hps.scot.nhs.uk).

Northern Ireland:
Public Health Laboratory, Belfast City Hospital
(Tel: 01232 329241)

References

ACIP (1998) Measles, mumps, and rubella – vaccine use and strategies for elimination of measles, rubella, and congenital rubella syndrome and control of mumps: recommendations of the Advisory Committee on Immunization Practices (ACIP) *MMWR* **47**(RR-8): 1–57. www.cdc.gov/mmwr/preview/mmwrhtml/00053391.htm (22 May 1998).

Afzal MA, Ozoemena LC, O'Hare A *et al.* (2006) Absence of detectable measles virus genome sequence in blood of autistic children who have had their MMR vaccination during the routine childhood immunisation schedule of the UK. *J Med Virol* **78**: 623–30.

Aickin R, Hill D and Kemp A (1994) Measles immunisation in children with allergy to egg. *BMJ* **308**: 223–5.

Alcardi J, Goutieres F, Arsenio-Nunes ML and Lebon P (1997) Acute measles encephalitis in children with immunosuppression. *Pediatrics* **59**(2): 232–9.

American Academy of Pediatrics (2003) Active immunization. In: Pickering LK (ed.) *Red Book: 2003 Report of the Committee on Infectious Diseases,* 26th edition. Elk Grove Village, IL: American Academy of Pediatrics.

Angel JB, Udem SA, Snydman DR *et al.* (1996) Measles pneumonitis following measles-mumps-rubella vaccination of patients with HIV infection, 1993. *MMWR* **45**: 603–6.

Babad HR, Nokes DJ, Gay N *et al.* (1995) Predicting the impact of measles vaccination in England and Wales: model validation and analysis of policy options. *Epidemiol Infect* **114**: 319–44.

Barthez Carpentier MA, Billard C, Maheut J *et al.* (1992) Acute measles encephalitis of the delayed type: neuroradiological and immunological findings. *Eur Neurol* **32**(4): 235–7.

Best JM, Cooray S and Banatvala JE (2004) Rubella. In: Mahy BMJ and ter Meulen V (eds) *Topley and Wilson's Virology*, tenth edition. London: Hodder Arnold.

Bohlke K, Davis RL, Moray SH *et al.* (2003) Risk of anaphylaxis after vaccination of children and adolescents. *Pediatrics* **112**: 815–20.

British HIV Association (2006) *Immunisation guidelines for HIV-infected adults*. BHIVA. www.bhiva.org/pdf/2006/Immunisation506.pdf

Brown DW, Ramsay ME, Richards AF and Miller E (1994) Salivary diagnosis of measles: a study of notified cases in the United Kingdom, 1991–3. *BMJ* **308**(6935): 1015–17.

Buimovici-Klein E, Hite RL, Byrne T and Cooper LR (1997) Isolation of rubella virus in milk after postpartum immunization. *J Pediatr* **91**: 939–43.

Chen RT, Moses JM, Markowitz LE and Orenstein WA (1991) Adverse events following measles-mumps-rubella and measles vaccinations in college students. *Vaccine* **9**: 297–9.

Chin J (ed.) (2000) *Control of Communicable Diseases Manual*, 17th edition. Washington, DC: American Public Health Association.

Dales L, Hammer SJ and Smith NJ (2001) Time trends in autism and in MMR immunization coverage in California. *JAMA* **285**(22): 2852–3.

da Silveira CM, Salisbury DM and de Quadros CA (1997) Measles vaccination and Guillain-Barré syndrome. *Lancet* **349**(9044): 14–16.

Davis RL, Marcuse E, Black S *et al.* (1997) MMR2 immunization at 4 to 5 years and 10 to 12 years of age: a comparison of adverse clinical events after immunization in the Vaccine Safety Datalink project. The Vaccine Safety Datalink Team. *Pediatrics* **100**: 767–71.

Department of Health (1992) *Changes in Supply of Vaccine*. Circular (PL/CMO(92)11).

De Serres G, Boulianne N, Meyer F and Ward BJ (1995) Measles vaccine efficacy during an outbreak in a highly vaccinated population: incremental increase in protection with age at vaccination up to 18 months. *Epidemiol Infect* **115**: 315–23.

De Wilde S, Carey IM, Richards N *et al.* (2001) Do children who become autistic consult more often after MMR vaccination? *Br J General Practice* **51**: 226–7.

D'Souza RM, Campbell-Lloyd S, Isaacs D *et al.* (2000) Adverse events following immunisation associated with the 1998 Australian Measles Control Campaign. *Commun Dis Intell* **24**: 27–33.

D'Souza Y, Fombonne E and Ward BJ (2006) No evidence of persisting measles virus in peripheral blood mononuclear cells from children with autism spectrum disorder. *Pediatrics* **118**: 1664–75.

Farrington CP, Miller E and Taylor B (2001) MMR and autism: further evidence against a causal association. *Vaccine* **19**: 3632–5.

Fasano MB, Wood RA, Cooke SK and Sampson HA (1992) Egg hypersensitivity and adverse reactions to measles, mumps and rubella vaccine. *J Pediatr* **120**: 878–81.

Feeney M, Gregg A, Winwood P and Snook J (1997) A case-control study of measles vaccination and inflammatory bowel disease. The East Dorset Gastroenterology Group. *Lancet* **350**: 764–6.

Fombonne E (1998) Inflammatory bowel disease and autism. *Lancet* **351**: 955.

Fombonne E (2001) Is there an epidemic of autism? *Pediatrics* **107**: 411–12.

Fox A and Lack G (2003) Egg allergy and MMR vaccination. *Br J Gen Pract* **53**: 801–2.

Freigang B, Jadavji TP and Freigang DW (1994) Lack of adverse reactions to measles, mumps and rubella vaccine in egg-allergic children. *Ann Allergy* **73**: 486–8.

Gay NJ, Hesketh LM, Morgan-Capner P and Miller E (1995) Interpretation of serological surveillance data for measles using mathematical models: implications for vaccine strategy. *Epidemiol Infect* **115**: 139–56.

Gilat T, Hacohen D, Lilos P and Langman MJ (1987) Childhood factors in ulcerative colitis and Crohn's disease. An international co-operative study. *Scan J Gastroenterology* **22**: 1009–24.

Gillberg C and Heijbel H (1998) MMR and autism. *Autism* **2**: 423–4.

Gray HM, Hann IM, Glass S *et al.* (1987) Mortality and morbidity caused by measles in children with malignant disease attending four major treatment centres: a retrospective view. *BMJ* **295**: 19–22.

Harling R, White JM, Ramsay ME *et al.* (2005) The effectiveness of the mumps component of the MMR vaccine: a case control study. *Vaccine* **23**(31): 4070–4.

Health Protection Agency (2006) Measles deaths, England and Wales, by age group, 1980-2004. www.hpa.org.uk/infections/topics_az/measles/data_death_age.htm

Honda H, Shimizu J and Rutter M (2005) No effect of MMR withdrawal on the incidence of autism: a total population study. *J Child Psychol Psychiatry* **46**(6): 572–9.

Jin L, Beard S, Hunjan R *et al.* (2002) Characterization of measles virus strains causing SSPE: a study of 11 cases. *J Neurovirol* **8**(4): 335–44.

Kaye JA, del Mar Melero-Montes M and Jick H (2001) Mumps, measles and rubella vaccine and the incidence of autism recorded by general practitioners: a time trend analysis. *BMJ* **322**(7284): 460–3.

Khakoo GA and Lack G (2000) Recommendations for using MMR vaccine in children allergic to eggs. *BMJ* **320**: 929–32.

Kidd IM, Booth CJ, Rigden SP *et al.* (2003) Measles-associated encephalitis in children with renal transplants: a predictable effect of waning herd immunity? *Lancet* **362**: 832.

Landes RD, Bass JW, Millunchick EW and Oetgen WJ (1980) Neonatal rubella following postpartum maternal immunisation. *J Pediatr* **97**: 465–7.

Losonsky GA, Fishaut JM, Strussenberg J and Ogra PL (1982) Effect of immunization against rubella on lactation products. I. Development and characterization of specific immunologic reactivity in breast milk. *J Infect Dis* **145**: 654–60.

Madsen KM and Vestergaard M (2004) MMR vaccination and autism: what is the evidence for a causal association? *Drug Saf* **27**: 831–40.

Makela A, Nuorti JP and Peltola H (2002) Neurologic disorders after measles-mumps-rubella vaccination. *Pediatrics* **110**: 957–63.

McLean ME and Carter AO (1990) Measles in Canada – 1989. *Canada Diseases Weekly Report* **16**(42): 213–8.

Medical Research Council (1977) Clinical trial of live measles vaccine given alone and live vaccine preceded by killed vaccine. Fourth report of the Medical Research Council by the measles sub-committee on development of vaccines and immunisation procedures. *Lancet* **ii**: 571–5.

Miki K, Komase K, Mgone CS *et al.* (2002) Molecular analysis of measles virus genome derived from SSPE and acute measles patients in Papua, New Guinea. *J Med Virol* **68**(1): 105–12.

Miller CL (1978) Severity of notified measles. *BMJ* **1**(6122): 1253.

Miller CL (1985) Deaths from measles in England and Wales, 1970–83. *BMJ* (Clin Res Ed) **290**(6466): 443–4.

Miller C, Miller E, Rowe K *et al.* (1989) Surveillance of symptoms following MMR vaccine in children. *Practitioner* **233**(1461): 69–73.

Miller CL, Farrington CP and Harbert K (1992) The epidemiology of subacute sclerosing panencephalitis in England and Wales 1970–1989. *Int J Epidemiol* **21**(5): 998–1006.

Miller CL, Andrews N, Rush M *et al.* (2004) The epidemiology of subacute sclerosing panencephalitis in England and Wales 1990–2002. *Arch Dis Child* **89**(12): 1145–8.

Miller E, Goldacre M, Pugh S *et al.* (1993) Risk of aseptic meningitis after measles, mumps, and rubella vaccine in UK children. *Lancet* **341**(8851): 979–82.

Miller E, Waight P, Farrington P *et al.* (2001) Idiopathic thrombocytopenic purpura and MMR vaccine. *Arch Dis Child* **84**: 227–9.

Miller E, Andrews N, Waight P and Taylor B (2003) Bacterial infections, immune overload, and MMR vaccine. Measles, mumps, and rubella. *Arch Dis Child* **88**(3): 222–3.

Miller E, Andrews N, Grant A *et al.* (2005) No evidence of an association between MMR vaccine and gait disturbance. *Arch Dis Child* **90**(3): 292–6.

Morse D, O'Shea M, Hamilton G *et al.* (1994) Outbreak of measles in a teenage school population: the need to immunize susceptible adolescents. *Epidemiol Infect* **113**: 355–65.

Mullooly J and Black S (2001) Simultaneous administration of varicella vaccine and other recommended childhood vaccines – United States, 1995–1999. *MMWR* **50**(47): 1058–61.

Norrby E and Oxman MN (1990) Measles virus. In: Fields BN and Knipe DM (eds) *Virology*, 2nd edition. New York: Raven Press Ltd, pp 1013–44.

Offit PA, Quarles J, Gerber MA *et al.* (2002) Addressing parents' concerns: do multiple vaccines overwhelm or weaken the infant's immune system? *Pediatrics* **109**(1): 124–9.

Orenstein WA, Markowitz L, Preblud SR *et al.* (1986) Appropriate age for measles vaccination in the United States. *Dev Biol Stand* **65**: 13–21.

Patja A, Davidkin I, Kurki T *et al.* (2000) Serious adverse events after measles-mumps-rubella vaccination during a fourteen-year prospective follow-up. *Pediatr Infect Dis J* **19**(12): 1127–34.

Patja A, Paunio M, Kinnunen E *et al.* (2001) Risk of Guillaine-Barré syndrome after measles-mumps-rubella vaccination. *J Pediatr* **138**: 250–4.

Pebody RG, Paunio M and Ruutu P (1998) Measles, measles vaccination, and Crohn's disease has not increased in Finland. *BMJ* **316**(7146): 1745–6.

Peltola H, Heinonen OP and Valle M (1994) The elimination of indigenous measles, mumps and rubella from Finland by a 12-year two-dose vaccination program. *N Engl J Med* **331**(21): 1397–402.

Perry RT and Halsey NA (2004) The clinical significance of measles: a review. *J Infect Dis* **189**: S4–16.

Plotkin SA and Orenstein WA (eds) (2004) *Vaccines,* 4th edition. Philadelphia: WB Saunders Company, Chapter 19.

Pool V, Braun MM, Kelso JM *et al.* (2002) Prevalence of anti-gelatin IgE antibodies in people with anaphylaxis after measles-mumps-rubella vaccine in the United States. *Pediatrics* **110**(6): e71. www.pediatrics.org/cgi/content/full/110/6/e71

Ramsay ME, Brown DW, Eastcott HR and Begg NT (1991) Saliva antibody testing and vaccination in a mumps outbreak. *CDR (Lond Engl Rev)* **1**(9): R96–8.

Ramsay M, Gay N, Miller E *et al.* (1994) The epidemiology of measles in England and Wales; rationale for the 1994 national vaccination campaign. *CDR Review* **4**(12): R141–6.

Ramsay ME, Brugha R, Brown DW *et al.* (1998) Salivary diagnosis of rubella: a study of notified cases in the United Kingdom, 1991–4. *Epidemiol Infect* **120**(3): 315–19.

Ramsay ME, Jin Li, White J *et al.* (2003) The elimination of indigenous measles transmission in England and Wales. *J Infect Dis* **187**(suppl. 1): S198–207.

Redd SC, King GE, Heath JL *et al.* (2004) Comparison of vaccination with measles-mumps-rubella at 9, 12 and 15 months of age. *J Infect Dis* **189**: S116–22.

Seagroatt V (2005) MMR vaccine and Crohn's disease: ecological study of hospital admissions in England, 1991 to 2002. *BMJ* **330**(7500):1120–1.

Slater PE (1997) Chronic arthropathy after rubella vaccination in women. False alarm? *JAMA* **278**: 594–5.

Taylor B, Miller E, Farrington CP *et al.* (1999) Autism and measles, mumps and rubella: no epidemiological evidence for a causal association. *Lancet* **53**(9169): 2026–9.

Taylor B, Miller E, Langman R *et al.* (2002) Measles, mumps and rubella vaccination and bowel problems or developmental regression in children with autism population study. *BMJ* **324**(7334): 393–6.

Tischer A and Gerike E (2000) Immune response after primary and re-vaccination with different combined vaccines against measles, mumps, rubella. *Vaccine* **18**(14): 1382–92.

Tookey PA, Jones G, Miller BH and Peckham CS (1991) Rubella vaccination in pregnancy. *CDR (London Engl Rev)* **1**(8): R86–8.

Vestergaard M, Hviid A, Madsen KM *et al.* (2004) MMR vaccination and febrile seizures. Evaluation of susceptible subgroups and long-term prognosis. *JAMA* **292**(3): 351–7.

Vyse AJ, Gay NJ, White JM *et al.* (2002) Evolution of surveillance of measles, mumps, and rubella in England and Wales: providing the platform for evidence based vaccination policy. *Epidemiol Rev* **24**(2): 125–36.

WHO (2003) Eliminating measles and rubella and preventing congenital rubella infections. www.euro.who.int/vaccine/20030808_4

WHO (2005) Vaccine Preventable Diseases Monitoring System. Global summary. www-nt.who.int/immunization_monitoring/en/globalsummary/countryprofileselect.cfm

22

Meningococcal

MENINGOCOCCAL MENINGITIS AND SEPTICAEMIA NOTIFIABLE

The disease

Meningococcal disease is the result of a systemic bacterial infection by *Neisseria meningitidis*. Meningococci are gram-negative diplococci, divided into antigenically distinct groups. There are at least 13 serogroups, of which groups B and C are the most common in the UK. Other less common serogroups include A, Y, W135, 29E and Z. The 13 serogroups can be further subdivided by serotyping and serosubtyping and by sulphonamide sensitivity. Increasing use of molecular-based methods is allowing further classification of the organism and identification of specific clonal complexes that appear to be associated with invasive disease.

Meningococcal infection most commonly presents as either meningitis or septicaemia, or a combination of both. Less commonly, individuals may present with pneumonia, myocarditis, endocarditis, pericarditis, arthritis, conjunctivitis, urethritis, pharyngitis and cervicitis (Rosenstein *et al.*, 2001).

The incubation period is from two to seven days, and the onset of disease varies from fulminant with acute and overwhelming features, to insidious with mild prodromal symptoms. Early symptoms and signs are usually malaise, pyrexia and vomiting. Headache, neck stiffness, photophobia, drowsiness or confusion and joint pains may occur variably. In meningococcal septicaemia, a rash may develop, along with signs of advancing shock and isolated limb and/or joint pain. The rash may be non-specific early on but as the disease progresses the rash may become petechial or purpuric and may not blanch.This can readily be confirmed by gentle pressure with a glass (the 'glass' test) when the rash can be seen to persist (Figure 22.1). In young infants particularly, the onset may be insidious and the signs be non-specific without 'classical' features of meningitis.

Health professionals should be alert to the possibility of meningococcal infection in a young child presenting with vomiting, pyrexia and irritability and, if still patent, raised anterior fontanelle tension. Clinical deterioration may be very rapid with poor peripheral perfusion, pallor, tachypnoea, tachycardia and the emergence of the meningococcal rash. In severe cases, patients may present with hypotension or in a coma.

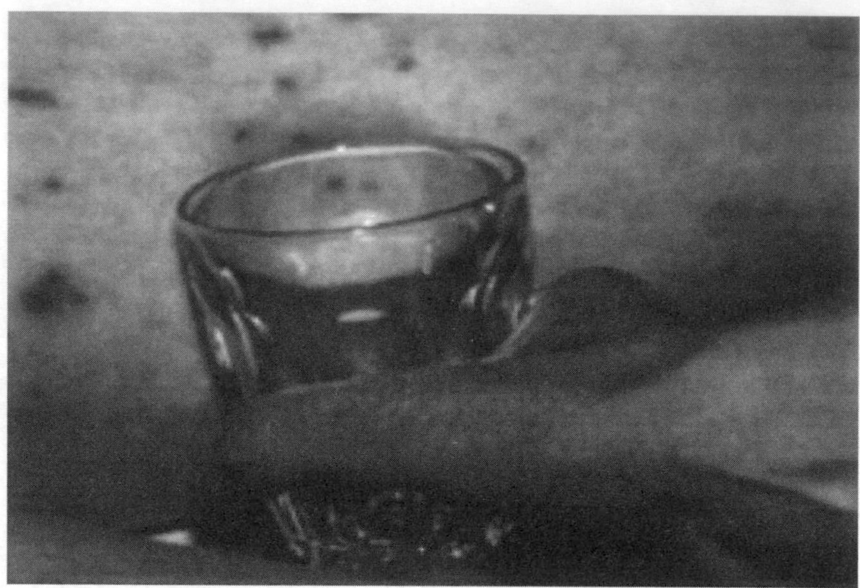

Figure 22.1 The 'glass' test (*picture courtesy of Meningitis Research Foundation)*

Meningococcal bacteria colonise the nasopharynx of humans and are frequently harmless commensals. Between 5 and 11% of adults and up to 25% of adolescents carry the bacteria without any signs or symptoms of the disease. In infants and young children, the carriage rate is low (Cartwright, 1995). It is not fully understood why the disease develops in some individuals but not in others. Age, season, smoking, preceding influenza A infection, and living in 'closed' or 'semi-closed' communities, such as university halls of residence or military barracks, have been identified as risk factors (Cartwright, 1995).

Transmission is by aerosol, droplets or direct contact with respiratory secretions of someone carrying the organism. Transmission usually requires either frequent or prolonged close contact. There is a marked seasonal variation in meningococcal disease, with peak levels in the winter months declining to low levels by late summer.

The incidence of meningococcal disease is highest in children aged one to five years followed by infants under one year of age. The next highest risk group is young people aged 15 to 19 years.

Overall mortality remains around 10% in the UK (Ramsay *et al.*, 1997; Goldacre *et al.*, 2003). Case fatality ratios increase with age and are higher in

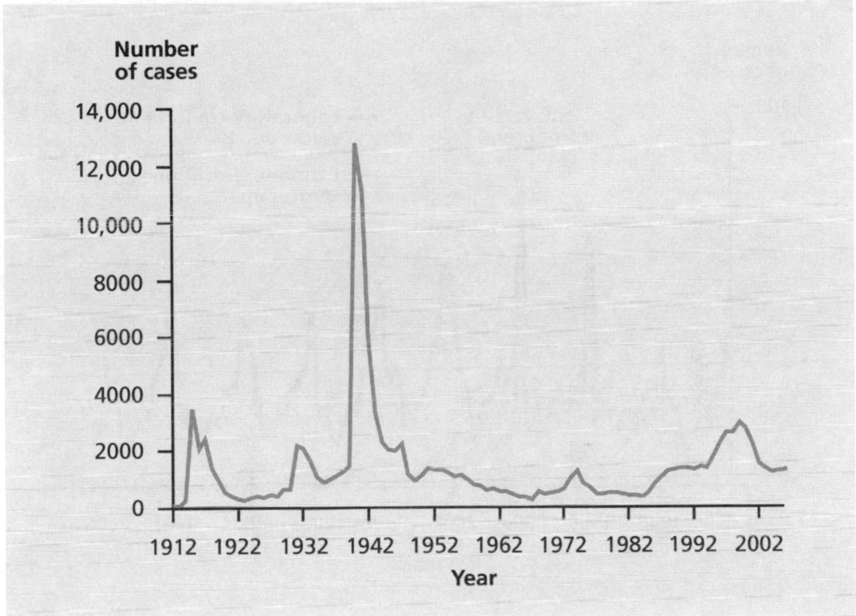

Figure 22.2 Notifications of meningococcal disease, England and Wales 1912–2004

individuals with serogroup C than with serogroup B infections (Ramsay *et al.*, 1997; Goldacre *et al.*, 2003) and also higher in those infected with strains with certain typing patterns (Trotter *et al.*, 2002). Mortality is higher in cases with septicaemia than in those with meningitis alone (Davison *et al.*, 2002). Recent studies in paediatric intensive care settings have indicated that prompt and active management may reduce fatality ratios (Booy *et al.*, 2001; Thorburn *et al.*, 2001). In those who survive, approximately 25% may experience a reduced quality of life, with 10–20% developing permanent sequelae (Erickson and De Wals, 1998; Granoff, *et al.*, 2004). The most common long-term effects are skin scars, limb amputation(s), hearing loss, seizures and brain damage (Steven and Wood, 1995; Lepow *et al.*, 1999).

History and epidemiology of the disease

Large epidemics of meningococcal disease caused by serogroup A infections coincided with each of the two world wars (Figure 22.2) (Jones, 1995). After the Second World War, incidence declined. However, between 1972 and 1975, incidence increased temporarily, associated with a serogroup B serotype 2a strain. In 1985, another hyperendemic period began, associated with increased circulation of a hypervirulent B15:P1.16 strain. A further hyperendemic period started in 1995–96, associated with an increased proportion of disease due to

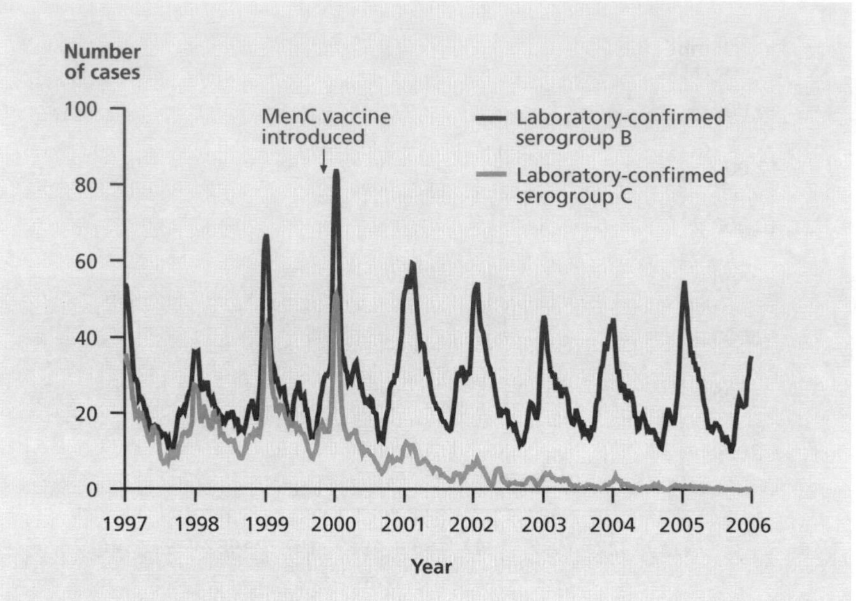

Figure 22.3 Laboratory-confirmed cases of meningococcal disease, England and Wales, five weekly moving averages: 1997 to 2006 (week 04)

serogroup C serotype 2a infection. There was a shift in age distribution towards teenagers and young adults, among whom case fatality rates are particularly high.

In the mid-1990s, vaccines based on the serogroup C polysaccharide provided only short-term protection to older children and adults and did not protect infants. New meningococcal C (MenC) conjugate vaccines were therefore developed that would provide longer-term protection and would be effective in infants. As the rate of meningococcal serogroup C infections continued to rise, the development of the new vaccines was accelerated.

In November 1999, a new MenC conjugate vaccine was introduced into the UK routine immunisation programme. All children and adolescents under the age of 18 years were immunised over a two-year period. In January 2002, the campaign was extended to include all adults under 25 years of age.

Following the MenC vaccine campaign, the number of laboratory-confirmed group C cases fell by over 90% in all age groups immunised (Figure 22.3) (Salisbury *et al.*, 2001; Trotter *et al.*, 2004). Cases in other age groups fell by approximately two-thirds as a result of reduced carriage rates and indirect protection (Trotter *et al.*, 2003).

In 2006, following studies that showed that protection against meningococcal group C waned during the second year of life (Trotter *et al.*, 2004), a booster dose (combined with Hib as Hib/MenC) was introduced at 12 months of age.

Group B strains now account for over 80% of laboratory-confirmed isolates submitted to the Health Protection Agency (HPA) Meningococcal Reference Unit (Health Protection Agency) www.hpa.org.uk/cdph/issues/CDPHVol15/no3/Meningococcal_ Guidelines.pdf

Meningococcal disease occurs in all countries. In the 'meningitis belt' of sub-Saharan Africa, the incidence of meningococcal infection rises sharply towards the end of the dry, dusty season when disease spreads rapidly, resulting in large epidemics within very short periods. These are predominantly due to serogroup A, but recent outbreaks have included serogroup W135.

There have been large epidemics of meningococcal disease linked to the annual hajj pilgrimage to Mecca in Saudi Arabia, resulting in importations into a number of countries, including the UK. These were predominantly serogroup A epidemics and immunisation against this strain became a requirement for entry to Saudi Arabia. In 2000 and 2001, there was an increase in W135 infections at the hajj and quadrivalent (serogroups A, C, Y, W135) vaccine became an entry requirement in 2002. Following this recommendation, W135 cases returned to very low levels in the UK.

The meningococcal vaccination

MenC conjugate vaccine

The MenC conjugate vaccines are made from capsular polysaccharide that has been extracted from cultures of group C *Neisseria meningitidis*. The polysaccharide is linked (conjugated) to a carrier protein, according to the manufacturer's method. In the UK, MenC vaccines have been used that have been conjugated with either CRM_{197} (a non-toxic variant of diphtheria toxin) or tetanus toxoid. The conjugation increases the immunogenicity, especially in young children in whom the plain polysaccharide vaccines are less immunogenic.

MenC vaccine confers no protection against other types of meningococcal disease, such as serogroups B, A or W135.

Hib/MenC conjugate vaccine

The Hib/MenC conjugate vaccine is made from capsular polysaccharides of *Haemophilus influenzae* type b and group C *Neisseria meningitidis*, which are conjugated to tetanus toxoid. The vaccine has been shown to elicit booster responses to both Hib and MenC when given in the second year of life to children who were primed in infancy with Hib and MenC conjugate vaccines.

Quadrivalent (ACWY) polysaccharide vaccine

The polysaccharide (non-conjugated) vaccine is made from the outer capsules of serogroups A, C, W135 and Y *Neisseria meningitidis* organisms.

Young infants respond to group A, Y and W135 polysaccharide from three months of age. However, protection is not long-lasting (Cadoz *et al.*, 1985; Peltola *et al.*, 1985; Al-Mazrou *et al.*, 2005).

Vaccine-induced immunity lasts approximately three to five years in older children and adults; in younger children, a more rapid decline in antibody has been noted (Frasch, 1995). The response is strictly serogroup-specific and confers no protection against group B organisms.

The above vaccines do not contain thiomersal. They are inactivated, do not contain live organisms and cannot cause the diseases against which they protect.

At present there is no available vaccine effective against group B organisms.

Storage

Vaccines should be stored in the original packaging at +2˚C to +8˚C and protected from light. All vaccines are sensitive to some extent to heat and cold. Heat speeds up the decline in potency of most vaccines, thus reducing their shelf life. Effectiveness cannot be guaranteed for vaccines unless they have been stored at the correct temperature. Freezing may cause increased reactogenicity and loss of potency for some vaccines. It can also cause hairline cracks in the container, leading to contamination of the contents.

Presentation

MenC conjugate

The MenC conjugate vaccine is available either as a lyophilised powder for reconstitution with a diluent or as a suspension in a syringe. After reconstitution of the lyophilised suspension, the vaccine must be used within one hour.

Discard any vaccine that is unused one hour following reconstitution.
Note: The diluent must not be frozen.

Hib/MenC conjugate

Hib/MenC is supplied as a vial of white powder and 0.5ml of solvent in a pre-filled syringe. The vaccine must be reconstituted by adding the entire contents of the pre-filled syringe to the vial containing the powder. After addition of the solvent, the mixture should be well shaken until the powder is completely dissolved. After reconstitution, the vaccine should be administered promptly, or allowed to stand between +2° and +8° and be used within 24 hours.

Quadrivalent (ACW135Y) polysaccharide vaccine

The quadrivalent A, C, W135 and Y polysaccharide vaccine should be reconstituted immediately before use with the diluent supplied by the manufacturer. After reconstitution, the vaccine must be used within one hour. Discard any vaccine that is unused one hour following reconstitution.
Note: The diluent must not be frozen.

Dosage and schedule

MenC vaccine

Infants under one year of age:

- First dose of 0.5ml of MenC vaccine.
- Second dose of 0.5ml, one month after the first dose.
- A third dose of 0.5ml of MenC-containing vaccine should be given at the recommended interval (see below).

Children over one year and adults under 25 years of age should have a single dose of MenC-containing vaccine.

Quadrivalent (ACWY) polysaccharide vaccine

Children over three months of age and under two years:

- First dose of 0.5ml.
- Second dose of 0.5ml three months after the first dose.

Children over two years of age and adults:

- Single dose of 0.5ml.

Reinforcing doses should be given at recommended intervals (see below).

Administration

The vaccines are routinely given intramuscularly into the upper arm or anterolateral thigh. This is to reduce the risk of localised reactions, which are more common when the vaccine is given subcutaneously (Mark *et al.*, 1999; Diggle and Deeks, 2000; Zuckerman, 2000). However, for individuals with a bleeding disorder, vaccines should be given by deep subcutaneous injection to reduce the risk of bleeding.

Meningococcal vaccines can be given at the same time as other vaccines such as measles, mumps and rubella (MMR), diphtheria, tetanus, pertussis, polio and Hib. The vaccines should be given at a separate site, preferably a separate limb. If given in the same limb, they should be given at least 2.5cm apart (American Academy of Pediatrics, 2003). The site at which each vaccine is given should be noted in the child's record.

At the moment, there are no data on the administration of Hib/MenC vaccine at the same time as pneumococcal conjugate vaccine (PCV). Although there is no reason to think that this would cause any safety concerns, there is a theoretical possibility of reduced response to one or other vaccine. Therefore, as a precautionary measure, Hib/MenC should not be given routinely at the same time as the booster of PCV. However, where rapid protection is required, the two can be given on the same day or at any interval. As more data accumulates this advice may be modified.

Disposal

Equipment used for vaccination, including empty vials or ampoules, should be disposed of at the end of a session by sealing in a proper, puncture-resistant 'sharps' box (UN-approved, BS 7320).

Recommendations for the use of the MenC conjugate vaccines

The objective of the immunisation programme is to protect those under 25 years of age, and individuals outside this age range who may be at elevated risk from meningococcal C disease.

Primary immunisation

Infants under one year of age

The primary course of MenC vaccination consists of two doses, with an interval of one month between each dose. The recommended age for vaccination is at three and four months of age. If the primary course is interrupted it should be resumed but not repeated (see below).

The currently available MenC vaccines are now licensed for use in a two-dose schedule from two months of age. Although the licence states that two doses should be given at least two months apart, evidence from UK studies shows that immunogenicity is adequate in children immunised at a one-month interval (Southern *et al*., 2006).

Children from one year of age and adults

The primary course of MenC vaccine for this age group is one dose. If the primary course in children under one year was not completed, then a single booster dose of Hib/MenC vaccine should be given, at least one month after the last dose.

All individuals under 25 years and other individuals at elevated risk, regardless of their age, should be immunised with a single dose of MenC. Any unprotected individual attending university, irrespective of age, should be immunised before they enrol or as soon as possible thereafter.

Reinforcing immunisation

A reinforcing (booster) dose of Hib/MenC is recommended at 12 months of age for children who have received a complete primary course of two doses of MenC vaccine. It should be given one month before pneumococcal conjugate and MMR vaccines.

Individuals with unknown or incomplete vaccination histories

Where a child born in the UK presents with an inadequate immunisation history, every effort should be made to clarify what immunisations they may have had (see Chapter 11). Children coming to the UK who have a history of completing immunisation in their country of origin may not have been offered protection against all the antigens currently used in the UK, and they may not have received MenC-containing vaccines in their country of origin (www-nt.who.int/immunization_monitoring/en/globalsummary/countryprofileselect.cfm).

Children coming from developing countries, from areas of conflict, or from hard-to-reach population groups may not have been fully immunised. Where there is no reliable history of previous immunisation, it should be assumed that they are unimmunised and the full UK recommendations should be followed (see Chapter 11).

A child who has not completed the primary course (and is under one year of age) should have the outstanding doses at appropriate intervals (see above). If an individual is coming into the UK to attend university and has not previously been immunised against group C disease (with either polysaccharide or conjugate vaccine) they should receive one dose of MenC vaccine as soon as possible.

Children and adults with asplenia or splenic dysfunction

Children and adults with asplenia or splenic dysfunction may be at increased risk of invasive meningococcal infection. Such individuals, irrespective of age or interval from splenectomy, may have a sub-optimal response to the vaccine (Balmer *et al.*, 2004).

Children under one year of age should be vaccinated according to the UK schedule, receiving two doses in infancy and a booster dose at 12 months of age.

Children over one year of age and adults should be given two doses of Hib/MenC vaccine two months apart.

Children and adults who have been fully immunised with MenC as part of the routine programme, but who then develop splenic dysfunction, should be offered an additional dose of MenC (usually as combined Hib/MenC vaccine).

If travelling to a country where there is an increased risk of serogroup A, W135 or Y disease, such individuals should also receive the quadrivalent polysaccharide vaccine (see below).

Recommendations for the use of the quadrivalent (ACWY) polysaccharide vaccine

Primary immunisation

Children over three months and under two years of age

The primary course consists of two doses with an interval of three months between doses.

Children over two years of age and adults

The primary course consists of a single dose.

Reinforcing immunisation

A reinforcing dose should be given every five years to those at continued risk.

Children who were under five years when they were first vaccinated, should be given a booster dose after 2–3 years if they remain at high risk.

Visa entry requirements should be checked for travel to individual countries.

Individuals who are travelling or going to reside abroad

In some areas of the world the risk of acquiring meningococcal infection particularly of developing group A disease, is much higher than in the UK. Individuals who are particularly at risk are visitors who live or travel 'rough', such as backpackers, and those living or working with local people. Large epidemics of both group A and group W135 meningococcal infection have occurred in association with hajj pilgrimages to Saudi Arabia, and vaccination against A, C, W135 and Y serogroups is now a visa entry requirement.

Epidemics, mainly group A and more recently W135 infections, occur throughout tropical Africa, particularly in the savannah during the dry season, which varies from country to country and can be unpredictable. Immunisation is recommended for long-stay or high-risk visitors to sub-Saharan Africa, for example those who will be living or working closely with local people, or those who are backpacking.

From time to time, outbreaks of meningococcal infection may be reported from other parts of the world, including the Indian sub-continent and other parts of Asia (see, for example, www.hpa.org.uk/cdr/archives/2005/cdr1905.pdf www.who.int/csr/don/2005_01_28a/en/index.html). Where such outbreaks are shown to be due to vaccine-preventable serogroups, vaccination may be recommended for certain travellers to the affected areas. More detailed country by country information is contained in *Health information for overseas travel* (Department of Health, 2001).

Note. MenC conjugate vaccine protects against group C disease only. Individuals travelling abroad (see above) should be immunised with the quadrivalent polysaccharide vaccine, even if they have previously received the MenC conjugate vaccine.

Contraindications

There are very few individuals who cannot receive meningococcal vaccines. When there is doubt, appropriate advice should be sought from a consultant paediatrician, immunisation co-ordinator or consultant in communicable disease control, rather than withhold immunisation.

The vaccines should not be given to those who have had:

- a confirmed anaphylactic reaction to a previous dose of the vaccine
- a confirmed anaphylactic reaction to any constituent of the vaccine, including meningococcal polysaccharide, diphtheria toxoid or the CRM_{197} carrier protein, or tetanus toxoid.

Confirmed anaphylaxis after immunisation is extremely rare, with anaphylaxis reactions reported in approximately one in every 500,000 doses (www.mhra.gov.uk/home/groups/pl-p/documents/websiteresources/con2022528.pdf). Other allergic conditions, may occur more commonly and are not contraindications to further immunisation. A careful history of the event will often distinguish between anaphylaxis and other events that are either not due to the vaccine or not life threatening. In the latter circumstance, it may be possible to continue the immunisation course. Specialist advice must be sought on the vaccines and circumstances in which they could be given. The risk to the individual of not being immunised must be taken into account.

Precautions

Minor illnesses without fever or systemic upset are not valid reasons to postpone immunisation. If an individual is acutely unwell, immunisation may be postponed until they have recovered fully. This is to avoid confusing the differential diagnosis of any acute illness by wrongly attributing any signs or symptoms to the adverse effects of the vaccine.

Pregnancy and breast-feeding

Meningococcal vaccines may be given to pregnant women when clinically indicated. There is no evidence of risk from vaccinating pregnant women or those who are breast-feeding with inactivated virus or bacterial vaccines or toxoids (Granoff *et al.*, 2004). In cases where meningococcal immunisation has been inadvertently given in pregnancy, there has been no evidence of fetal problems.

Premature infants

It is important that premature infants have their immunisations at the appropriate chronological age, according to the schedule. There is no evidence that premature babies are at increased risk of adverse reactions from vaccines (Slack *et al.,* 2001).

Immunosuppression and HIV infection

Individuals with immunosuppression and human immunodeficiency virus (HIV) infection (regardless of CD4 count) should be given meningococcal vaccines in accordance with the routine schedule. These individuals may not make a full antibody response. Re-immunisation should be considered after treatment is finished and recovery has occurred. Specialist advice may be required.

Further guidance is provided by the Royal College of Paediatrics and Child Health (www.rcpch.ac.uk), the British HIV Association (BHIVA) *Immunisation guidelines for HIV-infected adults* (BHIVA, 2006) and the Children's HIV Association of UK and Ireland (CHIVA) immunisation guidelines (www.bhiva.org/chiva).

Adverse reactions

MenC conjugate vaccine

Pain, tenderness, swelling or redness at the injection site, and mild fevers are common in all age groups. In infants and toddlers, crying, irritability, drowsiness, impaired sleep, reduced eating, diarrhoea and vomiting are commonly seen. In older children and adults, headaches, myalgia and drowsiness may be seen.

Confirmed anaphylaxis after immunisation is extremely rare, with anaphylaxis reactions reported approximately one in every 500,000 doses (www.mhra.gov.uk/home/groups/pl-p/documents/websiteresources/con 2022528.pdf). Other allergic conditions may occur more commonly and are not contraindications to further immunisation.

Neurological reactions such as dizziness, febrile/afebrile seizures, faints, numbness and hypotonia following MenC are very rare.

Hib/MenC conjugate

Mild side effects such as irritability, loss of appetite, pain, swelling or redness at the site of the injection, and slightly raised temperature commonly occur. Less commonly crying, diarrhoea, vomiting, atopic dermatitis, malaise and fever over 39.5°C have been reported.

Quadrivalent (ACW135Y) polysaccharide vaccine

Generalised reactions are rare although pyrexia occurs more frequently in young children than in adults.

Injection site reactions occur in approximately 10% of recipients and last for approximately 24 to 48 hours.

Confirmed anaphylaxis after immunisation is extremely rare, with anaphylactoid reactions reported approximately one in every 500,000 doses (www.mhra.gov.uk/home/groups/pl-p/documents/websiteresources/con2022528.pdf). All suspected adverse reactions to vaccines occurring in children after the administration of the MenC conjugate vaccine should be reported to the Commission on Human Medicines using the Yellow Card scheme (see Chapter 9 for more information). Serious suspected adverse reactions to vaccines in adults should be reported through the Yellow Card scheme.

All suspected adverse reactions to vaccines occurring in children, or in individuals of any age after vaccination with vaccines labelled with a black triangle (▼), should be reported to the Commission on Human Medicines using the Yellow Card scheme. Serious suspected adverse reactions to vaccines in adults should be reported through the Yellow Card scheme.

Management of suspected cases, contacts, carriers and outbreaks

Management of cases

Current expert advice endorses the importance of early recognition, prompt antibiotic treatment and speedy referral to hospital for all suspected cases. Benzylpenicillin is the antibiotic of choice and should be administered by the general practitioner before transfer to hospital, unless there is a history of immediate allergic reactions after previous penicillin administration. The recommended dose is 1200mg for adults and children aged 10 years or over, 600mg for children aged one to nine years, and 300mg for those aged under one year. Although benzylpenicillin may reduce the chance of isolating the causative organism, this is outweighed by the benefit to the patient, and new techniques are available that facilitate the diagnosis of meningococcal disease even after antibiotics have been given.

Guidelines for the management of meningococcal disease are available at www.hpa.org.uk/cdph/issues/CDPHVol5/no3/Meningococcal_Guidelines.pdf

Management of contacts

For public health management of contacts of cases and outbreaks, advice must be sought from your local health protection unit.

Household contacts of cases of meningococcal infection are at increased risk of developing the disease. This risk is highest in the first seven days following onset in the index case but persists for at least four weeks. Immediate risk can be reduced by the administration of antibiotic prophylaxis to the whole contact group.

The recommended schedule for prophylaxis is:

Rifampicin 600mg every 12 hours for two days in adults, 10mg/kg dose for children over one year of age, and 5mg/kg for children less than one year.

Ciprofloxacin as a single dose of 500mg is an alternative for adults (250mg for children aged five to 12 years) but is not yet licensed in the UK for this purpose.

Rifampicin 600mg twice daily for two days or intramuscular ceftriaxone 250mg should be given to pregnant contacts.

Unless the index case received ceftriaxone treatment in hospital, chemoprophylaxis should also be given to the patient before discharge.

For confirmed serogroup C infection, MenC vaccination should be offered to all close contacts (of all ages) previously unimmunised with MenC vaccine. Close contacts who are not, or are only partially, immunised should complete a course of MenC vaccination. Those who completed a course more than one year before should be offered a booster.

If the index case has been previously vaccinated, a booster dose of MenC vaccine is recommended.

For confirmed serogroup A infection, vaccination with quadrivalent (ACW135Y) polysaccharide vaccine should be offered to all close contacts over two months of age.

For confirmed serogroup W135 or Y infections, vaccination with quadrivalent (ACW135Y) polysaccharide vaccine should be offered to all close contacts over two years of age.

For probable cases with serogroup A, C, W135 or Y isolated from nasopharyngeal swab, quadrivalent vaccine should be offered to close contacts. Individuals should be immunised with either the quadrivalent vaccine (group A, W135 and Y infection) or MenC vaccine (group C infection) as appropriate.

Chemoprophylaxis should be given first, and the decision to offer vaccine should be made when the results of serogrouping are available. **Vaccine does not protect against serogroup B meningococcal infection, but any case provides an opportunity to check the MenC vaccine status of the index case and contacts, and to ensure that individuals under the age of 25 years have been fully immunised according to the UK schedule.**

Management of local outbreaks

In addition to sporadic cases, outbreaks of meningococcal infections can occur particularly in closed or semi-closed communities such as schools, military establishments and universities. Advice on the management of such outbreaks should be obtained from the local health protection unit.

Advice on the use of meningococcal vaccines in outbreaks is available from:

Health Protection Agency
(Tel: 020 8200 6868)
or HPA regional units
Health Protection Agency,
Meningococcal Reference Unit
(Tel: 0161 276 5698)
Health Protection Scotland
(Tel: 0141 300 1100)
Scottish Meningococcal and Pneumococcal Reference Laboratory
(Tel: 0141 201 3836).

Meningococcal vaccine has no part to play in the management of outbreaks of group B meningococcal meningitis.

Supplies

Meningitis C conjugate:

- Meningitec – manufactured by Wyeth Pharmaceuticals
- Menjugate – manufactured by Novartis Vaccines
- NeisVac-C – manufactured by Baxter Healthcare
- Menitorix (Hib/MenC) – manufactured by GlaxoSmithKline.

These vaccines are supplied by Healthcare Logistics (Tel: 0870 871 1890) as part of the national childhood immunisation programme.

In Scotland, supplies should be obtained from the local childhood vaccine holding centres. Details of these are available from Scottish Healthcare Supplies (Tel: 0141 282 2240).

Quadrivalent A,C,W,Y polysaccharide vaccine – manufactured by GlaxoSmithKline (Tel: 0808 100 9997).

References

Al-Mazrou Y, Khalil M, Borrow R *et al.* (2005) Serologic responses to ACYW135 polysaccharide meningococcal vaccine in Saudi children under 5 years of age. *Infect Immun* **73**(5). 2932–9.

American Academy of Pediatrics (2003) Active immunization. In: Pickering LK (ed.) *Red Book: 2003 Report of the Committee on Infectious Diseases,* 26th edition. Elk Grove Village, IL: American Academy of Pediatrics, p 33.

Balmer P, Falconer M, McDonald P *et al.* (2004) Immune response to meningococcal serogroup C conjugate vaccine in asplenic individuals. *Infect Immun* **72**(1): 332–7.

Bohlke K, Davis RL, Marcy SH *et al.* (2003) Risk of anaphylaxis after vaccination of children and adolescents. *Pediatrics* **112**: 815–20.

Booy R, Habibi P, Nadel S *et al.* (2001) Reduction in case fatality rates from meningococcal disease associated with improved healthcare delivery. *Arch Dis Child* **85**: 386–90.

British HIV Association (2006) *Immunisation guidelines for HIV-infected adults:* www.bhiva.org/pdf/2006/Immunisation506.pdf.

Cadoz M, Armand J, Arminjon F *et al.* (1985) Tetravalent (ACYW135) meningococcal vaccine in children: immunogenicity and safety. *Vaccine* **3**(3): 340–2.

Canadian Medical Association (1998) Pertussis vaccine. In: *Canadian Immunisation Guide,* 5th edition. Canadian Medical Association.

Cartwright K (1995) Meningococcal carriage and disease. In: Cartwright K (ed.) *Meningococcal disease.* Chichester, UK: John Wiley & Sons, pp 115–46.

Davison KL, Ramsay ME, Crowcroft NS *et al.* (2002) Estimating the burden of serogroup C meningococcal disease in England and Wales. *Commun Dis Public Health* **3**: 213–19.

Committee on Safety of Medicines (2002) Report of the Committee on Safety of Medicines Expert Working Group on Meningococcal Group C Conjugate Vaccines. www.mhra.gov.uk/home/groups/pl-p/documents/websiteresources/con2022528.pdf

Diggle L and Deeks J (2000) Effect of needle length on incidence of local reactions to routine immunisation in infants aged 4 months: randomised controlled trial. *BMJ* **321**(7266): 931–3.

Department of Health (2001) *Health information for overseas travel,* 2nd edition. London: TSO.

Erickson L and De Wals P (1998) Complications and sequelae of meningococcal disease in Quebec, Canada, 1990–1994. *Clin Infect Dis* **26**(5): 1159–64.

Frasch CE (1995) Meningococcal vaccines: past, present and future. In: Cartwright K (ed.) *Meningococcal disease.* Chichester, UK: John Wiley & Sons pp 245–83.

Goldacre MJ, Roberts SE and Yeates D (2003) Case fatality rates for meningococcal disease in an English population, 1963–98: database study. *BMJ* **327**: 596–7.

Granoff DM, Feavers IM and Borrow R (2004) Meningococcal vaccines. In: Plotkin SA and Orenstein WA (eds) *Vaccines.* 4th edition. Philadelphia: WB Saunders Company, pp 959–88.

Jones D (1995) Epidemiology of meningococcal disease in Europe and the USA. In: Cartwright K (ed.) *Meningococcal disease*. Chichester, UK: John Wiley & Sons, pp 147–58.

Lepow ML, Perkins BA, Hughes PA and Poolman JT (1999) Meningococcal vaccines. In: Plotkin SA and Orenstein WA (eds) *Vaccines,* 3rd edition. Philadelphia: WB Saunders Company, pp 711–27.

Mark A, Carlsson RM and Granstrom M (1999) Subcutaneous versus intramuscular injection for booster DT vaccination of adolescents. *Vaccine* **17**(15–16): 2067–72.

Peltola H, Safary A, Kayhty H *et al.* (1985) Evaluation of two tetravalent (ACYW135) meningococcal vaccines in infants and small children: a clinical study comparing immunogenicity of O-acetyl-negative and O-acetyl-positive group C polysaccharides. *Pediatrics* **76**(1): 91–6.

Plotkin SA and Orenstein WA (eds) (2004) *Vaccines,* 4th edition. Philadelphia: WB Saunders Company, pp 959–88.

Ramsay M, Kaczmarski E, Rush M *et al.* (1997) Changing patterns of case ascertainment and trends in meningococcal disease in England and Wales. *Commun Dis Rep CDR Rev* **7**(4): R49–54.

Ramsay ME, Andrews NJ, Trotter CL *et al.* (2003) Herd immunity from meningococcal serogroup C conjugate vaccination in England: database analysis. *BMJ* **326**(7385): 365–6.

Rosenstein NE, Perkins BA, Stephens DS *et al.* (2001) Meningococcal disease. *NEJM* **344**: 1378–88.

Salisbury D, Miller E and Ramsay M (2001) Planning, registration, and implementation of an immunisation campaign against meningococcal serogroup C disease in the UK: a success story. *Vaccine* **20** (Suppl 1): S58–67.

Slack MH, Schapira D, Thwaites RJ *et al.* (2001) Immune response of premature infants to meningococcal serogroup C and combined diphtheria-tetanus toxoids-acellular pertussis-*Haemophilus influenzae* type b conjugate vaccines. *J Infect Dis* **184**(12):1617–20.

Southern J, Crowley-Luke A, Barrow R *et al.* (2006) Immunogenicity of one, two and three doses of a meningococcal C conjugate to tetanus toxoid, given as a three-dose primary vaccination course in UK infants at 2, 3 and 4 months of age with acellular pertussis-containing DTP/Hib vaccine. *Vaccine* **24**: 215–19.

Steven N and Wood M (1995) The clinical spectrum of meningococcal disease. In: Cartwright K (ed.) *Meningococcal disease*. Chichester, UK: John Wiley & Sons, pp 177–206.

Thornburn K, Baines P, Thomson A and Hart CA (2001) Mortality in severe meningococcal disease. *Arch Dis Child* **85**: 382–5.

Trotter CL, Fox AJ, Ramsay ME, et al. (2002) Fatal outcome from meningococcal disease – an association with meningococcal phenotype but not with reduced susceptibility to bentylpenicillin. *J Med Microbiol* **51**(10): 855–60.

Trotter CL and Gay NJ (2003) Analysis of longitudinal carriage studies accounting for sensitivity of swabbing: an application to *Neisseria meningitidis*. *Epidemiol Infect* **130**(2): 201-5.

Trotter CL, Andrews NJ, Kaczmarski EB *et al.* (2004) Effectiveness of meningococcal serogroup C conjugate vaccine 4 years after introduction. *Lancet* **364**(9431): 365–7.

Zuckerman JN (2000) The importance of injecting vaccines into muscle. Different patients need different needle sizes. *BMJ* **321**(7271): 1237–8.

23

Mumps

NOTIFIABLE

The disease

Mumps is an acute viral illness caused by a paramyxovirus. It is usually characterised by bilateral parotid swelling, although it may present with unilateral swelling. Parotitis may be preceded by several days of non-specific symptoms such as fever, headache, malaise, myalgias and anorexia. Asymptomatic mumps infection is common, particularly in children (Plotkin and Orenstein, 2004).

Mumps is spread by airborne or droplet transmission. The incubation period is around 17 days, with a range of 14 to 25 days. Individuals with mumps are infectious from several days before the parotid swelling to several days after it appears.

Mumps virus frequently affects the nervous system and may be symptomatic or asymptomatic. Meningism (headache, photophobia, neck stiffness) occurs in up to 15% of cases and mumps viruses are often identified in the cerebrospinal fluid. Neurological complications, including meningitis and encephalitis, may precede or follow parotitis and can also occur in its absence.

Other common complications include pancreatitis (4%), oophoritis (5% of post-pubertal women) and orchitis (around 25% of post-pubertal men) (Falk *et al.*, 1989; Plotkin and Orenstein, 2004; Philip *et al.*, 1959). Sub-fertility following bilateral orchitis has rarely been reported (Bjorvatn *et al.*, 1973; Dejucq and Jegou, 2001). Sensorineural deafness (bilateral or unilateral) is a well-recognised complication of mumps, with estimates of its frequency varying from one in 3400 cases to one in 20,000 (Garty *et al.*, 1988). Nephritis, arthropathy, cardiac abnormalities and, rarely, death have been reported.

History and epidemiology of the disease

Before the introduction of the measles, mumps and rubella (MMR) vaccine in 1988, mumps occurred commonly in school-age children, and more than 85% of adults had evidence of previous mumps infection (Morgan Capner *et al.*, 1988). Mumps was the cause of about 1200 hospital admissions each year in

England and Wales and was the commonest cause of viral meningitis in children (Galbraith *et al.*, 1984; Communicable Disease Surveillance Centre, 1985).

Mumps was made a notifiable disease in the UK in October 1988 at the time of the introduction of the MMR vaccine. High coverage of MMR vaccine resulted in a substantial reduction in mumps transmission in the UK and the incidence declined in all age groups, including those too old to have been immunised. From 1989, reports of both clinically diagnosed and laboratory-confirmed mumps cases fell dramatically. In November 1994, to prevent a predicted epidemic of measles, children aged between five and 16 years were immunised with measles-rubella (MR) vaccine. At that time, insufficient stocks of MMR were available to vaccinate all of these children against mumps. Younger members of this age group, however, were unlikely to have been exposed to mumps infection and many remained susceptible into early adulthood.

In October 1996, a two-dose MMR schedule was introduced. A single dose of a mumps-containing vaccine used in the UK confers between 61% and 91% protection against mumps (Plotkin and Orenstein, 2004). Two doses are therefore needed for both individual and population protection.

In Finland, a two-dose MMR schedule was introduced in 1982; high coverage of each dose has been achieved consistently. Indigenous measles, mumps and rubella have been eliminated since 1994 (Peltola *et al.*, 1994). The United States introduced its two-dose schedule in 1989 and, in 2000, announced that it had interrupted endemic transmission (Plotkin and Orenstein, 2004). MMR is now routinely given in over 100 countries, including those in the European Union, North America and Australasia.

Since 1999, there has been a considerable increase in confirmed mumps cases. Most of these cases have occurred in adolescents or young adults who were too old to have been offered MMR when it was introduced in 1988 or to have had a second dose when this was introduced in 1996. They had not previously been exposed to natural mumps infection as children and so remained susceptible. In late 2004, a further increase in clinically diagnosed and confirmed mumps infections was observed. The vast majority of confirmed cases were in those born between 1980 and 1987 and outbreaks occurred mainly in higher education institutions.

Many of the individuals in the cohorts recently affected by mumps believe that they had been immunised with mumps-containing vaccine in the past.

However, before 1988, there was no routine immunisation against mumps in the UK, and the campaign in 1994 used MR vaccine because sufficient quantities of MMR vaccine were not available. Young people may therefore have had two doses of measles-containing vaccine and one of rubella, but no mumps vaccine. Others have had only one dose of mumps vaccine in MMR (see Figure 23.1).

The MMR vaccination

MMR vaccines are freeze-dried preparations containing live, attenuated strains of measles, mumps and rubella viruses. The three attenuated virus strains are cultured separately in appropriate media and mixed before being lyophilised. These vaccines contain the following:

Priorix®

Each 0.5ml dose of reconstituted vaccine contains:

not less than $10^{3.0}$ cell culture infective $dose_{50}$ ($CCID_{50}$) of the Schwarz measles virus
not less than $10^{3.7}$ $CCID_{50}$ of the RIT 4385 mumps virus
not less than $10^{3.0}$ $CCID_{50}$ of the Wistar RA 27/3 rubella virus strains.

M-M-R™II

Each 0.5ml dose when reconstituted contains not less than the equivalent of:

1000 tissue culture infective $dose_{50}$ ($TCID_{50}$) of the more attenuated Enders line of the Edmonston strain of measles virus
20,000 $TCID_{50}$ of mumps virus (Jeryl Lynn® Level B strain)
1000 $TCID_{50}$ of rubella virus (Wistar RA 27/3 strain).

MMR vaccine does not contain thiomersal or any other preservatives. The vaccine contains live organisms that have been attenuated (modified). MMR is recommended when protection against measles, mumps and/or rubella is required.

Storage

The unreconstituted vaccine and its diluent should be stored in the original packaging at +2˚C to +8˚C and protected from light. All vaccines are sensitive to some extent to heat and cold. Heat speeds up the decline in potency of most vaccines, thus reducing their shelf life. Effectiveness cannot be guaranteed for vaccines unless they have been stored at the correct temperature. Freezing may cause increased reactogenicity and loss of potency for some vaccines. It can also cause hairline cracks in the container, leading to contamination of the contents.

Measles vaccine																										
*MR (%)																					92					
*Second dose catch up MMR (%)															60											
First dose catch up MMR																					Not known					
†Routine second dose MMR (%)							73	75	75	74	75	76														
†Routine first dose MMR (%)				81	80	82	84	87	88	88	91	92	92	91	91	92	90	86	68	7						
Age in 2006	1	2	3	4	5	6	7	8	9	10	11	12	13	14	15	16	17	18	19	20	21	22	23	24	25	26
Year of birth	2005	2004	2003	2002	2001	2000	1999	1998	1997	1996	1995	1994	1993	1992	1991	1990	1989	1988	1987	1986	1985	1984	1983	1982	1981	1980

* The percentages shown for the second dose catchup MMR and MR relate to the coverage for the whole campaign cohort
† The percentages shown for the routine first and second dose of MMR are coverage data for England only and are based on levels recorded when the birth cohort was aged between two and five years respectively

Figure 23.1 Opportunity for protection from mumps by vaccination in the UK immunsation programme

The vaccines should be reconstituted with the diluent supplied by the manufacturer and either used within one hour or discarded.

Presentation

Mumps vaccine is only available as part of a combined product (MMR).

Priorix is supplied as a whitish to slightly pink pellet of lyophilised vaccine for reconstitution with the diluent supplied. The reconstituted vaccine must be shaken well until the pellet is completely dissolved in the diluent.

M-M-R II is supplied as a lyophilised powder for reconstitution with the diluent supplied. The reconstituted vaccine must be shaken gently to ensure thorough mixing. The reconstituted vaccine is yellow in colour and should only be used if clear and free from particulate matter.

Dosage and schedule

Two doses of 0.5ml at the recommended interval (see below).

Administration

Vaccines are routinely given intramuscularly into the upper arm or anterolateral thigh. However, for individuals with a bleeding disorder, vaccines should be given by deep subcutaneous injection to reduce the risk of bleeding.

MMR vaccine can be given at the same time as other vaccines such as DTaP/IPV, MenC, PCV and hepatitis B. The vaccine should be given at a separate site, preferably in a different limb. If given in the same limb, they should be given at least 2.5cm apart (American Academy of Pediatrics, 2003). If MMR cannot be given at the same time as an inactivated vaccine, it can be given at any interval before or after.

MMR should ideally be given at the same time as other live vaccines, such as BCG. If live vaccines are given simultaneously, then each vaccine virus will begin to replicate and an appropriate immune response is made to each vaccine. After a live vaccine is given, natural interferon is produced in response to that vaccine. If a second live vaccine is given during this response, the interferon may prevent replication of the second vaccine virus. This may attenuate the response to the second vaccine. Based on evidence that MMR vaccine can lead to an attenuation of the varicella vaccine response (Mullooly and Black, 2001), the recommended interval between live vaccines is currently four weeks. For this reason, if live vaccines cannot be administered simultaneously, a four-week interval is recommended.

Four weeks should be left between giving MMR vaccine and carrying out tuberculin testing. The measles vaccine component of MMR can reduce the delayed-type hypersensitivity response. As this is the basis of a positive tuberculin test, this could give a false negative response.

When MMR is given within three months of receiving blood products, such as immunoglobulin, the response to the measles component may be reduced. This is because such blood products may contain significant levels of measles-specific antibody, which could then prevent vaccine virus replication. Where possible, MMR should be deferred until three months after receipt of such products. If immediate measles protection is required in someone who has recently received a blood product, MMR vaccine should still be given. To confer longer-term protection, MMR should be repeated after three months.

Disposal

Equipment used for vaccination, including used vials or ampoules, should be disposed of at the end of a session by sealing in a proper, puncture-resistant 'sharps' box (UN-approved, BS 7320).

Recommendations for the use of the vaccine

The objective of the immunisation programme is to provide two doses of MMR vaccine at appropriate intervals for all eligible individuals.

Over 90% of individuals will seroconvert to measles, mumps and rubella antibodies after the first dose of the MMR vaccines currently used in the UK (Tischer and Gerike, 2000). Antibody responses from pre-licence studies may be higher, however, than clinical protection under routine use. Evidence shows that a single dose of measles-containing vaccine confers protection in around 90% of individuals for measles (Morse *et al.*, 1994; Medical Research Council, 1977). A single dose of a rubella-containing vaccine confers around 95 to 100% protection (Plotkin and Orenstein, 2004). A single dose of a mumps-containing vaccine used in the UK confers between 61% and 91% protection against mumps (Plotkin and Orenstein, 2004). A more recent study in the UK suggested that a single dose of MMR is around 64% effective against mumps (Harling *et al.*, 2005). Therefore, two doses of MMR are required to produce satisfactory protection against measles, mumps and rubella.

MMR is recommended when protection against measles, mumps and/or rubella is required. MMR vaccine can be given irrespective of a history of measles, mumps or rubella infection. There are no ill effects from immunising such individuals because they have pre-existing immunity that inhibits replication of the vaccine viruses.

Children under ten years of age

The first dose of MMR should be given at any time after the first birthday, ideally at 13 months of age. Immunisation before 13 months of age provides earlier protection in localities where the risk of measles is higher, but residual maternal antibodies may reduce the response rate to the vaccine. The optimal age chosen for scheduling children is therefore a compromise between risk of disease and level of protection.

If a dose of MMR is given before the first birthday, either because of travel to an endemic country, or because of a local outbreak, then this dose should be ignored, and two further doses given at the recommended times after the first birthday and pre-school.

A second dose is normally given before school entry but can be given routinely at any time from three months after the first dose. Allowing three months between doses is likely to maximise the response rate, particularly in young children under the age of 18 months where maternal antibodies may reduce the response to vaccination (Orenstein *et al.*, 1986; Redd *et al.*, 2004; de Serres *et al.*, 1995). Where protection against measles is urgently required, the second dose can be given one month after the first (ACIP, 1998). If the child is given the second dose less than three months after the first dose and at less than 18 months of age, then the routine pre-school dose (a third dose) should be given in order to ensure full protection.

Children aged ten years or over and adults

All children should have received two doses of MMR vaccine before they leave school. The teenage (school-leaving) booster session or appointment is an opportunity to ensure that unimmunised or partially immunised children are given MMR. If two doses of MMR are required, then the second dose should be given one month after the first.

MMR vaccine can be given to individuals of any age. Entry into college, university or other higher education institutions, prison or military service provides an opportunity to check an individual's immunisation history. Those who have not received MMR should be offered appropriate MMR immunisation.

The decision on when to vaccinate adults needs to take into consideration the past vaccination history, the likelihood of an individual remaining susceptible and the future risk of exposure and disease:

- individuals who were born between 1980 and 1990 may not be protected against mumps but are likely to be vaccinated against measles and rubella. They may never have received a mumps-containing vaccine or had only one dose of MMR, and had limited opportunity for exposure to natural mumps. They should be recalled and given MMR vaccine. If this is their first dose, a further dose of MMR should be given from one month later
- individuals born between 1970 and 1979 may have been vaccinated against measles and many will have been exposed to mumps and rubella during childhood. However, this age group should be offered MMR wherever feasible, particularly if they are considered to be at high risk of exposure. Where such adults are being vaccinated because they have been demonstrated to be susceptible to at least one of the vaccine components, then either two doses should be given, or there should be evidence of seroconversion to the relevant antigen
- individuals born before 1970 are likely to have had all three natural infections and are less likely to be susceptible. MMR vaccine should be offered to such individuals on request or if they are considered to be at high risk of exposure. Where such adults are being vaccinated because they have been demonstrated to be susceptible to at least one of the vaccine components, then either two doses should be given or there should be evidence of seroconversion to the relevant antigen.

Individuals with unknown or incomplete vaccination histories

Children coming from developing countries will probably have received a measles-containing vaccine in their country of origin but may not have received mumps or rubella vaccines (www-nt.who.int/immunization_monitoring/en/globalsummary/countryprofileselect.cfm). Unless there is a reliable history of appropriate immunisation, individuals should be assumed to be unimmunised and the recommendations above should be followed. Individuals aged 18 months and over who have not received MMR should receive two doses at least one month apart. An individual who has already received one dose of MMR should receive a second dose to ensure that they are protected.

Healthcare workers

Protection of healthcare workers is especially important in the context of their ability to transmit measles, mumps or rubella infections to vulnerable groups. While they may need MMR vaccination for their own benefit, on the grounds outlined above, they also should be immune to measles, mumps and rubella for the protection of their patients.

Satisfactory evidence of protection would include documentation of:

- having received two doses of MMR, or
- positive antibody tests for measles and rubella.

Individuals who are travelling or going to reside abroad

All travellers to epidemic or endemic areas should ensure that they are fully immunised according to the UK schedule (see above). Infants from six months of age travelling to mumps endemic areas or to an area where there is a current outbreak should receive MMR. As the response to MMR in infants is sub-optimal where the vaccine has been given before one year of age, immunisation with two further doses of MMR should be given at the recommended ages. Children who are travelling who have received one dose of MMR at the routine age should have the second dose brought forward to at least one month after the first. If the child is under 18 months of age when the second dose is given, then the routine pre-school dose (a third dose) should be given in order to ensure full protection.

Contraindications

There are very few individuals who cannot receive MMR vaccine. When there is doubt, appropriate advice should be sought from a consultant paediatrician, immunisation co-ordinator or consultant in communicable disease control rather than withholding the vaccine.

The vaccine should not be given to:

- those who are immunosuppressed (see Chapter 6 for more detail)
- those who have had a confirmed anaphylactic reaction to a previous dose of a measles-, mumps- or rubella-containing vaccine
- those who have had a confirmed anaphylactic reaction to neomycin or gelatin
- pregnant women.

Anaphylaxis after MMR is extremely rare (3.5 to 14.4 per million doses) (Bohlke *et al*., 2003; Patja *et al*., 2000; Pool *et al*., 2002; D'Souza *et al*., 2000). Minor allergic conditions may occur and are not contraindications to further immunisation with MMR or other vaccines. A careful history of that event will often distinguish between anaphylaxis and other events that are either not due to the vaccine or are not life-threatening. In the latter circumstances, it may be possible to continue the immunisation course. Specialist advice must be sought on the vaccines and circumstances in which they could be given. The lifelong risk to the individual of not being immunised must be taken into account.

Precautions

Minor illnesses without fever or systemic upset are not valid reasons to postpone immunisation. If an individual is acutely unwell, immunisation should be postponed until they have fully recovered. This is to avoid confusing the differential diagnosis of any acute illness by wrongly attributing any signs or symptoms to the adverse effects of the vaccine.

Idiopathic thrombocytopaenic purpura

Idiopathic thrombocytopaenic purpura (ITP) has occurred rarely following MMR vaccination, usually within six weeks of the first dose. The risk of developing ITP after MMR vaccine is much less than the risk of developing it after infection with wild measles or rubella virus.

If ITP has occurred within six weeks of the first dose of MMR, then blood should be taken and tested for measles, mumps and rubella antibodies before a second dose is given. Serum should be sent to the Health Protection Agency (HPA) Virus Reference Laboratory (Colindale), which offers free, specialised serological testing for such children. If the results suggest incomplete immunity against measles, mumps or rubella, then a second dose of MMR is recommended.

Allergy to egg

Children with egg allergy should have MMR vaccine. Recent data suggest that anaphylactic reactions to MMR vaccine are not associated with hypersensitivity to egg antigens but to other components of the vaccine (such as gelatin) (Fox and Lack, 2003). In three large studies with a combined total of over 1000 patients with egg allergy, no severe cardiorespiratory reactions were reported after MMR vaccination (Fasano *et al*., 1992; Freigang *et al*., 1994; Aickin *et al*., 1994; Khakoo and Lack, 2000).

If there is a history of confirmed anaphylactic reaction to egg-containing food, paediatric advice should be sought with a view to immunisation under controlled conditions such as admission to hospital as a day case.

Pregnancy and breast-feeding

There is no evidence that rubella-containing vaccines are teratogenic. In the USA, UK and Germany, 661 women were followed through active surveillance, including 293 who were vaccinated (mainly with single rubella vaccine) in the high-risk period (i.e. the six weeks after the last menstrual period). Only 16 infants had evidence of infection and none had permanent abnormalities compatible with congenital rubella syndrome (Best *et al.*, 2004). However, as a precaution, MMR vaccine should not be given to women known to be pregnant. If MMR vaccine is given to adult women, they should be advised to guard against pregnancy for one month.

Termination of pregnancy following inadvertent immunisation should not be recommended (Tookey *et al.*, 1991). The potential parents should be given information on the evidence of lack of risk from vaccination in pregnancy. Surveillance of inadvertent MMR administration in pregnancy is being conducted by the HPA Immunisation Department, to whom such cases should be reported (Tel: 020 8200 4400).

Breast-feeding is not a contraindication to MMR immunisation, and MMR vaccine can be given to breast-feeding mothers without any risk to their baby. Very occasionally, rubella vaccine virus has been found in breast milk, but this has not caused any symptoms in the baby (Buimovici-Klein *et al.*, 1997; Landes *et al.*, 1980; Losonsky *et al.*, 1982). The vaccine does not work when taken orally. There is no evidence of mumps and measles vaccine viruses being found in breast milk.

Premature infants

It is important that premature infants have their immunisations at the appropriate chronological age, according to the schedule (see Chapter 11).

Immunosuppression and HIV

MMR vaccine is not recommended for patients with severe immunosuppression (see Chapter 6) (Angel *et al.*, 1996). MMR vaccine can be given to HIV-positive patients without or with moderate immunosuppression (as defined in Table 23.1).

Table 23.1 CD4 count/μl (% of total lymphocytes)

Age	<12 months	1–5 years	6–12 years	>12 years
No suppression	⩾1500 (⩾25%)	⩾1000 (15–24%)	⩾500 (⩾25%)	⩾500 (⩾25%)
Moderate suppression	750–1499 (15–24%)	500–999 (15–24%)	200–499 (15–24%)	200–499 (15–24%)
Severe suppression	<750 (<15%)	<500 (<15%)	<200 (<15%)	<200 (<15%)

Further guidance is provided by the Royal College of Paediatrics and Child Health (www.rcpch.ac.uk), the British HIV Association (BHIVA) *Immunisation guidelines for HIV-infected adults* (BHIVA, 2006) and the Children's HIV Association of UK and Ireland (CHIVA) immunisation guidelines (www.bhiva.org/chiva).

Neurological conditions

The presence of a neurological condition is not a contraindication to immunisation. If there is evidence of current neurological deterioration, including poorly controlled epilepsy, immunisation should be deferred until the condition has stabilised. Children with a personal or close family history of seizures should be given MMR vaccine. Advice about likely timing of any fever and management of a fever should be given. Doctors and nurses should seek specialist paediatric advice rather than refuse immunisation.

Adverse reactions

Adverse reactions following the MMR vaccine (except allergic reactions) are due to effective replication of the vaccine viruses with subsequent mild illness. Such events are to be expected in some individuals. Events due to the measles component occur six to 11 days after vaccination. Events due to the mumps and rubella components usually occur two to three weeks after vaccination but may occur up to six weeks after vaccination. These events only occur in individuals who are susceptible to that component, and are therefore less common after second and subsequent doses. Individuals with vaccine-associated symptoms are not infectious to others.

Common events

Following the first dose of MMR vaccine, malaise, fever and/or a rash may occur, most commonly about a week after immunisation, and last about two to three days. In a study of over 6000 children aged one to two years, the symptoms reported were similar in nature, frequency, time of onset and duration to those commonly reported after measles vaccine alone (Miller *et al.*, 1989). Parotid swelling occurred in about 1% of children of all ages up to four years, usually in the third week.

Adverse reactions are considerably less common after a second dose of MMR vaccine than after the first dose. One study showed no increase in fever or rash after re-immunisation of college students compared with unimmunised controls (Chen *et al.*, 1991). An analysis of allergic reactions reported through the US Vaccine Adverse Events Reporting System in 1991–93 showed fewer reactions among children aged six to 19 years, considered to be second-dose recipients, than among those aged one to four years, considered to be first-dose recipients (Chen *et al.*, 1991). In a study of over 8000 children, there was no increased risk of convulsions, rash or joint pain in the months after the second dose of the MMR vaccination given between four and six years of age (Davis *et al.*, 1997).

Rare and more serious events

Febrile seizures are the most commonly reported neurological event following measles immunisation. Seizures occur during the sixth to eleventh day in one in 1000 children vaccinated with MMR – a rate similar to that reported in the same period after measles vaccine. The rate of febrile seizures following MMR is lower than that following infection with measles disease (Plotkin and Orenstein, 2004). There is good evidence that febrile seizures following MMR immunisation do not increase the risk of subsequent epilepsy compared with febrile seizures due to other causes (Vestergaard *et al.*, 2004).

One strain of mumps virus (Urabe) in an MMR vaccine previously used in the UK was associated with an increased risk of aseptic meningitis (Miller *et al.*, 1993). This vaccine was replaced in 1992 (Department of Health,1992) and is no longer licensed in the UK. A study in Finland using MMR containing a different mumps strain (Jeryl Lynn), similar to those strains used currently in MMR in the UK, did not identify any association between MMR and aseptic meningitis (Makela *et al.*, 2002).

Because MMR vaccine contains live, attenuated viruses, it is biologically plausible that it may cause encephalitis. A recent large record-linkage study in Finland looking at over half a million children aged between one and seven years did not identify any association between MMR and encephalitis (Makela *et al.*, 2002).

ITP is a condition that may occur following MMR and is most likely due to the rubella component. This usually occurs within six weeks and resolves spontaneously. ITP occurs in about one in 22,300 children who are given a first dose of MMR in the second year of life (Miller *et al.*, 2001). If ITP has occurred within six weeks of the first dose of MMR, then blood should be taken and tested for measles, mumps and rubella antibodies before a second dose is given (see above).

Arthropathy (arthralgia or arthritis) has also been reported to occur rarely after MMR immunisation, probably due to the rubella component. If it is caused by the vaccine, it should occur between 14 and 21 days after immunisation. Where it occurs at other times, it is highly unlikely to have been caused by vaccination. Several controlled epidemiological studies have shown no excess risk of chronic arthritis in women (Slater, 1997).

All suspected adverse reactions to vaccines occurring in children, or in individuals of any age after vaccines labelled with a black triangle (▼), should be reported to the Commission on Human Medicines using the Yellow Card scheme. Serious, suspected adverse reactions to vaccines in adults should be reported through the Yellow Card scheme.

Other conditions reported after vaccines containing measles, mumps and rubella

Following the November 1994 MR immunisation campaign, only three cases of Guillain-Barré syndrome (GBS) were reported. From the background rate, between one and eight cases would have been expected in this population over this period. Therefore, it is likely that these three cases were coincidental and not caused by the vaccine. Analysis of reporting rates of GBS from acute flaccid paralysis surveillance undertaken in the WHO Region of the Americas has shown no increase in rates of GBS following measles immunisation campaigns when 80 million children were immunised (da Silveira *et al.*, 1997). In a population that received 900,000 doses of MMR, there was no increased risk of GBS at any time after vaccinations (Patja *et al.*, 2001). This evidence refutes the suggestion that MMR causes GBS.

Although gait disturbance has been reported after MMR, a recent epidemiological study showed no evidence of a causal association between MMR and gait disturbance (Miller *et al.*, 2005).

In recent years, the postulated link between measles vaccine and bowel disease has been investigated. There was no increase in the incidence of inflammatory bowel disorders in those vaccinated with measles-containing vaccines when compared with controls (Gilat *et al.*, 1987; Feeney *et al.*, 1997). No increase in the incidence of inflammatory bowel disease has been observed since the introduction of MMR vaccination in Finland (Pebody *et al.*, 1998) or in the UK (Seagroatt, 2005).

There is overwhelming evidence that MMR does not cause autism (www.iom.edu/report.asp?id=20155). Over the past seven years, a large number of studies have been published looking at this issue. Such studies have shown:

- no increased risk of autism in children vaccinated with MMR compared with unvaccinated children (Farrington *et al.*, 2001; Madsen and Vestergaard, 2004)
- no clustering of the onset of symptoms of autism in the period following MMR vaccination (Taylor *et al.*, 1999; De Wilde *et al.*, 2001; Makela *et al.*, 2002)
- that the increase in the reported incidence of autism preceded the use of MMR in the UK (Taylor *et al.*, 1999)
- that the incidence of autism continued to rise after 1993, despite the withdrawal of MMR in Japan (Honda *et al.*, 2005)
- that there is no correlation between the rate of autism and MMR vaccine coverage in either the UK or the USA (Kaye *et al.*, 2001; Dales *et al.*, 2001)
- no difference between the proportion of children developing autism after MMR who have a regressive form compared with those who develop autism without vaccination (Fombonne, 2001; Taylor *et al.*, 2002; Gillberg and Heijbel, 1998)
- no difference between the proportion of children developing autism after MMR who have associated bowel symptoms compared with those who develop autism without vaccination (Fombonne, 1998; Fombonne, 2001; Taylor *et al.*, 2002)
- that no vaccine virus can be detected in children with autism using the most sensitive methods available (Afzal *et al.*, 2006).

For the latest evidence see the Department of Health's website www.mmrthe facts.nhs.uk.

It has been suggested that combined MMR vaccine could potentially overload the immune system. From the moment of birth, humans are exposed to countless numbers of foreign antigens and infectious agents in their everyday environment. Responding to the three viruses in MMR would use only a tiny proportion of the total capacity of an infant's immune system (Offit *et al.*,

2002). The three viruses in MMR replicate at different rates from each other and would be expected to reach high levels at different times.

A study examining the issue of immunological overload found a lower rate of admission for serious bacterial infection in the period shortly after MMR vaccination compared with other time periods. This suggests that MMR does not cause any general suppression of the immune system (Miller *et al.*, 2003).

Management of cases, contacts and outbreaks

Diagnosis

Prompt notification of measles, mumps and rubella to the local health protection unit (HPU) is required to ensure that public health action can be taken promptly. Notification should be based on clinical suspicion and should not await laboratory confirmation. Since 1994, few clinically diagnosed cases have been subsequently confirmed to be true measles, mumps or rubella. Confirmation rates do increase, however, during outbreaks and epidemics.

The diagnosis of measles, mumps and rubella can be confirmed through non-invasive means. Detection of specific IgM in oral fluid (saliva) samples, ideally between one and six weeks after the onset of rash or parotid swelling, has been shown to be highly sensitive and specific for confirmation of these infections (Brown *et al.*, 1994; Ramsay *et al.*, 1991; Ramsay *et al.*, 1998). It is recommended that oral fluid samples should be obtained from all notified cases, other than during a large epidemic. Advice on this procedure can be obtained from the local HPU.

Protection of contacts with MMR

Antibody response to the mumps component of MMR vaccine does not develop soon enough to provide effective prophylaxis after exposure to suspected mumps. Even where it is too late to provide effective post-exposure prophylaxis with MMR, the vaccine can provide protection against future exposure to all three infections. Therefore, contact with suspected measles, mumps or rubella provides a good opportunity to offer MMR vaccine to previously unvaccinated individuals. If the individual is already incubating measles, mumps or rubella, MMR vaccination will not exacerbate the symptoms. In these circumstances, individuals should be advised that a mumps-like illness occurring shortly after vaccination is likely to be due to natural infection. If there is doubt about an individual's vaccination status, MMR should still be given as there are no ill effects from vaccinating those who are already immune.

Protection of contacts with immunoglobulin

Human normal immunoglobulin is not routinely used for post-exposure protection from mumps since there is no evidence that it is effective.

Supplies

- M-M-R II – manufactured by Sanofi Pasteur MSD.
- Priorix – manufactured by GlaxoSmithKline.

These vaccines are supplied by Healthcare Logistics (Tel: 0870 871 1890) as part of the national childhood immunisation programme.

In Scotland, supplies should be obtained from local childhood vaccine holding centres. Details of these are available from Scottish Healthcare Supplies (Tel: 0131 275 6154).

In Northern Ireland, supplies should be obtained from local childhood vaccine holding centres. Details of these are available from the regional pharmaceutical procurement service
(Tel: 02890 552368).

References

ACIP (1998) Measles, mumps, and rubella – vaccine use and strategies for elimination of measles, rubella, and congenital rubella syndrome and control of mumps: recommendations of the Advisory Committee on Immunization Practices (ACIP). *MMWR* **47**(RR-8):1–57. www.cdc.gov/mmwr/preview/mmwrhtml/00053391.htm (22 May 1998).

Afzal MA, Ozoemena LC, O'Hare A *et al.* (2006) Absence of detectable measles virus genome sequence in blood of autistic children who have had their MMR vaccination during the routine childhood immunisation schedule of the UK. *J Med Virol* **78**: 623–30.

Aickin R, Hill D and Kemp A (1994) Measles immunisation in children with allergy to egg. *BMJ* **308**: 223–5

American Academy of Pediatrics (2003) Active immunization. In: Pickering LK (ed.) *Red Book: 2003 Report of the Committee on Infectious Diseases,* 26th edition. Elk Grove Village, IL: American Academy of Pediatrics.

Angel JB, Udem SA, Snydman DR *et al.* (1996) Measles pneumonitis following measles-mumps-rubella vaccination of patients with HIV infection, 1993. *MMWR* **45**: 603–6.

Best JM, Cooray S and Banatvala JE (2004) Rubella. In: Mahy BMJ and ter Meulen V (eds) *Topley and Wilson's Virology*, 10th edition. London: Hodder Arnold.

Bjorvatn B *et al.* (1973) Mumps virus recovered from testicles by fine-needle aspiration biopsy in cases of mumps orchitis. *Scand J Infect Dis* **5**: 3–5.

Bohlke K, Davis RL, Moray SH *et al.* (2003) Risk of anaphylaxis after vaccination of children and adolescents. *Pediatrics* **112**: 815–20.

British HIV Association (2006) *Immunisation guidelines for HIV-infected adults*. BHIVA. www.bhiva.org/pdf/2006/Immunisation506.pdf

Brown DW, Ramsay ME, Richards AF and Miller E (1994) Salivary diagnosis of measles: a study of notified cases in the United Kingdom, 1991–3. *BMJ* **308**(6935): 1015–17.

Buimovici-Klein E, Hite RL, Byrne T and Cooper LR (1997) Isolation of rubella virus in milk after postpartum immunization. *J Pediatr* **91**: 939–43.

Chen RT, Moses JM, Markowitz LE and Orenstein WA (1991) Adverse events following measles-mumps-rubella and measles vaccinations in college students. *Vaccine* **9**: 297–9.

Communicable Disease Surveillance Centre (1985) Virus meningitis and encephalitis. *BMJ* **290**: 921–2.

da Silveira CM, Salisbury DM and de Quadros CA (1997) Measles vaccination and Guillain-Barré syndrome. *Lancet* **349**(9044): 14–16.

Dales L, Hammer SJ and Smith NJ (2001) Time trends in autism and in MMR immunization coverage in California. *JAMA* **285**(22): 2852–3.

Davis RL, Marcuse E, Black S *et al.* (1997) MMR2 immunization at 4 to 5 years and 10 to 12 years of age: a comparison of adverse clinical events after immunization in the Vaccine Safety Datalink project. *Pediatrics* **100**: 767–71.

de Serres G, Boulianne N, Meyer F and Ward BJ (1995) Measles vaccine efficacy during an outbreak in a highly vaccinated population: incremental increase in protection with age at vaccination up to 18 months. *Epidemiol Infect* **115**: 315–23

De Wilde S, Carey IM, Richards N *et al.* (2001) Do children who become autistic consult more often after MMR vaccination? *Br J General Practice* **51**: 226–7.

Dejucq N and Jegou B (2001) Viruses in the mammalian male genital tract and their effects on the reproductive system. *Microbiol Mol Biol Rev* **65**: 208–31.

Department of Health (1992) *Changes in supply of vaccine*. Circular (PL/CMO(92)11).

D'Souza RM, Campbell-Lloyd S, Isaacs D *et al.* (2000) Adverse events following immunisation associated with the 1998 Australian Measles Control Campaign. *Commun Dis Intell* **24**: 27–33.

Feeney M, Gregg A, Winwood P and Snook J (1997) A case-control study of measles vaccination and inflammatory bowel disease. The East Dorset Gastroenterology Group. *Lancet* **350**: 764–6.

Falk WA , Buchan K, Dow M *et al.* (1989) The epidemiology of mumps in southern Alberta, 1980–1982. *Am J Epidemiol* **130**(4): 736–49.

Farrington CP, Miller E and Taylor B (2001) MMR and autism: further evidence against a causal association. *Vaccine* **19**: 3632–5.

Fasano MB, Wood RA, Cooke SK and Sampson HA (1992) Egg hypersensitivity and adverse reactions to measles, mumps and rubella vaccine. *J Pediatr* **120**: 878–81.

Fombonne E (1998) Inflammatory bowel disease and autism. *Lancet* **351**: 955.

Fombonne E (2001) Is there an epidemic of autism? *Pediatrics* **107**: 411–12.

Fox A and Lack G (2003) Egg allergy and MMR vaccination. *Br J Gen Pract* **53**: 801–2.

Freigang B, Jadavji TP and Freigang DW (1994) Lack of adverse reactions to measles, mumps and rubella vaccine in egg-allergic children. *Ann Allergy* **73**: 486–8.

Galbraith NS, Young SEJ, Pusey JJ *et al.* (1984) Mumps surveillance in England and Wales 1962–1981. *Lancet* **14**: 91–4.

Garty BBZ, Danon YL and Nitzan M (1988) Hearing loss due to mumps. *Arch Dis Child* **63**(1): 105–6. Correspondence on Hall paper.

Gilat T, Hacohen D, Lilos P and Langman MJ (1987) Childhood factors in ulcerative colitis and Crohn's disease. An international co-operative study. *Scan J Gastroenterology* **22**: 1009–24.

Gillberg C and Heijbel H (1998) MMR and autism. *Autism* **2**: 423–4.

Harling R, White JM, Ramsay ME, Macsween KF and van den Bosch C (2005) The effectiveness of the mumps component of the MMR vaccine: a case control study. *Vaccine* **23**(31): 4070–4.

Kaye JA, del Mar Melero-Montes M and Jick H (2001) Mumps, measles and rubella vaccine and the incidence of autism recorded by general practitioners: a time trend analysis. *BMJ* **322**(7284): 460–3.

Khakoo GA and Lack G (2000) Recommendations for using MMR vaccine in children allergic to eggs. *BMJ* **320**: 929–32.

Landes RD, Bass JW, Millunchick EW and Oetgen WJ (1980) Neonatal rubella following postpartum maternal immunisation. *J Pediatr* **97**: 465–7.

Losonsky GA, Fishaut JM, Strussenberg J and Ogra PL (1982) Effect of immunization against rubella on lactation products. Development and characterization of specific immunologic reactivity in breast milk. *J Infect Dis* **145**: 654–60.

Madsen KM and Vestergaard M (2004) MMR vaccination and autism: what is the evidence for a causal association? *Drug Saf* **27**: 831–40.

Makela A, Nuorti JP and Peltola H (2002) Neurologic disorders after measles-mumps-rubella vaccination. *Pediatrics* **110**: 957–63.

Medical Research Council (1977) Clinical trial of live vaccine given alone and live vaccine preceded by killed vaccine. Fourth report of the Medical Research Council by the measles sub-committee on development of vaccines and immunisation procedures. *Lancet* **ii**: 571–5.

Miller C, Miller E, Rowe K *et al.* (1989) Surveillance of symptoms following MMR vaccine in children. *Practitioner* **233**(1461): 69–73.

Miller E, Goldacre M, Pugh S *et al.* (1993) Risk of aseptic meningitis after measles, mumps, and rubella vaccine in UK children. *Lancet* **341**(8851): 979–82.

Miller E, Waight P, Farrington P *et al.* (2001) Idiopathic thrombocytopenic purpura and MMR vaccine. *Arch Dis Child* **84**: 227–9.

Miller E, Andrews N, Waight P and Taylor B (2003) Bacterial infections, immune overload, and MMR vaccine. Measles, mumps, and rubella. *Arch Dis Child* **88**(3): 222–3.

Miller E, Andrews N, Grant A *et al.* (2005) No evidence of an association between MMR vaccine and gait disturbance. *Arch Dis Child*, **88**(3): 292–6.

Morgan Capner P, Wright J, Miller CL and Miller E (1988) Surveillance of antibody to measles, mumps and rubella by age. *BMJ* **297**: 770–2.

Morse D, O'Shea M, Hamilton G *et al.* (1994) Outbreak of measles in a teenage school population: the need to immunize susceptible adolescents. *Epidemiol Infect* **113**: 355–65.

Mullooly J and Black S (2001) Simultaneous administration of varicella vaccine and other recommended childhood vaccines – United States, 1995–1999. *MMWR* **50**(47): 1058–61.

Offit PA, Quarles J, Gerber MA *et al.* (2002) Addressing parents' concerns: do multiple vaccines overwhelm or weaken the infant's immune system? *Pediatrics* **109**(1): 124–9.

Orenstein WA, Markowitz L, Preblud SR *et al.* (1986) Appropriate age for measles vaccination in the United States. *Dev Biol Stand* **65**: 13–21.

Patja A, Davidkin I, Kurki T *et al.* (2000) Serious adverse events after measles-mumps-rubella vaccination during a fourteen-year prospective follow-up. *Pediatr Infect Dis J.* **19**: 1127–34.

Patja A, Paunio M, Kinnunen E *et al.* (2001) Risk of Guillain-Barré syndrome after measles-mumps-rubella vaccination. *J Pediatr* **138**: 250–4.

Pebody RG, Paunio M and Ruutu P (1998) Measles, measles vaccination, and Crohn's disease has not increased in Finland. *BMJ* **316**(7146): 1745–6.

Peltola H, Heinonen OP and Valle M (1994) The elimination of indigenous measles, mumps and rubella from Finland by a 12-year two-dose vaccination program. *NEJM* **331**(21): 1397–402.

Philip RN, Reinhard KR and Lackman DB (1959) Observations on a mumps epidemic in a 'virgin' population. *Am J Hyg* **69**: 91–111.

Plotkin SA and Orenstein WA (eds) (2004) *Vaccines,* 4th edition. Philadelphia: WB Saunders Company, Chapters 19, 20 and 26.

Pool V, Braun MM, Kelso JM *et al.* (2002) Prevalence of anti-gelatin IgE antibodies in people with anaphylaxis after measles-mumps-rubella vaccine in the United States. *Pediatrics* **110**(6):e71. www.pediatrics.org/cgi/content/full/110/6/e71

Ramsay ME, Brown DW, Eastcott HR and Begg NT (1991) Saliva antibody testing and vaccination in a mumps outbreak. *CDR (Lond Engl Rev)* **1**(9): R96–8.

Ramsay ME, Brugha R, Brown DW *et al.* (1998) Salivary diagnosis of rubella: a study of notified cases in the United Kingdom, 1991–4. *Epidemiol Infect* **120**(3): 315–19.

Redd SC, King GE, Heath JL *et al.* (2004) Comparison of vaccination with measles-mumps-rubella at 9, 12 and 15 months of age. *J Infect Dis* **189**: S116–22

Schlegel M, Osterwalder JJ, Galeazzi RL and Vernazza PL (1999) Comparative efficacy of three mumps vaccines during disease outbreak in eastern Switzerland: cohort study. *BMJ* **319**: 352–3.

Seagroatt V (2005) MMR vaccine and Crohn's disease: ecological study of hospital admissions in England, 1991 to 2002. *BMJ* **330**: 1120–1.

Slater PE (1997) Chronic arthropathy after rubella vaccination in women. False alarm? *JAMA* **278**: 594–5.

Taylor B, Miller E, Farrington CP *et al.* (1999) Autism and measles, mumps and rubella: no epidemiological evidence for a causal association. *Lancet* **353**(9169): 2026–9.

Taylor B, Miller E, Langman R *et al.* (2002) Measles, mumps and rubella vaccination and bowel problems or developmental regression in children with autism: population study. *BMJ* **324**(7334): 393–6.

Tischer A and Gerike E (2000) Immune response after primary and re-vaccination with different combined vaccines against measles, mumps, rubella. *Vaccine* **18**(14): 1382–92.

Tookey PA, Jones G, Miller BH and Peckham CS (1991) Rubella vaccination in pregnancy. *CDR* **1**(8): R86–8.

Vestergaard M, Hviid A, Madsen KM *et al.* (2004) MMR vaccination and febrile seizures. Evaluation of susceptible subgroups and long-term prognosis. *JAMA* **292**: 351–7.

WHO (2003) Eliminating measles and rubella and preventing congenital rubella infection. www.euro.who.int/vaccine/20030808_4

WHO (2005) Vaccine Preventable Disease Monitoring System. Global summary. www-nt.who.int/immunization_monitoring/en/globalsummary/countryprofileselect.cfm)

24

Pertussis

NOTIFIABLE

The disease

Whooping cough is a highly infectious disease that is usually caused by *Bordetella pertussis*. A similar illness is caused by *B. parapertussis*, but this is not preventable with presently available vaccines.

There is an initial catarrhal stage, followed by an irritating cough that gradually becomes paroxysmal, usually within one to two weeks. The paroxysms are often followed by a characteristic 'whoop', often accompanied by vomiting. In young infants, the typical 'whoop' may never develop and coughing spasms may be followed by periods of apnoea. The illness often lasts for two to three months. In older children and adults, the disease may be mild and not recognised as whooping cough.

Pertussis may be complicated by bronchopneumonia, repeated vomiting leading to weight loss, and cerebral hypoxia with a resulting risk of brain damage. Severe complications and deaths occur most commonly in infants under six months of age. Minor complications include subconjunctival haemorrhages, epistaxis (nosebleeds), facial oedema, ulceration of the tongue or surrounding area, and suppurative otitis media.

Transmission of the infection is by droplet, and cases are most infectious during the early catarrhal phase. The incubation period is between six and 20 days and cases are infectious from six days after exposure to three weeks after the onset of typical paroxysms.

History and epidemiology of the disease

Before the introduction of pertussis immunisation in the 1950s, the average annual number of notifications exceeded 120,000 in the UK.

By 1972, when vaccine coverage was around 80%, there were only 2069 notifications of pertussis. Because of professional and public anxiety about the safety and efficacy of the vaccine, coverage fell to about 30% in 1975 and major epidemics occurred in 1977–79 and 1981–83. In 1978, there were over 68,000 notifications and 14 deaths. The actual number of deaths due to

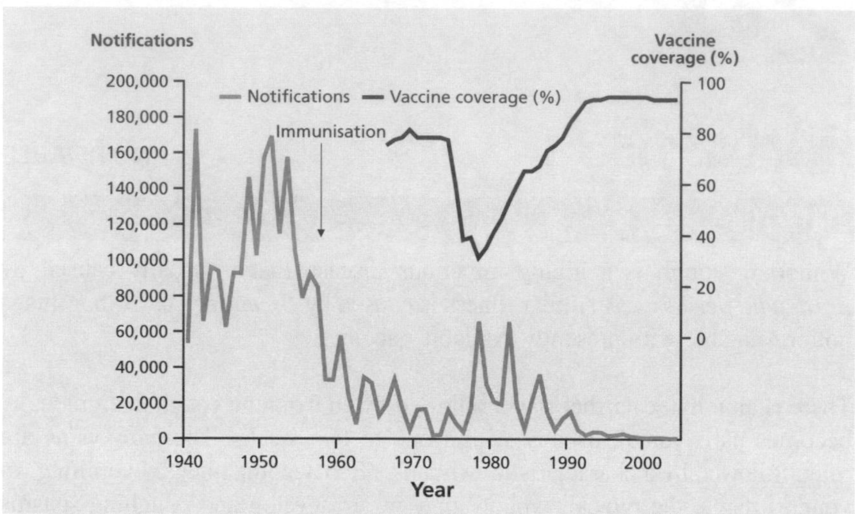

Figure 24.1 Pertussis notifications and vaccine coverage of children by their second birthday, England and Wales (1940–2003)

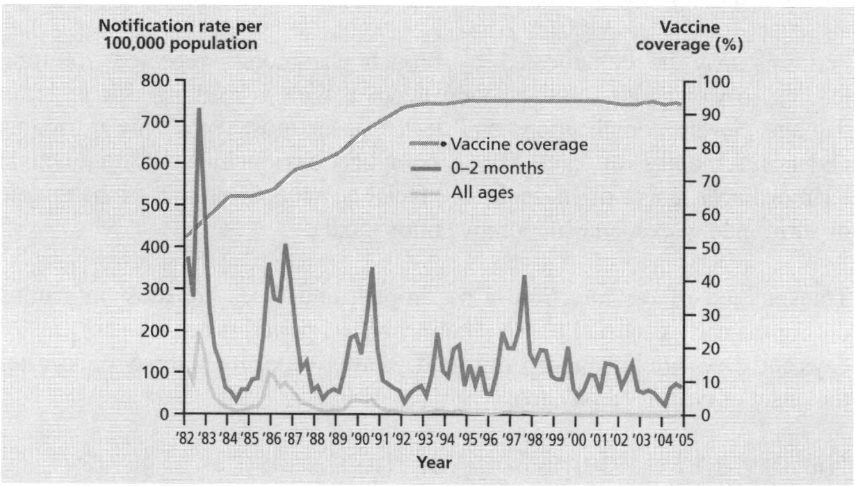

Figure 24.2 Notification rates of whooping cough (in all ages and infants aged under three months) and vaccine coverage at two years of age, England and Wales (1982–2005)

pertussis is higher, since not all cases in infants are recognised (Miller and Fletcher, 1976). These two major epidemics illustrate the impact of the fall in coverage of an effective vaccine.

The return of professional and public confidence resulted in increased vaccine uptake. Since the mid-1990s, coverage has been consistently over 90% by the second birthday, with fewer than 6000 notifications per year. In 2002, only 1051 cases were reported. The most recent estimate of deaths in England is nine deaths per year (Crowcroft *et al.*, 2002).

Despite the current low levels of disease, pertussis in the very young remains a significant cause of illness and death. The majority of hospitalisations following pertussis have occurred in those under six months of age, some of whom were seriously ill and required admission to paediatric intensive care units (Crowcroft *et al.*, 2003).

As the morbidity and mortality are highest in infants, high coverage must be maintained to protect those who are too young to be immunised. Adults and older children may infect younger members of their family who are too young to be immunised (Crowcroft *et al.*, 2003).

The pertussis vaccination

The acellular vaccines are made from highly purified selected components of the *Bordetella pertussis* organism. These components are treated with formaldehyde or glutaraldehyde and then adsorbed onto adjuvants, either aluminium phosphate or aluminium hydroxide, to improve immunogenicity.

Acellular vaccines differ in source, number of components, amount of each component, and method of manufacture, resulting in differences in efficacy and in the frequency of adverse effects (Edwards and Decker, 2004). The vaccine chosen for primary immunisation in the UK programme (Pediacel) contains five purified pertussis components. This vaccine has been shown to offer equal or better protection against clinically typical pertussis disease than the whole-cell pertussis vaccine previously used in the UK (Miller, 1999). The incidence of local and systemic reactions is lower with acellular pertussis vaccines than with whole-cell pertussis vaccines (Miller, 1999). The five-component vaccine contains pertussis toxoid (PT), filamentous haemagglutinin (FHA), fimbrial agglutinogens (FIM) 2 and 3, and pertactin (PRN). The three-component vaccine contains PT, FHA and PRN.

Three- and five-component pertussis-containing vaccines are provided according to their suitability for pre-school boosting. The pre-school vaccines are not provided for the purpose of primary immunisation. The three-component preparation (DTaP/IPV – Infanrix-IPV) does not provide the same level of protection against whooping cough in primary immunisation. The five-component pre-school preparation (dTaP/IPV– Repevax) does not contain the recommended strength of diphtheria vaccine for primary immunisation.

The pertussis vaccines are only given as part of combined products:

- diphtheria/tetanus/acellular pertussis/inactivated polio vaccine/ *Haemophilus influenzae* type b (DTaP/IPV/Hib)
- diphtheria/tetanus/acellular pertussis/inactivated polio vaccine/ (DTaP/IPV or dTaP/IPV).

The above vaccines are thiomersal-free. They are inactivated, do not contain live organisms and cannot cause the diseases against which they protect.

Monovalent pertussis vaccine is not available.

Storage

Vaccines should be stored in the original packaging at +2˚C to +8˚C and protected from light. All vaccines are sensitive to some extent to heat and cold. Heat speeds up the decline in potency of most vaccines, thus reducing their shelf life. Effectiveness cannot be guaranteed for vaccines unless they have been stored at the correct temperature. Freezing may cause increased reactogenicity and loss of potency for some vaccines. It can also cause hairline cracks in the container, leading to contamination of the contents.

Presentation

Pertussis-containing vaccines are available only as part of combined products. It is supplied as a cloudy white suspension either in a single-dose ampoule or in a pre-filled syringe. The suspension may sediment during storage and should be shaken to distribute the suspension uniformly before administration.

Dosage and schedule

- First dose of 0.5ml of a pertussis-containing vaccine.
- Second dose of 0.5ml, one month after the first dose.
- Third dose of 0.5ml, one month after the second dose.
- A fourth dose of 0.5ml should be given at the recommended interval.

Administration

Vaccines are routinely given intramuscularly into the upper arm or antero-lateral thigh. This is to reduce the risk of localised reactions, which are more common when vaccines are given subcutaneously (Mark *et al.*, 1999; Diggle and Deeks, 2000; Zuckerman, 2000). However, for individuals with a bleeding disorder, vaccines should be given by deep subcutaneous injection to reduce the risk of bleeding.

Pertussis-containing vaccines can be given at the same time as other vaccines such as MMR, MenC and hepatitis B. The vaccines should be given at a separate site, preferably in a different limb. If given in the same limb, they should be given at least 2.5cm apart (American Academy of Pediatrics, 2003). The site at which each vaccine was given should be noted in the patient's records.

Disposal

Equipment used for vaccination, including used vials or ampoules, should be disposed of at the end of a session by sealing in a proper, puncture-resistant 'sharps' box (UN-approved, BS 7320).

Recommendations for the use of the vaccine

The objective of the immunisation programme is to provide a minimum of four doses of a pertussis-containing vaccine at appropriate intervals for all individuals up to ten years of age.

To fulfil this objective, the appropriate vaccine for each age group is determined also by the need to protect individuals against diphtheria, tetanus, Hib and polio.

Primary immunisation

Infants and children under ten years of age

The primary course of pertussis vaccination consists of three doses of a pertussis-containing product with an interval of one month between each dose. DTaP/IPV/Hib is recommended for all infants from two months up to ten years of age. If the primary course is interrupted it should be resumed but not repeated, allowing an interval of one month between the remaining doses. DTaP/IPV/Hib should be used to complete a primary course that has been started with a whole-cell or another acellular pertussis preparation.

Children of one to ten years who have completed a primary course (which includes three doses of diphtheria, tetanus and polio), but have not received three doses of a pertussis-containing vaccine should be offered a dose of combined DTaP/IPV (or DTaP/IPV/Hib) vaccine to provide some priming against pertussis. The DTaP/IPV vaccine, which contains a lower dose of pertussis antigen, should only be used as a booster in fully primed children. They should then receive the first reinforcing dose as scheduled, also as DTaP/IPV (or DTaP/IPV/Hib), preferably allowing a minimum interval of one year.

Similarly, children who present first for the pre-school booster without any pertussis, should also receive DTaP/IPV (or DTaP/IPV/Hib) as priming and reinforcing doses, preferably allowing a minimum interval of one year.

Children of one to ten years who have completed the primary course plus a reinforcing dose (which includes four doses of diphtheria, tetanus and polio), but have not received four doses of pertussis-containing vaccine, may be offered a dose of combined DTaP/IPV or DTaP/IPV/Hib (if appropriate) to provide some or additional protection against pertussis, preferably allowing an interval of one year from the previous dose.

These children will therefore receive an extra dose of diphtheria, tetanus or polio vaccines. Such additional doses are unlikely to produce an unacceptable rate of reactions (Ramsay *et al.*, 1997).

Children aged ten years or over, and adults

Currently immunisation against pertussis is not recommended.

Reinforcing immunisation

Children under ten years of age should receive the first pertussis booster combined with diphtheria, tetanus and polio vaccines. Either of the recommended pre-school vaccines should be used to boost a primary course of whole-cell or acellular pertussis preparations. The first booster of pertussis-containing vaccine should ideally be given three years after completion of the primary course, normally between three years and four months to five years of age.

When primary vaccination has been delayed, this first booster dose may be given at the scheduled visit provided it is one year since the third primary dose. This will re-establish the child in the routine schedule. dTaP/IPV or DTaP/IPV should be used in this age group. Td/IPV should not be used routinely for this purpose in this age group because it does not contain pertussis and has not been shown to give an equivalent diphtheria antitoxin response to other recommended preparations.

If a child attends for a booster dose and has a history of receiving a vaccine following a tetanus-prone wound, attempts should be made to identify which vaccine was given. If the vaccine given was the same as that due at the current visit and at an appropriate interval, then the booster dose is not required. Otherwise, the dose given at the time of injury should be discounted as it may not provide satisfactory protection against all antigens, and the scheduled immunisation should be given. Such additional doses are unlikely to produce an unacceptable rate of reactions (Ramsay *et al.*, 1997).

Individuals aged ten years or over who have only had three doses of pertussis vaccine do not need further doses of pertussis-containing vaccine.

Vaccination of children with unknown or incomplete immunisation status

Where a child born in the UK presents with an inadequate immunisation history, every effort should be made to clarify what immunisations they may have had (see Chapter 11). A child who has not completed the primary course should have the outstanding doses at monthly intervals. Children may receive the first booster dose as early as one year after the third primary dose to re-establish them on the routine schedule.

Children coming to the UK who have a history of completing immunisation in their country of origin may not have been offered protection against all the antigens currently used in the UK. They will probably have received pertussis-containing vaccines in their country of origin (www-nt.who.int/immunization_monitoring/en/globalsummary/countryprofileselect.cfm).

Children coming from developing countries, from areas of conflict or from hard-to-reach population groups may not have been fully immunised. Where there is no reliable history of previous immunisation, it should be assumed that they are unimmunised, and the full UK recommendations should be followed (see Chapter 11 on vaccine schedules).

Children coming to the UK may have had a fourth dose of a pertussis-containing vaccine that is given at around 18 months in some countries. This dose should be discounted as it may not provide satisfactory protection until the time of the teenage booster. The routine pre-school and subsequent boosters should be given according to the UK schedule.

Contraindications

There are very few individuals who cannot receive pertussis-containing vaccines. When there is doubt, appropriate advice should be sought from a consultant paediatrician, immunisation co-ordinator or consultant in communicable disease control rather than withhold vaccine.

The vaccines should not be given to those who have had:

- a confirmed anaphylactic reaction to a previous dose of a pertussis-containing vaccine, or
- a confirmed anaphylactic reaction to neomycin, streptomycin or polymyxin B (which may be present in trace amounts).

Confirmed anaphylaxis occurs extremely rarely. Data from the UK, Canada and the US point to rates of 0.65 to 3 anaphylaxis events per million doses of vaccine given (Bohlke *et al.,* 2003; Canadian Medical Association, 2002). Other allergic conditions may occur more commonly and are not contraindications to further immunisation. A careful history of the event will often distinguish between anaphylaxis and other events that are either not due to the vaccine or not life-threatening. In the latter circumstance, it may be possible to continue the immunisation course. Specialist advice must be sought on the vaccines and circumstances in which they could be given. The risk to the individual of not being immunised must be taken into account.

Precautions

Minor illnesses without fever or systemic upset are not valid reasons to postpone immunisation. If an individual is acutely unwell, immunisation should be postponed until they have fully recovered. This is to avoid confusing the differential diagnosis of any acute illness by wrongly attributing any signs or symptoms to the adverse effects of the vaccine.

Systemic and local reactions following a previous immunisation

This section gives advice on the immunisation of children with a history of a severe or mild systemic or local reaction within 72 hours of a preceding vaccine. Immunisation with pertussis-containing vaccine **should** continue following a history of:

- fever, irrespective of its severity
- hypotonic-hyporesponsive episodes (HHE)

- persistent crying or screaming for more than three hours
- severe local reaction, irrespective of extent.

Previous experience suggested that the above events occurred more often after whole-cell DTP vaccine than after DT alone or after DTaP. Following the replacement of whole-cell pertussis vaccine with an acellular pertussis vaccine (DTaP/IPV/Hib) in Canada, there was a significant reduction in the number of reports of febrile seizures collected through the Immunization Monitoring Program – ACTive (IMPACT) (Le Saux *et al.*, 2003). When DTaP vaccines were compared with DT alone, severe general and local reactions occurred at the same rate (Tozzi and Olin, 1997). Therefore, these reactions were not due to the acellular pertussis components.

Children who have had severe reactions, as above, have continued and completed immunisation with pertussis-containing vaccines without recurrence of these reactions (Vermeer-de Bondt *et al.*, 1998; Gold *et al.*, 2000).

In Canada, a severe general or local reaction to DTaP/IPV/Hib is not a contra-indication to further doses of the vaccine (Canadian Medical Association, 1998). Adverse events after childhood immunisation are carefully monitored in Canada (Le Saux *et al.*, 2003), and experience there suggests that further doses are not associated with recurrence or worsening of the preceding events (S Halperin and R Pless, pers. comm., 2003).

Since local or general reactions are less frequent after acellular than whole-cell pertussis vaccines, the number of children with such events will be small. There is no benefit in withholding acellular pertussis-containing vaccines in order to reduce the risks of adverse events, and there is additional protection from completing pertussis immunisation; this should be carried out in accordance with the routine immunisation schedule. Children who have had a local or general reaction after whole-cell pertussis vaccine should complete their immunisation with acellular pertussis preparations.

Pregnancy and breast-feeding

Pertussis-containing vaccines may be given to pregnant women when protection is required without delay. There is no evidence of risk from vaccinating pregnant women or those who are breast-feeding with inactivated viral or bacterial vaccines or toxoids (Plotkin and Orenstein, 2004).

Premature infants

It is important that premature infants have their immunisations at the appropriate chronological age, according to the schedule. There is no evidence that premature babies are at an increased risk of adverse reactions from vaccines (Slack *et al.*, 2001).

Immunosuppression and HIV infection

Individuals with immunosuppression and HIV infection (regardless of CD4 count) should be given pertussis-containing vaccines in accordance with the routine recommended schedule. These individuals may not make a full antibody response. Re-immunisation should be considered after treatment is finished and recovery has occurred. Specialist advice may be required.

Further guidance is provided by the Royal College of Paediatrics and Child Health (www.rcpch.ac.uk), the British HIV Association (BHIVA) *Immunisation guidelines for HIV-infected adults* (BHIVA, 2006) and the Children's HIV Association of UK and Ireland (CHIVA) immunisation guidelines (www.bhiva.org/chiva).

Neurological conditions

Pre-existing neurological conditions

The presence of a neurological condition is not a contraindication to immunisation. Where there is evidence of a neurological condition in a child, the advice given in the flow chart in Figure 24.3 should be followed.

If a child has a stable pre-existing neurological abnormality, such as spina bifida, congenital abnormality of the brain or perinatal hypoxic ischaemic encephalopathy, they should be immunised according to the recommended schedule. When there has been a documented history of cerebral damage in the neonatal period, immunisation should be carried out unless there is evidence of an evolving neurological abnormality.

If there is evidence of current neurological deterioration, including poorly controlled epilepsy, immunisation should be deferred and the child should be referred to a child specialist for investigation to see if an underlying cause can be identified. If a cause is not identified, immunisation should be deferred until the condition has stabilised. If a cause is identified, immunisation should proceed as normal.

A family history of seizures is not a contraindication to immunisation. When there is a personal or family history of febrile seizures, there is an increased

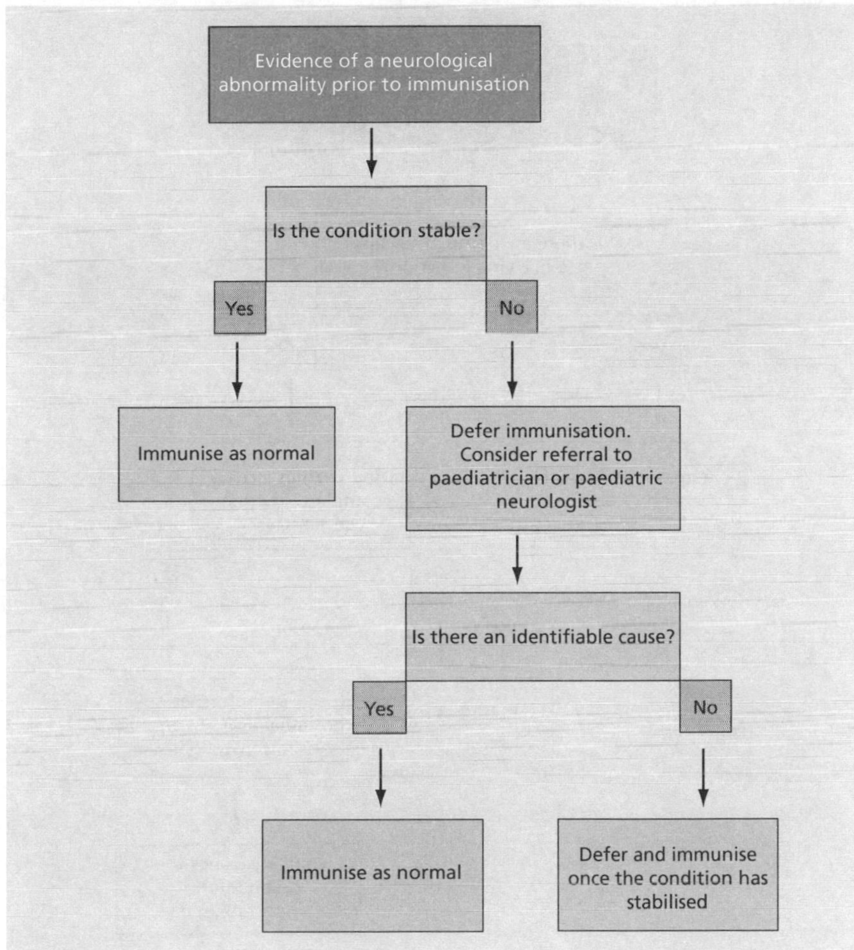

Figure 24.3 Flow chart for evidence of a neurological condition before immunisation

risk of these occurring after any fever, including that caused by immunisation. Seizures associated with fever are rare in the first six months of life and most common in the second year of life. After this age the frequency falls and they are rare after five years of age.

When a child has had a seizure associated with fever in the past, with no evidence of neurological deterioration, immunisation should proceed as recommended. Advice on the prevention and management of fever should be given before immunisation.

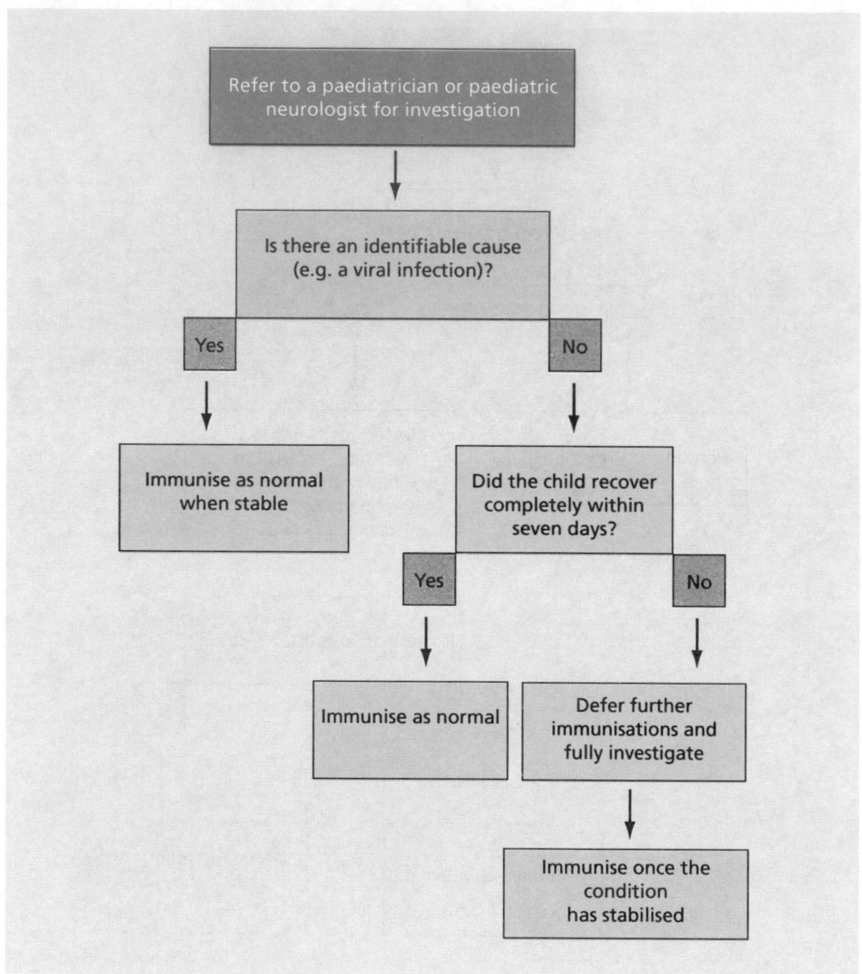

Figure 24.4 Flow chart for encephalitis or encephalopathy occurring within seven days of immunisation

When a child has had a seizure that is not associated with fever, and there is no evidence of neurological deterioration, immunisation should proceed as recommended. When immunised with DTP vaccine, children with a family or personal history of seizures had no significant adverse events and their developmental progress was normal (Ramsay *et al.*, 1994).

Neurological abnormalities following immunisation

If a child experiences encephalopathy or encephalitis within seven days of immunisation, the advice in the flow chart in Figure 24.4 should be followed.

It is unlikely that these conditions will have been caused by the vaccine and they should be investigated by a specialist. Immunisation should be deferred until the condition has stabilised in children where no underlying cause was found **and** the child did not recover completely within seven days. If a cause is identified or the child recovers within seven days, immunisation should proceed as recommended.

If a seizure associated with a fever occurs within 72 hours of an immunisation, further immunisation should be deferred until the condition is stable if no underlying cause has been found **and** the child did not recover completely within 24 hours. If a cause is identified or the child recovers within 24 hours, immunisation should continue as recommended.

Deferral of immunisation

There will be very few occasions when deferral of immunisation is required (see above). Deferral leaves the child unprotected; the period of deferral should be minimised so that immunisation can commence as soon as possible. If a specialist recommends deferral, this should be clearly communicated to the general practitioner, who must be informed as soon as the child is fit for immunisation.

Adverse reactions

Pain, swelling or redness at the injection site are common and may occur more frequently following subsequent doses. A small painless nodule may form at the injection site; this usually disappears and is of no consequence. The incidence of local reactions is lower with vaccines combined with acellular pertussis than with whole-cell pertussis, and is similar to that after DT vaccine (Miller, 1999; Tozzi and Olin, 1997).

Fever, convulsions, high-pitched screaming and episodes of pallor, cyanosis and limpness (HHE) occur with equal frequency after both DTaP and DT vaccines (Tozzi and Olin, 1997).

Confirmed anaphylaxis occurs extremely rarely. Data from the UK, Canada and the US point to rates of 0.65 to 3 anaphylaxis events per million doses (Bohlke *et al.*, 2003; Canadian Medical Association, 2002). Other allergic conditions may occur more commonly and are not contraindications to further immunisation.

All suspected adverse reactions to vaccines occurring in children, or in individuals of any age after vaccines labelled with a black triangle (▼), should be reported to the Commission on Human Medicines using the Yellow Card scheme. Serious suspected adverse reactions to vaccines in adults should be reported through the Yellow Card scheme.

Conditions historically associated with pertussis vaccine

In the past, there was public and professional anxiety that whole-cell pertussis vaccine contributed to the onset of neurological problems in young children. Between 1976 and 1979, a total of 1182 children with serious neurological illnesses were reported to the National Childhood Encephalopathy Study (NCES). Only 39 of these children had recently received whole-cell pertussis vaccine. The study concluded that whole-cell pertussis vaccine may very rarely be associated with the development of severe acute neurological illness in children who were previously apparently normal; most of these children suffered no apparent harm. The occurrence of a severe encephalopathy after whole-cell pertussis immunisation was sometimes associated with long-term residual neurological damage, but the evidence was insufficient to indicate whether or not whole-cell DTP increased the overall risk of chronic neurological dysfunction.

A major review of studies on adverse events after pertussis vaccine was published by the United States Institute of Medicine in 2001 (Howson *et al.*, 2001). This concluded that the evidence did not indicate a causal relationship between pertussis vaccine and infantile spasms, hypsarrhythmia, Reye's syndrome and sudden infant death syndrome (SIDS).

Cot deaths (SIDS) occur most commonly during the first year of life and may therefore coincide with the giving of pertussis-containing vaccines. Studies have established that this association is not causal (Fleming *et al.*, 2001).

It has been suggested that pertussis vaccine is linked with the development of asthma and allergy (Odent *et al.*, 1994). A recent double-blind study of pertussis vaccines found no significant differences in wheezing, itchy rash or sneezing between DTP-immunised children and controls (Nilsson *et al.*, 2003; DeStefano *et al.*, 2002). Asthma or allergy are not contraindications to the completion of pertussis immunisation.

Management of outbreaks and contacts of cases

Because three injections are required to protect against pertussis, the vaccine cannot be used to control outbreaks (Dodhia *et al.*, 2002). In outbreaks affecting children under ten years of age, those who have not received four doses of pertussis-containing vaccines should receive an additional dose(s) of dTaP/IPV (DTaP/IPV may be used if there is no dTaP/IPV available).

Antibiotic prophylaxis should be offered to unimmunised or partially immunised vulnerable contacts of cases after discussion with the local health protection unit (Dodhia *et al.*, 2002).

Supplies

- Pediacel (diphtheria/tetanus/5-component acellular pertussis/inactivated polio vaccine/*Haemophilus influenzae* type b (DTaP/IPV/Hib) – manufactured by Sanofi Pasteur MSD.
- Repevax (diphtheria/tetanus/5-component acellular pertussis/ inactivated polio vaccine (dTaP/IPV)) – manufactured by Sanofi Pasteur MSD.
- Infanrix IPV (diphtheria/tetanus/3-component acellular pertussis/ inactivated polio vaccine (DTaP/IPV)) – manufactured by GlaxoSmithKline.

These vaccines are supplied by Healthcare Logistics (Tel: 0870 871 1890) as part of the national childhood immunisation programme.

In Scotland, supplies should be obtained from local childhood vaccine holding centres. Details of these are available from Scottish Healthcare Supplies (Tel: 0141 282 2240).

In Northern Ireland, supplies should be obtained from local childhood vaccine holding centres. Details of these are available from the regional pharmaceutical procurement service (Tel: 02890 552368).

References

American Academy of Pediatrics (2003) Active immunization. In: Pickering LK (ed.) *Red Book: 2003 Report of the Committee on Infectious Diseases* 26th edition. Elk Grove Village, IL: American Academy of Pediatrics, p 33.

Bohlke K, Davis RL, Marcy SH *et al.* (2003) Risk of anaphylaxis after vaccination of children and adolescents. *Pediatrics* **112**: 815–20.

British HIV Association (2006) *Immunisation guidelines for HIV-infected adults:* www.bhiva.org/pdf/2006/Immunisation506.pdf.

Canadian Medical Association (1998) Pertussis vaccine. In: *Canadian Immunisation Guide*, 5th edition. Canadian Medical Association, p 133.

Canadian Medical Association (2002) General considerations. In: *Canadian Immunisation Guide*, 6th edition. Canadian Medical Association, p 14.

Crowcroft NS, Andrews N, Rooney C *et al.* (2002) Deaths from pertussis are underestimated in England. *Arch Dis Child* **86**: 336–8.

Crowcroft NS, Booy R, Harrison T *et al.* (2003) Severe and unrecognised: pertussis in UK infants. *Arch Dis Child* **88**: 802–6.

Department of Health (2001) *Health information for overseas travel,* 2nd edition. London: TSO.

DeStefano F, Gu D, Kramarz P *et al.* (2002) Childhood vaccinations and risk of asthma. *Pediatr Infect Dis J* **21**: 498–504.

Diggle L and Deeks J (2000) Effect of needle length on incidence of local reactions to routine immunisation in infants aged 4 months: randomised controlled trial. *BMJ* **321**: 931–3.

Dodhia H, Crowcroft NS, Bramley JC and Miller E (2002) UK guidelines for the use of erythromycin chemoprophylaxis in persons exposed to pertussis. *J Public Health Med* **24**: 200–6.

Edwards KM and Decker MD (2004) Pertussis vaccine. In: Plotkin SA and Orenstein WA (eds) *Vaccines,* 4th edition. Philadelphia: WB Saunders Company.

Fleming PJ, Blair PS and Platt MW *et al.* (2001) The UK accelerated immunisation programme and sudden unexpected death in infancy: case-control study. *BMJ* **322**: 1–5.

Gold M, Goodwin H, Botham S *et al.* (2000) Re-vaccination of 421 children with a past history of an adverse reaction in a specialised service. *Arch Dis Child* **83**: 28–31.

Howson CP, Howe CJ and Fineberg HV (eds) (2001) *Adverse effects of pertussis and rubella vaccines. A report of the committee to review the adverse consequences of pertussis and rubella vaccines.* Institute of Medicine Report. Washington, DC: National Academy Press.

Le Saux N, Barrowman NJ, Moore DL *et al.* (2003) Canadian Paediatric Society/Health Canada Immunization Monitoring Program – ACTive (IMPACT). Decrease in hospital admissions for febrile seizures and reports of hypotonic-hyporesponsive episodes presenting to hospital emergency departments since switching to acellular pertussis vaccine in Canada: a report from IMPACT. *Pediatrics* **112**(5): e348.

Mark A, Carlsson RM and Granstrom M (1999) Subcutaneous versus intramuscular injection for booster DT vaccination in adolescents. *Vaccine* **17**: 2067–72.

Miller E (1999) Overview of recent clinical trials of acellular pertussis vaccines. *Biologicals* **27**: 79–86.

Miller CL and Fletcher WB (1976) Severity of notified whooping cough. *BMJ* **1**: 117–19.

Nilsson L, Kjellman NI and Bjorksten B (2003) Allergic disease at the age of 7 years after pertussis vaccination in infancy: results from the follow-up of a randomised controlled trial of 3 vaccines. *Arch Pediatr Adolesc Med* **157**: 1184–9.

Odent MR, Culpin EE and Kimmel T (1994) Pertussis vaccination and asthma: is there a link? *JAMA* **272**: 592–3.

Plotkin SA and Orenstein WA (eds) (2004) *Vaccines,* 4th edition. Philadelphia: WB Saunders Company, Chapter 8.

Ramsay M, Begg N, Holland B and Dalphinis J (1994) Pertussis immunisation in children with a family or personal history of convulsions: a review of children referred for specialist advice. *Health Trends* **26**: 23–4.

Ramsay M, Joce R and Whalley J (1997) Adverse events after school leavers received combined tetanus and low-dose diphtheria vaccine. *CDR Review* **5**: R65–7.

Slack MH, Schapira D, Thwaites RJ *et al.* (2001) Immune response of premature infants to meningococcal serogroup C and combined diphtheria-tetanus toxoids-acellular pertussis-*Haemophilus influenzae* type b conjugate vaccines. *J Infect Dis* **184**(12): 1617–20.

Tozzi AE and Olin P (1997) Common side effects in the Italian and Stockholm 1 Trials. *Dev Biol Stand* **89**: 105– 8.

Vermeer-de Bondt PE, Labadie J and Rümke HC (1998) Rate of recurrent collapse after vaccination with whole-cell pertussis vaccine: follow up study. *BMJ* **316**: 902.

Zuckerman JN (2000) The importance of injecting vaccines into muscle. *BMJ* **321**: 1237–8.

25

Pneumococcal

PNEUMOCOCCAL MENINGITIS NOTIFIABLE

The disease

Pneumococcal disease is the term used to describe infections caused by the bacterium *Streptococcus pneumoniae* (also called pneumococcus).

S. pneumoniae is an encapsulated gram-positive coccus. The capsule is the most important virulence factor of *S. pneumoniae*; pneumococci that lack the capsule are normally not virulent. Over 90 different capsular types have been characterised. About 66% of the serious infections in adults and about 80% of invasive infections in children are caused by eight to ten capsular types (Health Protection Agency, 2003).

Some serotypes of the pneumococcus may be carried in the nasopharynx without symptoms, with disease occurring in a small proportion of infected individuals. Other serotypes are rarely identified in the nasopharynx but are associated with invasive disease. The incubation period for pneumococcal disease is not clearly defined but it may be as short as one to three days. The organism may spread locally into the sinuses or middle ear cavity, causing sinusitis or otitis media. It may also affect the lungs to cause pneumonia, or cause systemic (invasive) infections including bacteraemic pneumonia, bacteraemia and meningitis.

Transmission is by aerosol, droplets or direct contact with respiratory secretions of someone carrying the organism. Transmission usually requires either frequent or prolonged close contact. There is a seasonal variation in pneumococcal disease, with peak levels in the winter months.

Invasive pneumococcal disease is a major cause of morbidity and mortality. It particularly affects the very young, the elderly, those with an absent or non-functioning spleen and those with other causes of impaired immunity. Recurrent infections may occur in association with skull defects, cerebrospinal fluid (CSF) leaks, cochlear implants or fractures of the skull.

History and epidemiology of the disease

Currently, the pneumococcus is one of the most frequently reported causes of bacteraemia and meningitis. During 2005, 6207 laboratory isolates from blood,

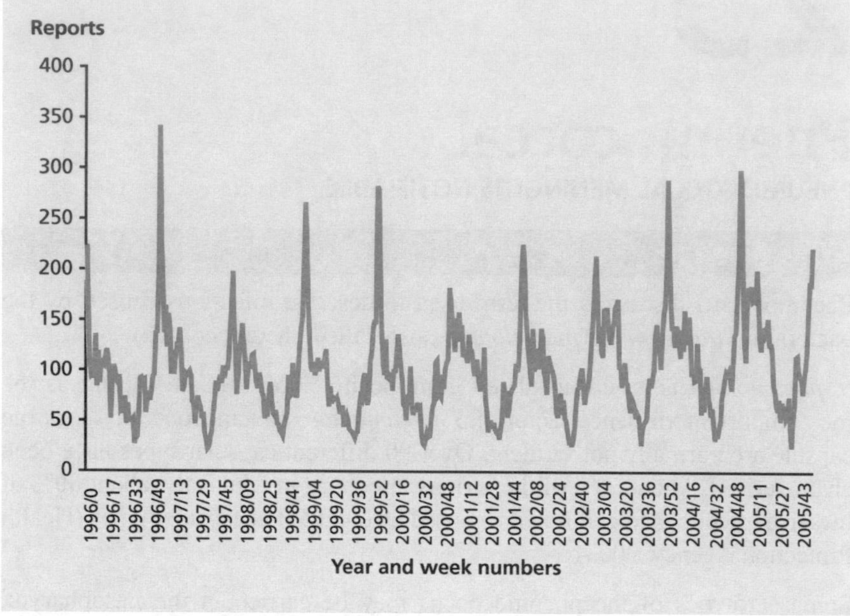

Figure 25.1 Weekly number of invasive pneumococcal disease cases in England and Wales (1996–2005)

CSF or other normally sterile sites were reported to the Health Protection Agency Centre for Infection (HPA CfI) from laboratories in England and Wales (Health Protection Agency, 2006). Figure 25.1 shows the weekly number of invasive pneumococcal disease cases in England and Wales between 1996 and 2005. The pneumococcus is also the commonest cause of community-acquired pneumonia (Bartlett and Mundy, 1995). Pneumococcal pneumonia is estimated to affect one in a thousand adults each year and has a case fatality ratio of 10 to 20% (World Health Organization, 1999).

Antimicrobial resistance among pneumococci occurs and susceptibility to macrolide antimicrobials, penicillin and cephalosporin can no longer be assumed. In 2000, 13% of invasive isolates in England and Wales reported to the HPA CDSC were resistant to erythromycin and 7% showed full or intermediate resistance to penicillin (George and Melegaro, 2001, 2003). An increase in pneumococcal antibiotic resistance has been reported worldwide (Appelobaum, 1992; Butler *et al.*, 1996; Davies *et al.*, 1999).

Since 1992, pneumococcal polysaccharide immunisation (see below) has been recommended for people with medical conditions for whom pneumococcal infection was likely to be more common or serious.

In recent years, the pneumococcal recommendations have undergone a number of changes:

- in 2002, a pneumococcal conjugate vaccine (see below) became available and was recommended for immunisation of at-risk groups under the age of two years
- in 2003, pneumococcal polysaccharide immunisation was recommended for all people aged 65 and over
- in 2004, the conjugate vaccine policy was extended to at-risk children under five years of age
- in 2006, pneumococcal conjugate vaccine was added to the routine childhood immunisation programme.

The pneumococcal vaccination

There are two types of pneumococcal vaccine:

- pneumococcal polysaccharide vaccine (PPV) contains purified capsular polysaccharide from each of 23 capsular types* of pneumococcus
- pneumococcal conjugate vaccine (PCV) contains polysaccharide from seven common capsular types.† These are conjugated to protein (CRM_{197}) using similar manufacturing technology to that for *Haemophilus influenzae* type b (Hib) and meningococcal C conjugate vaccines.

The pneumococcal polysaccharide and pneumococcal conjugate vaccines do not contain thiomersal. The vaccines are inactivated, do not contain live organisms and cannot cause the diseases against which they protect.

Pneumococcal polysaccharide vaccine (PPV)

Most healthy adults develop a good antibody response to a single dose of PPV by the third week following immunisation. Antibody response may be reduced in those with immunological impairment and those with an absent or dysfunctional spleen. Children younger than two years of age show poor antibody responses to immunisation with PPV.

It is difficult to reach firm conclusions about the effectiveness of PPV, but overall efficacy in preventing pneumococcal bacteraemia is probably 50 to 70% (Mangtani *et al.*, 2003; Fedson, 1999; Fine *et al.*, 1994; Butler *et al.*, 1993;

---

* 1, 2, 3, 4, 5, 6B, 7F, 8, 9N, 9V, 10A, 11A, 12F, 14, 15B, 17F, 18C, 19F, 19A, 20, 22F, 23F, 33F
† 4, 6B, 9V, 14, 18C, 19F, 23F

Melegaro and Edmunds, 2004). Current evidence suggests that PPV is not effective in protecting against non-bacteraemic pneumococcal pneumonia (Jackson *et al.*, 2003). It does not prevent otitis media or exacerbations of chronic bronchitis. The vaccine is relatively ineffective in patients with multiple myeloma, Hodgkin's and non-Hodgkin's lymphoma (especially during treatment) and chronic alcoholism.

The vaccine does not protect against pneumococcal infection due to capsular types not contained in the vaccine, but the 23 types included account for about 96% of the pneumococcal isolates that cause serious infection in the UK (Health Protection Agency, 2003).

The length of protection is not known and may vary between capsular types. Post-immunisation antibody levels usually begin to wane after about five years, but may decline more rapidly in asplenic patients and children with nephrotic syndrome (Butler *et al.*, 1993).

There is no evidence of effectiveness of PPV in children under two years of age (Fedson *et al.*, 1999).

Pneumococcal conjugate vaccine (PCV)

The antibody response in young children can be improved by conjugating the polysaccharide to proteins such as CRM_{197}. The conjugated vaccine is immunogenic in children from two months of age. Data on efficacy comes from pre- and post-licensing studies in the US in which children were vaccinated at two, four and six months of age, with a fourth dose at 15 months. At the time of the pre-licence study, the serotypes included in the vaccine accounted for 89% of invasive pneumococcal infections in the US. The serotype-specific efficacy was 97% after the fourth dose had been given. The vaccine protects against pneumococcal meningitis, bacteraemia, pneumonia and otitis media (Black *et al.*, 2000; Black *et al.*, 2002).

Post-licensure surveillance, following introduction of PCV in the US in 1999 as part of a universal infant immunisation programme, has shown a large reduction in both invasive and non-invasive disease incidence due to vaccine serotypes in both vaccinated and older unvaccinated populations ('herd immunity'). This reduction in disease has also been accompanied by a fall in the rate of penicillin-resistant pneumococcal infections (Black *et al.*, 2004). However, a small increase in invasive disease due to non-vaccine serotypes (termed 'serotype replacement') has also been observed (Whitney *et al.*, 2003).

Storage

Vaccines should be stored in the original packaging at +2°C to +8°C and protected from light. All vaccines are sensitive to some extent to heat and cold. Heat speeds up the decline in potency of most vaccines, thus reducing their shelf life. Effectiveness cannot be guaranteed for vaccines unless they have been stored at the correct temperature. Freezing may cause increased reactogenicity and loss of potency for some vaccines. It can also cause hairline cracks in the container, leading to contamination of the contents.

Presentation

Both PCV and PPV are supplied as single doses of 0.5ml.

PCV

Storage can cause the vaccine to separate into a white deposit and clear supernatant. The vaccine should be shaken well to obtain a white homogeneous suspension and should not be used if there is any residual particulate matter after shaking.

PPV

The polysaccharide vaccine should be inspected before being given to check that it is clear and colourless.

Vaccines must not be given intravenously.

Dosage and schedule

PCV

For children under one year of age:

- First dose of 0.5ml of PCV.
- Second dose of 0.5ml, two months after the first dose.
- A third dose of 0.5ml should be given at the recommended interval (see below).

Children over one year of age and under five years of age:

- A single dose of 0.5ml of PCV if indicated (see recommendations below).

PPV

Adults over 65 years and at-risk groups aged two years or over:

- A single dose of 0.5ml of PPV.

Administration

Vaccines are routinely given into the upper arm in children and adults or the anterolateral thigh in infants under one year of age. This is to reduce the risk of localised reactions, which are more common when vaccines are given subcutaneously (Mark *et al.*, 1999; Diggle and Deeks, 2000; Zuckerman, 2000). However, for individuals with a bleeding disorder, vaccines should be given by deep subcutaneous injection to reduce the risk of bleeding.

Pneumococcal vaccines can be given at the same time as other vaccines such as DTaP/IPV/Hib, MMR, MenC and influenza. The vaccines should be given at separate sites, preferably in different limbs. If given in the same limb, they should be given at least 2.5cm apart (American Academy of Pediatrics, 2003). The site at which each vaccine was given should be noted in the individual's records.

At the moment, there are no data on the administration of pneumococcal vaccination at the same time as the conjugate Hib/MenC vaccine (Menitorix ▼). Although there is no reason to think that this would cause any safety concerns, there is a theoretical possibility of reduced response from giving Hib/MenC at the same time as PCV. Therefore, as a precautionary measure, PCV should not be given routinely at the same time as the Hib/MenC booster. However, where rapid protection is required, for example those children under five years of age with splenic dysfunction, the two can be given on the same day or at any interval. As more data accumulate, this advice may be modified.

Disposal

Equipment used for vaccination, including used vials or ampoules, should be disposed of at the end of a session by sealing in a proper puncture-resistant 'sharps' box (UN-approved, BS 7320).

Recommendations for the use of pneumococcal vaccine

The objective of the immunisation programme is to protect all of those for whom pneumococcal infection is likely to be more common and/or serious, i.e.:

- infants as part of the routine childhood immunisation programme
- those aged 65 years or over
- those aged two months and over in the clinical risk groups shown in Table 25.1.

Table 25.1 Clinical risk groups who should receive the pneumococcal immunisation

Clinical risk group	Examples (decision based on clinical judgement)
Asplenia or dysfunction of the spleen	This also includes conditions such as homozygous sickle cell disease and coeliac syndrome that may lead to splenic dysfunction.
Chronic respiratory disease	This includes chronic obstructive pulmonary disease (COPD), including chronic bronchitis and emphysema; and such conditions as bronchiectasis, cystic fibrosis, interstitial lung fibrosis, pneumoconiosis and bronchopulmonary dysplasia (BPD). Children with respiratory conditions caused by aspiration, or a neuromuscular disease (e.g. cerebral palsy) with a risk of aspiration. Asthma is not an indication, unless so severe as to require continuous or frequently repeated use of systemic steroids (as defined in Immunosuppression below).
Chronic heart disease	This includes those requiring regular medication and/or follow-up for ischaemic heart disease, congenital heart disease, hypertension with cardiac complications, and chronic heart failure.
Chronic renal disease	This includes nephrotic syndrome, chronic renal failure and renal transplantation.
Chronic liver disease	This includes cirrhosis, biliary atresia and chronic hepatitis.
Diabetes	Diabetes mellitus requiring insulin or oral hypoglycaemic drugs. This does not include diabetes that is diet controlled.
Immunosuppression	Due to disease or treatment, including asplenia or splenic dysfunction and HIV infection at all stages. Patients undergoing chemotherapy leading to immunosuppression. Individuals on or likely to be on systemic steroids for more than a month at a dose equivalent to prednisolone at 20mg or more per day (any age), or for children under 20kg, a dose of 1mg or more per kg per day. *However, some immunocompromised patients may have a suboptimal immunological response to the vaccine.*
Individuals with cochlear implants	*It is important that immunisation does not delay the cochlear implantation.*
Individuals with cerebrospinal fluid leaks	This includes leakage of cerebrospinal fluid such as following trauma or major skull surgery.

Primary care staff should identify patients for whom vaccine is recommended and use all opportunities to ensure that they are appropriately immunised, for example:

- when immunising against influenza
- at other routine consultations, especially on discharge after hospital admission.

Primary immunisation

PCV

PCV is recommended for infants from two months of age as part of the routine childhood immunisation schedule and children under five years of age in a clinical risk group.

Infants under one year of age

The primary course of PCV vaccination consists of two doses with an interval of two months between each dose. The recommended age for vaccination is between two and four months. If the primary course is interrupted, it should be resumed but not repeated, allowing an interval of two months between doses. Although the currently available PCV is licensed for use as a three-dose primary course in infancy, evidence from UK immunogenicity studies shows that a two-dose primary immunisation course provides the same level of protection (Goldblatt *et al.*, 2006).

Children from one year to under two years of age

The primary course of PCV for this age group is one dose. If the primary course in children under one year was not completed, then a single booster dose of PCV should be given at least one month after the last dose to complete the course.

PPV

Adults 65 years or over

A single dose of PPV should be administered.

Risk groups

Children under two years of age

At-risk children (Table 25.1) should be given PCV according to the schedule for the routine immunisation programme, at 2, 4 and 13 months of age. At-risk children who present late for vaccination should be offered two doses of PCV*

* One month apart if necessary to ensure two doses are given before a dose at 13 months

Table 25.2 Vaccination schedule for those in a clinical risk group

Patient age at presentation	Vaccine given and when to immunise	
	7-valent PCV	**23-valent PPV**
At-risk children 2 months to under 12 months of age	Vaccination according to the routine immunisation schedule at 2, 4 and 13 months of age	One dose after the second birthday.
At-risk children 2 months to under 12 months of age who have asplenia or splenic dysfunction or who are immunosuppressed	Vaccination according to the routine immunisation schedule at 2, 4 and 13 months of age	One dose after the second birthday
At-risk children 12 months to under 5 years of age	One dose	One dose after the second birthday and at least 2 months after the final dose of PCV
At-risk children 12 months to under 5 years of age who have asplenia or splenic dysfunction or who are immunosuppressed	Two doses, with an interval of 2 months between doses	One dose after the second birthday and at least 2 months after the final dose of PCV
At-risk children aged over 5 years and at-risk adults	PCV is not recommended	One dose

before the age of 12 months, and a further dose at 13 months. At-risk children aged over 12 months who have either not been vaccinated or not completed a primary course should have a single dose of PCV.

For those children in this age group who have asplenia or splenic dysfunction, or who are immunocompromised and may have a sub-optimal immunological response to the first dose of vaccine, a second dose should be given two months after the first dose.

All at-risk children should be offered a single dose of PPV when they are two years of age or over (see below).

Children aged two to five years of age

A single dose of PPV should be given, at least two months after the final dose of PCV.

At-risk children under five years of age who have either not been vaccinated with PCV or not completed a primary course should have a single dose of PCV. For those children in this age group who have asplenia or splenic dysfunction, or who are immunocompromised and may have a sub-optimal immunological response to the first dose of PCV, a second dose should be given two months after the first dose. At-risk children under five years who have already received 23-valent PPV should receive a dose of PCV at least two months after the PPV.

Children between two and five years who have been fully immunised with PCV as part of the routine programme and who then develop splenic dysfunction or immunosuppression should be given an additional dose of PCV.

Children aged over five years and adults

A single dose of PPV should be given, at least two months after the final dose of PCV.

Reinforcing immunisation

PCV

A reinforcing (booster) dose of PCV is recommended at 13 months of age for children who have received a complete primary course of two PCVs. It should be given one month after the Hib/MenC vaccine.

PPV

Antibody levels are likely to decline rapidly in individuals with no spleen, splenic dysfunction or chronic renal disease (Giebink *et al.*, 1981; Rytel *et al.*, 1986) and therefore re-immunisation with 23-valent PPV is recommended every five years in these groups. Revaccination is well tolerated (Jackson *et al.*, 1999). Testing of antibody levels prior to vaccination is not required.

Although there is evidence of a decline in protection with time (Shapiro *et al.*, 1991), there are no studies showing additional protection from boosting individuals with other indications including age, and therefore routine revaccination is not currently recommended.

Individuals who have previously received 12- or 14-valent PPV or 7-valent PCV should be immunised with 23-valent PPV to gain protection from the additional serotypes.

Individuals with unknown or incomplete vaccination histories

Unless there is a reliable history of previous immunisation, individuals should be assumed to be unimmunised. The full UK recommendations should be followed. A child who has not completed the primary course (and is under one year of age) should have the outstanding doses at appropriate intervals (see above). A child aged one and under two years of age should have a single dose of PCV.

Children and adults requiring splenectomy or commencing immunosuppressive treatment

Previously unvaccinated children and adults requiring splenectomy or commencing immunosuppressive treatment may be at an increased risk of pneumococcal disease and should be vaccinated according to the schedule for this specific risk group. Children under five who have been fully immunised with PCV as part of the routine programme and who then develop splenic dysfunction more than one year after completing immunisation should be offered an additional dose of PCV.

Ideally, pneumococcal vaccine should be given four to six weeks before elective splenectomy or initiation of treatment such as chemotherapy or radiotherapy. Where this is not possible, it can be given up to two weeks before treatment. If it is not possible to vaccinate beforehand, splenectomy, chemotherapy or radiotherapy should never be delayed.

If it is not practicable to vaccinate two weeks before splenectomy, immunisation should be delayed until at least two weeks after the operation. This is because there is evidence that functional antibody responses may be better from this time (Shatz *et al.*, 1998). If it is not practicable to vaccinate two weeks before the initiation of chemotherapy and/or radiotherapy, immunisation can be delayed until at least three months after completion of therapy in order to maximise the response to the vaccine. Immunisation of these patients should not be delayed if this is likely to result in a failure to vaccinate.

Contraindications

There are very few individuals who cannot receive pneumococcal vaccines. When there is doubt, appropriate advice should be sought from a consultant paediatrician, immunisation co-ordinator or consultant in communicable disease control rather than withholding the vaccine.

The vaccines should not be given to those who have had:

- a confirmed anaphylactic reaction to a previous dose of the vaccines
- a confirmed anaphylactic reaction to any component of the vaccines.

Confirmed anaphylaxis is rare. Other allergic conditions, such as rashes, may occur more commonly and are not contraindications to further immunisation. A careful history of the event will often distinguish between true anaphylaxis and other events that are either not due to the vaccine or not life-threatening. In the latter circumstance, it may be possible to continue the immunisation course. Specialist advice must be sought on the vaccines and the circumstances in which they could be given. The risk to the individual of not being immunised must be taken into account.

Precautions

Minor illnesses without fever or systemic upset are not valid reasons to postpone immunisation. If an individual is acutely unwell, immunisation should be postponed until they have fully recovered. This is to avoid confusing the differential diagnosis of any acute illness by wrongly attributing any signs or symptoms to the adverse effects of the vaccine.

Pregnancy and breast-feeding

Pneumococcal-containing vaccines may be given to pregnant women when the need for protection is required without delay. There is no evidence of risk from vaccinating pregnant women or those who are breast-feeding with inactivated viral or bacterial vaccines or toxoids (Plotkin and Orenstein, 2004).

Premature infants

It is important that premature infants have their immunisation at the appropriate chronological age, according to the recommendation. There is no evidence that premature babies are at an increased risk of adverse reactions from vaccines (Slack *et al.*, 2001).

Immunosuppression and HIV infection

Individuals with immunosuppression and HIV infection (regardless of CD4 count) should be given pneumococcal vaccines in accordance with the recommendations above. These individuals may not make a full antibody response, and so an additional dose of PCV is recommended. Specialist advice may be required.

Studies on the clinical efficacy of PPV in HIV-infected adults have reported inconsistent findings, including one study from the developing world where a higher risk of pneumonia was observed in vaccinees (Watera *et al.*, 2004). Observational studies in developed countries have not confirmed this finding, and most experts believe that the potential benefit of pneumococcal vaccination outweighs the risk in developed countries (USPHS/IDSA, 2001).

Further guidance is provided by the Royal College of Paediatrics and Child Health (www.rcpch.ac.uk), the British HIV Association (BHIVA) *Immunisation guidelines for HIV-infected adults* (BHIVA, 2006) and the Children's HIV Association of UK and Ireland (CHIVA) immunisation guidelines (www.bhiva.org/chiva).

Adverse reactions

PCV

Swelling and redness at the injection site and low grade fever are among the most commonly reported adverse reactions (10–20%) (Black *et al.*, 2000). No increased local or systemic reactions have been reported with repeated doses during the primary series, although a higher rate of transient tenderness has been reported after a fourth dose.

PPV

Mild soreness and induration at the site of injection lasting one to three days and, less commonly, a low grade fever may occur. More severe systemic reactions are infrequent. In general, local and systemic reactions are more common in people with higher concentrations of antibodies to pneumococcal polysaccharides.

Management of cases, contacts and outbreaks

Cases of invasive pneumococcal disease (IPD)

Any case of invasive pneumococcal infection or lobar pneumonia believed to be due to *S. pneumoniae* should prompt a review of the patient's medical history to establish whether they are in a recognised risk group and whether they have been vaccinated. Patients with risk factors who have not previously been vaccinated should be given vaccination on discharge from hospital.

Children under five years of age

All children under five years of age who have had IPD, for example pneumocococcal meningitis or pneumococcal bacteraemia, should be given a dose of PCV irrespective of previous vaccination history. Children under

13 months who are unvaccinated or partially vaccinated should complete the immunisation schedule.

These children should be investigated for immunological risk factors to seek a possible treatable condition predisposing them to pneumococcal infection. If they are found to fall into one of the risk groups in Table 25.1, they should continue vaccination as for other at-risk children (see section on Recommendations for the use of pneumococcal vaccine).

All new cases of IPD in children eligible for routine PCV will be followed up by the Health Protection Agency in England and Wales and Health Protection Scotland. These cases will be offered antibody testing against each of the seven vaccine serotypes and advice on clinical and immunological investigation (see www.hpa.org.uk/infections/topics_az/vaccination/vacc_menu.htm).

Contacts

Close contacts of pneumococcal meningitis or other invasive pneumococcal disease are not normally at an increased risk of pneumococcal infection and therefore antibiotic prophylaxis is not indicated. Clusters of invasive pneumococcal disease should be discussed with local health protection teams.

Outbreaks

Outbreaks of pneumococcal respiratory disease in hospitals and residential care homes need prompt investigation. Control measures including vaccination may be appropriate; these should be agreed in discussion with local health protection or infection control teams.

Supplies

- 7-valent PCV (Prevenar™) is manufactured by Wyeth Vaccines (medical information: 01628 415330). It is supplied by Healthcare Logistics (Tel: 0870 871 1890) as part of the national childhood immunisation programme.

- 23-valent plain PPV (Pneumovax® II) is manufactured by Sanofi Pasteur MSD
(Tel: 0800 085 5511)
(Fax: 0800 085 8958).

In Northern Ireland, supplies should be obtained from local childhood vaccine-holding centres. Details of these are available from the regional pharmaceutical procurement service
(Tel: 028 9055 2368).

A patient card and information sheet for asplenic and hyposplenic patients is available from:
Department of Health Publications
(Tel: 08701 555 455).
(E-mail: dh@prolog.uk.com).

or in Wales from:
Welsh Assembly Publications Centre
(Tel: 029 2082 3683).
(E-mail: assembly-publications@wales.gsi.gov.uk).

or in Scotland from:

Chris Sinclair
Public Health Division 1
Health Department
Scottish Executive
Room 3ES
St Andrew's House
Regent Road
Edinburgh EH1 3DG
(Tel: 0131 244 2241).
(Fax: 0131 244 2157).
E-mail: chris.sinclair@scotland.gsi.gov.uk).

References

American Academy of Pediatrics (2003) Active immunization. In: Pickering LK (ed.) *Red Book: 2003 Report of the Committee on Infectious Diseases*, 26th edition. Elk Grove Village, IL: American Academy of Pediatrics, p 33.

Appelobaum PC (1992) Antimicrobial resistance in *Streptococcus pneumoniae*: an overview. *Clin Infect Dis* **15**: 77–83.

BHIVA (2006) *Immunisation guidelines for HIV-infected adults:* www.bhiva.org/pdf/2006/Immunisation506.pdf.

Bartlett JG and Mundy LM (1995) Community acquired pneumonia. *N Engl J Med* **333**: 1618–24.

Black S, Shinefield H, Fireman B *et al.* (2000) Efficacy, safety, and immunogenicity of heptavalent pneumococcal conjugate vaccine in children. *Pediatr Infect Dis J* **19**: 187–95.

Black S, Shinefield HR, Ling S *et al.* (2002) Effectiveness of heptavalent pneumococcal conjugate vaccine in children younger than five years of age for prevention of pneumonia. *Pediatr Infect Dis J* **21**: 810–15.

Black S *et al.* (2004) Post licensure surveillance for pneumococcal invasive disease after use of heptavalent pneumococcal conjugate vaccine in Northern California Kaiser Permanente. *Pediatr Infect Dis J* **23**: 485–9.

British Committee for Standards in Haematology (2002) Update on guidelines for the prevention and treatment of infection in patients with absent or dysfunctional spleen. *Clin Med* **5**: 440–3 (www.bcshguidelines.com/pdf/SPLEEN21.pdf).

Butler JC, Breiman RF, Campbell JF *et al.* (1993) Pneumococcal polysaccharide vaccine efficacy: an evaluation of current recommendations. *JAMA* **270**: 1826–31.

Butler JC, Dowell SF and Breiman RF (1998) Epidemiology of emerging pneumococcal drug resistance: implications for treatment and prevention. *Vaccine* **16**: 1693–7.

Clinical Haematology Task Force (1996) Guidelines for the prevention and treatment of infection in patients with an absent or dysfunctional spleen. Working Party of the British Committee for Standards in Haematology. *BMJ* **312**: 430–4.

Davies T, Goering RV, Lovgren M *et al.* (1999) Molecular epidemiological survey of penicillin-resistant *Streptococcus pneumoniae* from Asia, Europe, and North America. *Diagn Microbiol Infect Dis* **34**: 7–12.

Diggle L and Deeks J (2000) Effect of needle length on incidence of local reactions to routine immunisation in infants aged 4 months: randomised controlled trial. *BMJ* **321**: 931–3.

Fedson DS (1999) The clinical effectiveness of pneumococcal vaccination: a brief review. *Vaccine* **17**: S85–90.

Fedson DS, Musher DM and Eskola J (1999) Pneumococcal vaccine. In: Plotkin SA and Orenstein WA (eds) *Vaccine,* 3rd edition. Philadelphia: WB Saunders Company.

Fine MJ, Smith MA, Carson CA *et al.* (1994) Efficacy of pneumococcal vaccination in adults: a meta-analysis of randomised controlled trials. *Arch Int Med* **154**: 2666–77.

George AC and Melegaro A (2001) Invasive pneumococcal infection, England and Wales 1999. *Commun Dis Rep CDR Wkly* **11** (21).

George AC and Melegaro A (2003) Invasive pneumococcal infection, England and Wales 2000. *CDR Wkly* 3-9. www.hpa.org.uk

Giebink GS, Le CT, Cosio FG *et al.* (1981) Serum antibody responses of high-risk children and adults to vaccination with capsular polysaccharides of *Streptococcus pneumoniae*. *Rev Infect Dis* **3**:168–78.

Goldblatt D, Southern J, Ashton L *et al.* (2006) Immunogenicity and boosting after a reduced number of doses of a pneumococcal conjugate vaccine in infants and toddlers. *Pediatr Infect Dis J* **25**: 312–9.

Health Protection Agency (2003) Invasive pneumococcal infection, England and Wales: 2000. *CDR Wkly* 2003: 3–9.

Health Protection Agency (2006) www.hpa.org.uk/cfl/sil/pneumococci.htm

Jackson LA, Benson P, Sneller VP *et al.* (1999) Safety of revaccination with pneumococcal polysaccharide vaccine. *JAMA* **281**: 243–8.

Jackson LA, Neuzil KM, Yu O *et al.* (2003) Effectiveness of pneumococcal polysaccharide vaccine in older adults. *N Engl J Med* **348**: 1747–55.

Mangtani P, Cutts F and Hall AJ (2003) Efficacy of polysaccharide pneumococcal vaccine in adults in more developed countries: the state of the evidence. *Lancet Infect Dis* **3**: 71–8.

Mark A, Carlsson RM and Granstrom M (1999) Subcutaneous versus intramuscular injection for booster DT vaccination in adolescents. *Vaccine* **17**: 2067–72.

Melegaro A and Edmunds WJ (2004) The 23-valent pneumococcal polysaccharide vaccine. Part I. Efficacy of PPV in the elderly: a comparison of meta-analyses. *Eur J Epidemiol* **19**: 353–63.

Plotkin SA and Orenstein WA (eds) (2004) *Vaccines*, 4th edition. Philadelphia: WB Saunders Company, Chapter 8.

Reefhuis J, Honein MA, Whitney CG *et al.* (2003) Risk of bacterial meningitis in children with cochlear implants. *N Engl J Med* **349**: 435–45.

Rytel MW, Dailey MP, Schiffman G *et al.* (1986) Pneumococcal vaccine in immunization of patients with renal impairment. *Proc Soc Exp Biol Med* **182**: 468–73.

Shapiro ED, Berg AT, Austrian R *et al.* (1991) The protective efficacy of polyvalent pneumococcal polysaccharide vaccine. *N Engl J Med* **325**: 1453–60.

Shatz DV, Schinsky MF, Pais LB *et al.* (1998) Immune responses of splenectomized trauma patients to the 23-valent pneumococcal polysaccharide vaccine at 1 versus 7 versus 14 days after splenectomy. *J Trauma* **44**: 760–5.

Slack MH, Schapira D, Thwaites RJ *et al.* (2001) Immune response of premature infants to meningococcal serogroup C and combined diphtheria-tetanus toxoids-acellular pertussis-*Haemophilus influenzae* type b conjugate vaccines. *J Infect Dis* **184**(12): 1617–20.

Summerfield AQ, Cirstea SE, Roberts KL *et al.* (2005) Incidence of meningitis and of death from all causes among users of cochlear implants in the United Kingdom. *J Public Health* **27**(1): 55–61.

USPHS/IDSA (2001) Guidelines for the prevention of opportunistic infections in persons infected with human immunodeficiency virus. www.guideline.gov/summary/summary.aspx?doc_id=3080

Watera C, Nakiyingi J, Miiro G *et al.* (2004) 23-valent pneumococcal polysaccharide vaccine in HIV-infected Ugandan adults: 6-year follow-up of a clinical trial cohort. *AIDS* **18**: 1210–3.

Whitney CG, Farley MM, Hadler J *et al.* (2003) Decline in invasive pneumococcal disease after the introduction of protein-polysaccharide conjugate vaccine. *N Engl J Med* **348**(18): 1737–46.

World Health Organization (1999) Pneumococcal vaccines. WHO position paper. *Wkly Epidemiol Rec* **74**: 177–83. www.who.int/wer/pdf/1999/wer7423.pdf

Zuckerman JN (2000) The importance of injecting vaccines into muscle. *BMJ* **321**: 1237–8.

26

Poliomyelitis

NOTIFIABLE

The disease

Poliomyelitis is an acute illness that follows invasion through the gastro intestinal tract by one of the three serotypes of polio virus (serotypes 1, 2 and 3). The virus replicates in the gut and has a high affinity for nervous tissue. Spread occurs by way of the bloodstream to susceptible tissues or by way of retrograde axonal transport to the central nervous system. The infection is most frequently clinically inapparent, or symptoms may range in severity from a fever to aseptic meningitis or paralysis. Headache, gastrointestinal disturbance, malaise and stiffness of the neck and back, with or without paralysis, may occur. The ratio of inapparent to paralytic infections may be as high as 1000 to 1 in children and 75 to 1 in adults, depending on the polio virus type and the social conditions (Sutter *et al.*, 2004).

Transmission is through contact with the faeces or pharyngeal secretions of an infected person. The incubation period ranges from three to 21 days. Polio virus replicates for longer periods and it can be excreted for three to six weeks in faeces and two weeks in saliva (Gelfand *et al.*, 1957). Cases are most infectious immediately before, and one to two weeks after the onset of paralytic disease (Sutter *et al.*, 2004).

When the infection is endemic, the paralytic disease is caused by naturally occurring polio virus – 'wild virus'. The live attenuated vaccine virus retains the potential to revert to a virulent form that can rarely cause paralytic disease. This is called vaccine-associated paralytic polio (VAPP). When wild viruses have been eliminated, VAPP cases can occur rarely where live attenuated vaccines are used.

History and epidemiology of the disease

During the early 1950s, there were epidemics of poliomyelitis infections with as many as 8000 annual notifications of paralytic poliomyelitis in the UK.

Routine immunisation with inactivated poliomyelitis vaccine (IPV – Salk) was introduced in 1956. This was replaced by live attenuated oral polio vaccine (OPV – Sabin) in 1962. The introduction of polio immunisation was

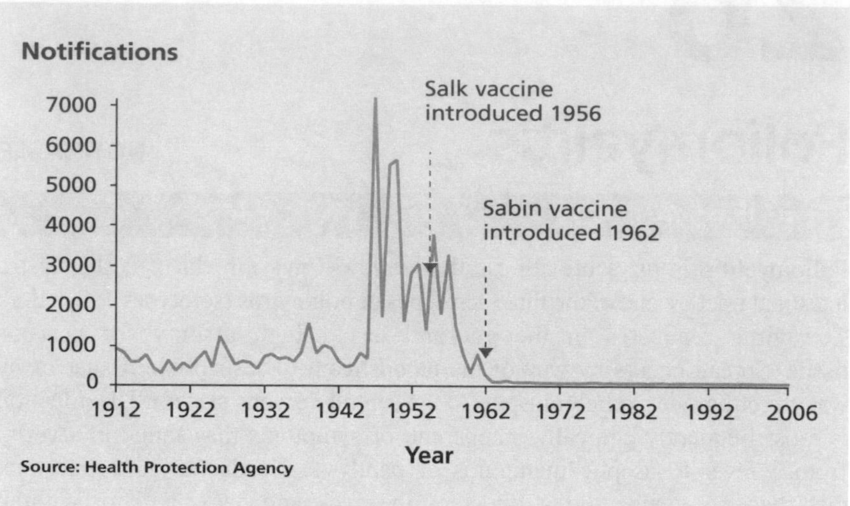

Figure 26.1 Polio notifications in England and Wales (1912–2006)

accompanied by mass campaigns targeted at all individuals aged less than 40 years.

Following the introduction of polio immunisation, cases fell rapidly to very low levels. The last outbreak of indigenous poliomyelitis was in the late 1970s. The last case of natural polio infection acquired in the UK was in 1984. Between 1985 and 2002, a total of 40 cases of paralytic polio were reported in the UK (Figure 26.2). Thirty cases were VAPP; six cases had wild virus infection acquired overseas; and in a further five cases, all occurring before 1993, the source of infection was unknown but wild virus was not detected.

The number of reported cases of polio worldwide fell from 35,251 in 1988 to 677 in 2003 (reported by January 2004) (WHO, 2004a). International commissions have certified that polio virus transmission has been interrupted in three World Health Organization (WHO) regions: the Americas, the Western Pacific and Europe. WHO has included the UK among the countries that are likely to have eliminated indigenous poliomyelitis due to wild virus (WHO, 2004b).

By 2004, poliomyelitis remained endemic in only a small number of developing countries and, therefore, the risk of importation to the UK had fallen to very low levels. Following a resurgence of polio in Nigeria, poliomyelitis was reported during 2005 and 2006 from several countries that

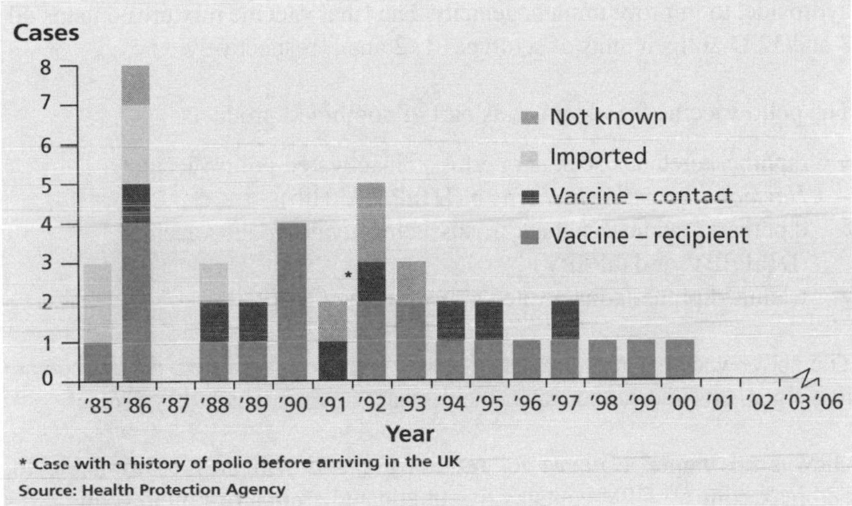

Figure 26.2 Reported cases of paralytic poliomyelitis by aetiology (all sources England and Wales 1985–2006)

have previously been polio-free. In these countries, intensive efforts to interrupt transmission and to establish control are being undertaken, and the risk of importation to the UK is still considered low.

Until 2004, OPV was used for routine immunisation in the UK because of the continuing risk of importation of wild virus. Both OPV and IPV provide excellent individual immunity. In addition, OPV provides community benefit as contacts of recently immunised children could be protected through acquisition of vaccine virus (Ramsay *et al.*, 1994a). OPV also promotes antibody formation in the gut, providing local resistance to subsequent infection with wild poliomyelitis virus. This reduces the frequency of symptomless excretion of wild viruses. The risks of wild polio virus being imported and the benefits of OPV need to be balanced against the risks of VAPP from OPV use and the efficacy of IPV. Since 2004, this balance favours the use of inactivated polio vaccine for routine immunisation in the UK.

The poliomyelitis vaccination

Inactivated polio vaccine (IPV) is made from polio virus strains Mahoney (Salk serotype 1), MEF-1 (Salk serotype 2) and Saukett (Salk serotype 3) grown in Vero cell culture. These components are treated with formaldehyde and then adsorbed onto adjuvants, either aluminium phosphate or aluminium hydroxide, to improve immunogenicity. The final vaccine mixture contains 40, 8 and 32 D-antigen units of serotypes 1, 2 and 3 respectively.

The polio vaccine is only given as part of combined products:

- diphtheria/tetanus/acellular pertussis/inactivated polio vaccine/ *Haemophilus influenzae* type b (DTaP/IPV/Hib)
- diphtheria/tetanus/acellular pertussis/inactivated polio vaccine (DTaP/IPV or dTaP/IPV)
- tetanus/diphtheria/inactivated polio vaccine (Td/IPV).

The above vaccines are thiomersal-free. They are inactivated, do not contain live organisms and cannot cause the diseases against which they protect.

OPV is no longer available for routine use and will only be available for outbreak control. OPV contains live attenuated strains of poliomyelitis virus types 1, 2 and 3 grown in cultures of monkey kidney cells or in human diploid (MRC-5) cells.

Td/IPV vaccine should be used where protection is required against tetanus, diphtheria or polio in order to provide comprehensive, long-term protection against all three diseases.

Storage

Vaccines should be stored in the original packaging at +2˚C to +8˚C and protected from light. All vaccines are sensitive to some extent to heat and cold. Heat speeds up the decline in potency of most vaccines, thus reducing their shelf life. Effectiveness cannot be guaranteed for vaccines unless they have been stored at the correct temperature. Freezing may cause increased reactogenicity and loss of potency for some vaccines. It can also cause hairline cracks in the container, leading to contamination of the contents.

Presentation

Polio vaccine is only available as part of combined products. It is supplied as a cloudy white suspension either in a single dose ampoule or in a pre-filled syringe. The suspension may sediment during storage and should be shaken to distribute the suspension uniformly before administration.

Dosage and schedule

- First dose of 0.5ml of a polio-containing vaccine.
- Second dose of 0.5ml, one month after the first dose.
- Third dose of 0.5ml, one month after the second dose.
- Fourth and fifth doses of 0.5ml should be given at the recommended intervals (see below).

Administration

Vaccines are routinely given intramuscularly into the upper arm or anterolateral thigh. This is to reduce the risk of localised reactions, which are more common when vaccines are given subcutaneously (Mark *et al.*, 1999; Diggle and Deeks, 2000; Zuckerman, 2000). However, for individuals with a bleeding disorder, vaccines should be given by deep subcutaneous injection to reduce the risk of bleeding.

IPV-containing vaccines can be given at the same time as other vaccines such as MMR, MenC and hepatitis B. The vaccines should be given at a separate site, preferably in a different limb. If given in the same limb, they should be given at least 2.5cm apart (American Academy of Pediatrics, 2003). The site at which each vaccine was given should be noted in the patient's records.

Disposal

Equipment used for vaccination, including used vials or ampoules, should be disposed of at the end of a session by sealing in a proper, puncture-resistant 'sharps' box (UN-approved, BS 7320).

Recommendations for the use of the vaccine

The objective of the immunisation programme is to provide a minimum of five doses of a polio-containing vaccine at appropriate intervals for all individuals. In most circumstances, a total of five doses of vaccine at the appropriate intervals are considered to give satisfactory long-term protection.

To fulfil this objective, the appropriate vaccine for each age group is determined also by the need to protect individuals against tetanus, pertussis, Hib and diphtheria.

Primary immunisation

Infants and children under ten years of age

The primary course of polio vaccination consists of three doses of an IPV-containing product with an interval of one month between each dose. DTaP/IPV/Hib is recommended to be given at two, three and four months of age but can be given at any stage from two months up to ten years of age. If the primary course is interrupted it should be resumed but not repeated, allowing an interval of one month between the remaining doses. Those who commenced vaccination with oral polio vaccine can complete the course with IPV-containing vaccines.

Children aged ten years or over, and adults

The primary course of polio vaccination consists of three doses of an IPV-containing product with an interval of one month between each dose. Td/IPV is recommended for all individuals aged ten years or over. If the primary course is interrupted it should be resumed but not repeated, allowing an interval of one month between the remaining doses. Those who commenced vaccination with oral polio vaccine can complete the course with IPV-containing vaccines.

Individuals born before 1962 may not have been immunised or may have received a low-potency polio vaccine; no opportunity should be missed to immunise them. Td/IPV is the appropriate vaccine for such use.

Reinforcing immunisation

Children under ten years should receive the first polio booster combined with diphtheria, tetanus, and pertussis vaccines. The first booster of an IPV-containing vaccine should ideally be given three years after completion of the primary course, normally between three years and four months and five years of age. When primary vaccination has been delayed, this first booster dose may be given at the scheduled visit provided it is one year since the third primary dose. This will re-establish the child on the routine schedule. DTaP/IPV or dTaP/IPV should be used in this age group. Td/IPV should not be used routinely for this purpose in this age group because it does not contain pertussis and has not been shown to give equivalent diphtheria antitoxin response compared with other recommended preparations.

Individuals aged ten years or over who have only had three doses of polio vaccine, of which the last dose was at least five years ago, should receive the first IPV booster combined with diphtheria and tetanus vaccines (Td/IPV).

The second booster dose of Td/IPV should be given to all individuals ideally ten years after the first booster dose. Where the previous doses have been delayed, the second booster should be given at the school session or scheduled appointment provided a minimum of five years have lapsed between the first and second boosters. This will be the last scheduled opportunity to ensure long-term protection.

If a person attends for a routine booster dose and has a history of receiving a vaccine following a tetanus-prone wound, attempts should be made to identify which vaccine was given. If the vaccine given at the time of the injury was the same as that due at the current visit and was given after an appropriate interval, then the routine booster dose is not required. Otherwise, the dose given at the time of injury should be discounted as it may not provide long-term protection against all antigens, and the scheduled immunisation should be given. Such additional doses are unlikely to produce an unacceptable rate of reactions (Ramsay *et al.*, 1997).

Vaccination of children with unknown or incomplete immunisation status

Where a child born in the UK presents with an inadequate immunisation history, every effort should be made to clarify what immunisations they may have had (see Chapter 11). A child who has not completed the primary course should have the outstanding doses at monthly intervals. Children may receive the first booster dose as early as one year after the third primary dose to re-establish them on the routine schedule. The second booster should be given at the time of leaving school to ensure long-term protection by this time. Wherever possible a minimum of five years should be left between the first and second boosters.

Children coming to the UK who have a history of completing immunisation in their country of origin may not have been offered protection against all the antigens currently used in the UK. They will probably have received polio-containing vaccines in their country of origin (www-nt.who.int/immunization_monitoring/en/globalsummary/countryprofileselect.cfm).

Children coming from developing countries, from areas of conflict or from hard-to-reach population groups may not have been fully immunised. Where there is no reliable history of previous immunisation, it should be assumed that they are unimmunised and the full UK recommendations should be followed (see Chapter 11).

Children coming to the UK may have had a fourth dose of a polio-containing vaccine that is given at around 18 months in some countries. This dose should be discounted as it may not provide satisfactory protection until the time of the teenage booster. The routine pre-school and subsequent boosters should be given according to the UK schedule.

Travellers and those going to reside abroad

All travellers to epidemic or endemic areas should ensure that they are fully immunised according to the UK schedule (see above). Additional doses of vaccines may be required according to the destination and the nature of travel intended (see Department of Health, 2001). Where tetanus, diphtheria or polio protection is required and the final dose of the relevant antigen was received more than ten years ago, Td/IPV should be given.

Polio vaccination in laboratory and healthcare workers

Individuals who may be exposed to polio in the course of their work, in microbiology laboratories and clinical infectious disease units, are at risk and must be protected (see Chapter 12).

Contraindications

There are very few individuals who cannot receive IPV-containing vaccines. When there is doubt, appropriate advice should be sought from a consultant paediatrician, immunisation co-ordinator or consultant in communicable disease control rather than withholding the vaccine.

The vaccines should not be given to those who have had:

- a confirmed anaphylactic reaction to a previous dose of IPV-containing vaccine, or
- a confirmed anaphylactic reaction to neomycin, streptomycin or polymyxin B (which may be present in trace amounts).

Confirmed anaphylaxis occurs extremely rarely. Data from the UK, Canada and the US point to rates of 0.65 to 3 anaphylaxis events per million doses of vaccine given (Bohlke *et al.*, 2003; Canadian Medical Association, 2002). Other allergic conditions may occur more commonly and are not contraindications to further immunisation. A careful history of the event will often distinguish between anaphylaxis and other events that either are not due to the vaccine or are not life-threatening. In the latter circumstance, it may be possible to continue the immunisation course. Specialist advice must be sought on the vaccines and circumstances in which they could be given. The risk to the individual of not being immunised must be taken into account.

Precautions

Minor illnesses without fever or systemic upset are not valid reasons to postpone immunisation.

If an individual is acutely unwell, immunisation should be postponed until they have fully recovered. This is to avoid confusing the differential diagnosis of any acute illness by wrongly attributing any sign or symptoms to the adverse effects of the vaccine.

Systemic and local reactions following a previous immunisation

This section gives advice on the immunisation of children with a history of a severe or mild systemic or local reaction within 72 hours of receiving a preceding vaccine. Immunisation with IPV-containing vaccine should continue following a history of:

- fever, irrespective of its severity
- hypotonic-hyporesponsive episodes (HHE)
- persistent crying or screaming for more than three hours
- severe local reaction, irrespective of extent.

In Canada, a severe general or local reaction to DTaP/IPV/Hib is not a contraindication to further doses of the vaccine (Canadian Medical Association, 1998). Adverse events after childhood immunisation are carefully monitored in Canada (Le Saux *et al.*, 2003), and experience there suggests that further doses were not associated with recurrence or worsening of the preceding events (S Halperin and R Pless, pers comm, 2003).

Pregnancy and breast-feeding

IPV-containing vaccines may be given to pregnant women when protection is required without delay. There is no evidence of risk from vaccinating pregnant women or those who are breast-feeding with inactivated virus or bacterial vaccines or toxoids (Plotkin and Orenstein, 2004).

Premature infants

It is important that premature infants have their immunisations at the appropriate chronological age, according to the schedule. There is no evidence that premature babies are at an increased risk of adverse reactions from vaccines (Slack *et al.*, 2001).

Immunosuppression and HIV infection

Individuals with immunosuppression and HIV infection (regardless of CD4 count) should be given IPV-containing vaccines in accordance with the recommendations above. These individuals may not make a full antibody response. Re-immunisation should be considered after treatment is finished and recovery has occurred. Specialist advice may be required.

Further guidance is provided by the Royal College of Paediatrics and Child Health (www.rcpch.ac.uk), the British HIV Association (BHIVA) *Immunisation guidelines for HIV-infected adults* (BHIVA, 2006) and the Children's HIV Association of UK and Ireland (CHIVA) immunisation guidelines (www.bhiva.org/chiva).

Neurological conditions

Pre-existing neurological conditions

The presence of a neurological condition is not a contraindication to immunisation. Where there is evidence of a neurological condition in a child, the advice given in the flow chart in Figure 26.3 should be followed.

If a child has a stable, pre-existing neurological abnormality such as spina bifida, congenital abnormality of the brain or perinatal hypoxic ischaemic encephalopathy, they should be immunised according to the recommended schedule. When there has been a documented history of cerebral damage in the neonatal period, immunisation should be carried out unless there is evidence of an evolving neurological abnormality.

If there is evidence of current neurological deterioration, including poorly controlled epilepsy, immunisation should be deferred and the child should be referred to a child specialist for investigation to see if an underlying cause can be identified. If a cause is not identified, immunisation should be deferred until the condition has stabilised. If a cause is identified, immunisation should proceed as normal.

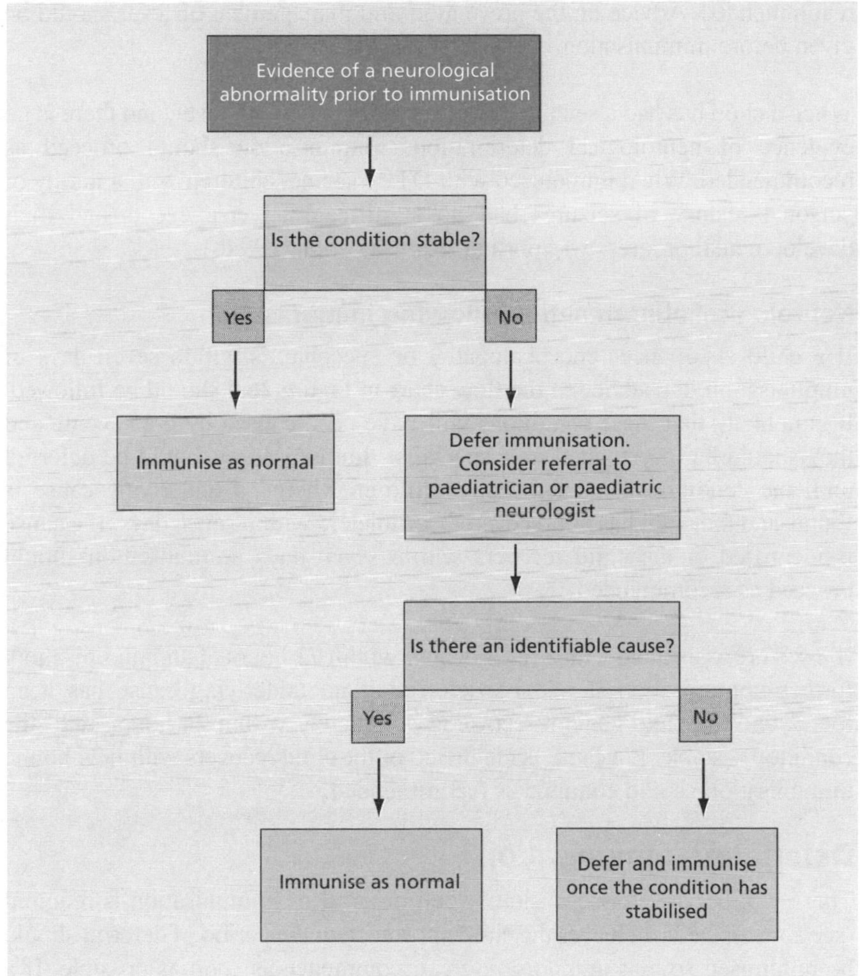

Figure 26.3 Flow chart for evidence of a neurological condition before immunisation

A family history of seizures is not a contraindication to immunisation. When there is a personal or family history of febrile seizures, there is an increased risk of these occurring after any fever, including that caused by immunisation. Seizures associated with fever are rare in the first six months of life and most common in the second year of life. After this age the frequency falls and they are rare after five years of age.

When a child has had a seizure associated with fever in the past, with no evidence of neurological deterioration, immunisation should proceed as recommended. Advice on the prevention and management of fever should be given before immunisation.

When a child has had a seizure that is not associated with fever, and there is no evidence of neurological deterioration, immunisation should proceed as recommended. When immunised with DTP vaccine, children with a family or personal history of seizures had no significant adverse events and their developmental progress was normal (Ramsay *et al.*, 1994b).

Neurological abnormalities following immunisation

If a child experiences encephalopathy or encephalitis within seven days of immunisation, the advice in the flow chart in Figure 26.4 should be followed. It is unlikely that these conditions will have been caused by the vaccine and they should be investigated by a specialist. Immunisation should be deferred until the condition has stabilised in children where no underlying cause is found, and the child has not recovered completely within seven days. If a cause is identified or the child recovers within seven days, immunisation should proceed as recommended.

If a seizure associated with a fever occurs within 72 hours of an immunisation, further immunisation should be deferred if no underlying cause has been found, and the child has not recovered completely within 24 hours, until the condition is stable. If a cause is identified or the child recovers within 24 hours, immunisation should continue as recommended.

Deferral of immunisation

There will be very few occasions when deferral of immunisation is required (see above). Deferral leaves the child unprotected; the period of deferral should be minimised so that immunisation can commence as soon as possible. If a specialist recommends deferral this should be clearly communicated to the general practitioner, who must be informed as soon as the child is fit for immunisation.

Adverse reactions

Pain, swelling or redness at the injection site are common and may occur more frequently following subsequent doses. A small, painless nodule may form at the injection site; this usually disappears and is of no consequence. The incidence of local reactions is lower with tetanus vaccines combined with acellular pertussis vaccines than with whole-cell pertussis vaccines and is similar to that after DT vaccine (Miller, 1999; Tozzi and Olin, 1997).

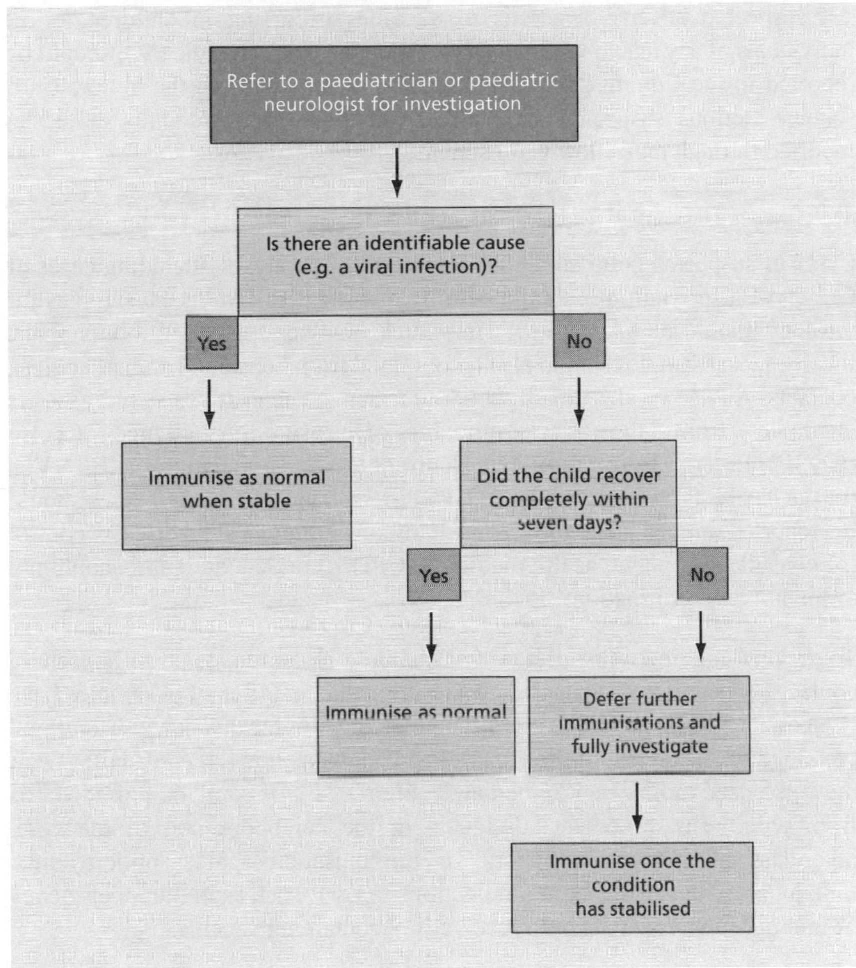

Figure 26.4 Flow chart for encephalitis or encephalopathy occurring within seven days of immunisation

Fever, convulsions, high-pitched screaming and episodes of pallor, cyanosis and limpness (HHE) occur with equal frequency after both DTaP and DT vaccines (Tozzi and Olin, 1997).

Confirmed anaphylaxis occurs extremely rarely. Data from the UK, Canada and the US point to rates of 0.65 to 3 anaphylaxis events per million doses of vaccine given (Bohlke *et al.*, 2003; Canadian Medical Association, 2002). Other allergic conditions may occur more commonly and are not contraindications to further immunisation.

All suspected adverse reactions to vaccines occurring in children, or in individuals of any age to vaccines labelled with a black triangle (▼), should be reported to the Commission on Human Medicines through the Yellow Card scheme. Serious, suspected adverse reactions to vaccines in adults should be reported through the Yellow Card scheme.

Management of suspected cases and outbreaks

Cases of suspected polio and other acute flaccid paralyses, including cases of Guillain-Barré syndrome, should be fully investigated. Two faecal samples for virology should be taken in the first week of illness, 24 to 48 hours apart. Ideally, faecal samples should also be obtained from household and other close contacts. Advice on the investigation and management of suspected cases is available from the Communicable Disease Surveillance Centre (CDSC)/Enteric, Respiratory and Neurological Virus Laboratory (ERNVL) (or the Health Protection Scotland (HPS) in Scotland). Suspected cases should be reported immediately to a consultant in communicable disease control (or consultant of public health medicine (CPHM) in Scotland) and should not await culture confirmation.

To prevent ongoing transmission, OPV should be administered to household contacts of people with suspected polio immediately (after stool samples have been obtained). A stock of OPV is retained centrally for this purpose, and will be issued on the advice of the Health Protection Agency (HPA) or HPS. OPV may also need to be given immediately, after a case of paralytic poliomyelitis from wild virus, to other individuals in the neighbourhood of the case, regardless of a previous history of immunisation against poliomyelitis. Individuals with genuine contraindications to OPV, such as immunodeficiency or immunosuppression, should receive IPV-containing vaccine.

Appropriate control measures should be instituted in discussion with ERNVL (HPS in Scotland) and will depend upon the nature of the case and the likely vaccine coverage in the locality.

Maintaining polio-free status

Continued demonstration of the adequacy of clinical surveillance in the UK is required by WHO. Information on all suspected cases of polio is therefore being collated by CDSC and HPS for the UK Eradication Panel.

Supplies

- Pediacel (diphtheria/tetanus/5-component acellular pertussis/ inactivated polio vaccine/*Haemophilus influenzae* type b (DTaP/IPV/Hib) – manufactured by Sanofi Pasteur MSD.
- Repevax (diphtheria/tetanus/5-component acellular pertussis/inactivated polio vaccine (dTaP/IPV)) – manufactured by Sanofi Pasteur MSD.
- Infanrix IPV (diphtheria/tetanus/3-component acellular pertussis/ inactivated polio vaccine (DTaP/IPV)) – manufactured by GlaxoSmithKline.
- Revaxis (diphtheria/tetanus/inactivated polio vaccine (Td/IPV)) – manufactured by Sanofi Pasteur MSD.

These vaccines are supplied by Healthcare Logistics (Tel: 0870 871 1890) as part of the national childhood immunisation programme.

In Scotland, supplies should be obtained from local childhood vaccine holding centres. Details of these are available from Scottish Healthcare Supplies (Tel: 0141 282 2240).

In Northern Ireland, supplies should be obtained from local childhood vaccine holding centres. Details of these are available from the regional pharmaceutical procurement service (Tel: 02890 552368).

References

American Academy of Pediatrics (2003) Active immunization. In: Pickering LK (ed.) *Red Book: 2003 Report of the Committee on Infectious Diseases*, 26th edition. Elk Grove Village, IL: American Academy of Pediatrics, p 33.

Bohlke K, Davis RL, Marcy SH *et al.* (2003) Risk of anaphylaxis after vaccination of children and adolescents. *Pediatrics* **112**: 815–20.

British HIV Association (2006) *Immunisation guidelines for HIV-infected adults:* www.bhiva.org/pdf/2006/Immunisation506.pdf.

Canadian Medical Association (1998) Pertussis vaccine. In *Canadian Immunisation Guide*, 5th edition. Canadian Medical Association, p 133.

Canadian Medical Association (2002) General considerations. In *Canadian Immunisation Guide*, 6th edition. Canadian Medical Association, p 14.

Department of Health (2001) *Health information for overseas travel*, 2nd edition. London: TSO.

Diggle L and Deeks J (2000) Effect of needle length on incidence of local reactions to routine immunisation in infants aged 4 months: randomised controlled trial. *BMJ* **321**: 931–3.

Gelfand HM, LeBlanc DR, Fox JP and Conwell DP (1957) Studies on the development of natural immunity to poliomyelitis in Louisiana II. Description and analysis of episodes of infection observed in study households. *Am J Hyg* **65**: 367– 85.

Le Saux N, Barrowman NJ, Moore DL *et al.* (2003) Canadian Paediatric Society/Health Canada Immunization Monitoring Program – Active (IMPACT). Decrease in hospital admissions for febrile seizures and reports of hypotonic-hyporesponsive episodes presenting to hospital emergency departments since switching to acellular pertussis vaccine in Canada: a report from IMPACT. *Pediatrics* **112**(5): e348.

Mark A, Carlsson RM and Granstrom M (1999) Subcutaneous versus intramuscular injection for booster DT vaccination in adolescents. *Vaccine* **17**: 2067–72

Miller E (1999) Overview of recent clinical trials of acellular pertussis vaccines. *Biologicals* **27**: 79–86.

Plotkin SA and Orenstein WA (eds) (2004) *Vaccines* 4th edition. Philadelphia: WB Saunders Company, Chapter 8.

Ramsay ME, Begg NT, Ghandi J and Brown D (1994a) Antibody response and viral excretion after live polio vaccine or a combined schedule of live and inactivated polio vaccines. *Pediatr Infect Dis J* **13**: 1117–21.

Ramsay M, Begg N, Holland B and Dalphinis J (1994b) Pertussis immunisation in children with a family or personal history of convulsions: a review of children referred for specialist advice. *Health Trends* **26**: 23–4.

Ramsay M, Joce R and Whalley J (1997) Adverse events after school leavers received combined tetanus and low dose diphtheria vaccine. *CDR Review* **5**: R65–7.

Slack MH, Schapira D, Thwaites RJ *et al.* (2001) Immune response of premature infants to meningococcal serogroup C and combined diphtheria-tetanus toxoids-acellular pertussis-*Haemophilus influenzae* type b conjugate vaccines. *J Infect Dis* **184**(12): 1617–20.

Sutter RW, Cochi S and Melnick JL (2004) Live attenuated polio virus vaccines. In: Plotkin SA and Orenstein WA (eds) *Vaccines*, 4th edition. Philadelphia: WB Saunders Company.

Tozzi AE and Olin P (1997) Common side effects in the Italian and Stockholm 1 Trials. *Dev Biol Stand* **89**: 105–8.

WHO (2004a)
www.polioeradication.org/casecount.asp (accessed October 2006).

WHO (2004b) *Polio News*, Issue 16, September 2002, p 1.
www.who.int/vaccines-documents/DocsPDF02/polio16.pdf (accessed 10 February 2004)

Zuckerman J N (2000) The importance of injecting vaccines into muscle. *BMJ* **321**: 1237–8.

27

Rabies

NOTIFIABLE

The disease

Rabies is an acute viral encephalomyelitis caused by members of the lyssavirus genus. The disease may be caused by rabies virus genotype 1 (classical rabies) or less commonly by rabies-related lyssaviruses. The presentations are clinically indistinguishable. Rabies-related lyssaviruses implicated in human disease include European bat lyssaviruses (EBLVs) and Australian bat lyssavirus (ABLV).

Infection is usually via the bite or scratch of a rabid animal, most frequently a dog. In some parts of the world, other animals such as bats, cats and monkeys are important sources of exposure. In parts of Europe (including the UK) EBLV-1 and EBLV-2 are found in insectivorous bats and have occasionally caused human disease.

On rare occasions, transmission of the virus has occurred through body fluids from an infectious animal coming into contact with an individual's mucous membranes. Exposure through mucous membranes has a low probability of infection but must be managed as a significant event. Infection does not occur through intact skin. Virus is present in some tissues and fluids of humans with rabies, but person-to-person spread of the disease has not been documented other than in exceptional circumstances. Cases have occurred rarely outside the UK through corneal grafts and other transplanted tissues taken from individuals with rabies.

The incubation period is generally between three and 12 weeks, but may range from four days to 19 years. In more than 93% of patients, the onset is within one year of exposure. The onset of illness is insidious. Early symptoms may include paraesthesiae around the site of the wound, fever, headache and malaise. The disease may then present with hydrophobia, hallucinations and maniacal behaviour progressing to paralysis and coma, or as an ascending flaccid paralysis and sensory disturbance. Rabies is almost always fatal, death resulting from respiratory paralysis. There is no specific treatment other than supportive care once clinical symptoms develop.

History and epidemiology of the disease

Rabies in animals occurs in all continents except Antarctica, although individual countries are reported to be rabies-free. In the US, classical rabies virus in animals has become more prevalent since the 1950s; skunks, raccoons and bats account for 85% of animal cases. In Asia, Africa, Central and South America, rabies (classical rabies virus, genotype 1) is endemic in feral dogs. In Mexico and Central and South America, vampire bats carry the classical rabies virus. Some countries that are declared rabies-free have rabies-related viruses in their bat populations, for example Australia and the UK. In the UK, rabies-related viruses have only been detected in Daubenton's bats. The virus has never been detected in the commonest bat species, the pipistrelles. In other parts of Europe and in Australia, other bat species have been affected.

During the twentieth century, rabies in wildlife has spread through parts of Central and Western Europe. Foxes have been the main host, but many other animals have also been infected, particularly dogs and cats. The incidence of endemic, fox-adapted rabies in Western Europe fell dramatically in the last years of the twentieth century. This has been largely due to the vaccination of wild and domestic animals. Rabies continues to be reported in domestic animals imported from non-rabies-free countries. Rabies remains prevalent in Eastern Europe and Turkey.

In humans, between 40,000 and 70,000 cases of rabies occur each year worldwide (World Health Organization, 2001). Most cases are in developing countries, particularly India (Plotkin and Orenstein, 2004). In the UK, deaths from classical rabies continue to occur in people infected abroad. Such instances are, however, rare, with 24 deaths having been reported since 1902. None had received appropriate post-exposure prophylaxis. A considerable number of people present for medical advice on their return to the UK with a history of exposure to an animal abroad. In 2000, 295 such people received prophylaxis in England and Wales (Hossain *et al.*, 2004).

No case of indigenous human rabies from animals other than bats has been reported in the UK since 1902. In 2002, a man died from rabies caused by EBLV-2 acquired in the UK from a bat (Fooks *et al.*, 2003). Only three other cases of EBLV infection (all fatal) have been reported in the past 30 years in Europe (Nathwani *et al.*, 2003).

The rabies vaccination

There are currently two rabies vaccines licensed for use in the UK – human diploid cell vaccine (HDCV) (Rabies Vaccine BP Pasteur Merieux) and purified chick embryo cell rabies vaccine (PCEC) (Rabipur®). Other cell-culture-derived vaccines are available in other countries and include rabies vaccine viruses grown in Vero cells.

The vaccines available in the UK are thiomersal-free. The vaccines are inactivated, do not contain live organisms and cannot cause the disease against which they protect.

HDCV is a freeze-dried suspension of Wistar rabies virus strain PM/WI 38 1503-3M cultured in human diploid cells and inactivated by betapropiolactone. The potency of the reconstituted vaccine is not less than 2.5IU per 1.0ml dose. It contains traces of neomycin, and human albumin is used as an excipient. The PCEC rabies vaccine is a freeze-dried suspension of the Flury LEP-25 rabies virus strain cultured in chick embryo cells and inactivated with beta-propiolactone. The potency of the reconstituted vaccine is not less than 2.5IU per 1.0ml dose. It contains traces of amphotericin B, chlortetracycline and neomycin.

These vaccines may be used interchangeably to provide protection pre- or post-exposure.

Storage

Vaccines should be stored in the original packaging at +2˚C to +8˚C and protected from light. All vaccines are sensitive to some extent to heat and cold. Heat speeds up the decline in potency of most vaccines, thus reducing their shelf life. Effectiveness cannot be guaranteed for vaccines unless they have been stored at the correct temperature. Freezing may cause increased reactogenicity and loss of potency for some vaccines. It can also cause hairline cracks in the container, leading to contamination of the contents.

Presentation

Rabies vaccines are white, lyophilised powder for reconstitution with the clear and colourless diluent supplied. The vaccines should only be reconstituted with the diluent supplied. On reconstitution Rabipur is a clear, colourless solution, and Rabies Vaccine BP is a pinkish-coloured solution.

They should be used immediately and no later than one hour after reconstitution with the diluent supplied.

Human rabies immunoglobulin (HRIG) should be stored in a refrigerator between +2°C and +8°C. These products are tolerant to ambient temperatures for up to one week. They can be distributed in sturdy packaging outside the cold chain if needed.

Dosage and schedule

For primary pre-exposure immunisation, three doses of 1.0ml of rabies vaccine should be given on days 0, 7 and 28. The third dose can be given from day 21 if there is insufficient time before travel.

Administration

Vaccines are routinely given intramuscularly into the upper arm or anterolateral thigh. However, for individuals with a bleeding disorder, vaccines should be given by deep subcutaneous injection to reduce the risk of bleeding.

The Joint Committee on Vaccination and Immunisation recommends the intramuscular rather than the intradermal route for rabies vaccine. The use of the intradermal route is not covered by the manufacturers' product licence and, if it is used, this is at the doctor's own responsibility.

Rabies vaccines can be given at the same time as other vaccines, including other travel vaccines. The vaccines should be given at separate sites, preferably in different limbs. If given in the same limb, they should be given at least 2.5cm apart (American Academy of Pediatrics, 2003). The site at which each vaccine was given should be noted in the individual's records. The vaccinee must keep a record of the vaccine and regimen received as it will influence future treatment.

Disposal

Equipment used for vaccination, including used vials or ampoules, should be disposed of at the end of a session by sealing in a proper, puncture-resistant 'sharps' box (UN-approved, BS 7320).

Rabies-specific immunoglobulin

HRIG is obtained from the plasma of immunised and screened human donors. Donors are selected from countries where there are no known cases of vCJD, and their plasma is comprehensively deactivated. HRIG is used after exposure to rabies to give rapid protection until rabies vaccine, which should be given at the same time at a separate site, becomes effective.

Administration

When indicated for post-exposure prophylaxis (see below), HRIG 20IU/kg body weight should be infiltrated in and around the cleansed wound. If infiltration of the whole volume is not possible or the wound is healed or not visible, any remaining HRIG should be given intramuscularly in the anterolateral thigh (not gluteal region), remote from the vaccination site. If vaccine is given but HRIG treatment is delayed, HRIG should still be given up to seven days after starting the course of vaccine.

Disposal

HRIG is for single use and any unused solution should be disposed of by incineration at a suitably approved facility.

Recommendations for use of the vaccine

The aim of the rabies immunisation programme is to protect those who are at most risk of exposure to rabies.

Pre-exposure (prophylactic) immunisation

Pre-exposure immunisation with rabies vaccine should be offered to:

- laboratory workers handling the virus
- those who, in the course of their work, regularly handle imported animals, for example:
  - at animal quarantine centres
  - at zoos
  - at research and acclimatisation centres where primates and other imported animals are housed
  - at ports, e.g. certain HM Revenue and Customs officers
  - at the premises of carrying agents authorised to carry imported animals
- veterinary and technical staff in the State Veterinary Service; the Department for Environment, Food and Rural Affairs; the Scottish Executive Environment and Rural Affairs Department; the Welsh Assembly Government Environment, Planning and Countryside Department; and the Northern Ireland Department of Agriculture and Rural Development
- inspectors appointed by local authorities under the Animal Health Act (2002). This only includes those local authority dog wardens who are also inspectors. Other dog wardens have a low risk of exposure, and post-exposure prophylaxis in the event of an incident is appropriate

- people who regularly handle bats in the UK
- those working abroad (e.g. veterinary staff or zoologists) who by the nature of their work are at risk of contact with rabid animals
- health workers who are about to be at risk of direct exposure to body fluids or other tissue from a patient with probable or confirmed rabies.

Pre-exposure immunisation is also recommended for some travellers, including:

- those living in or travelling for more than one month to rabies-enzootic areas, unless there is reliable access to prompt, safe medical care (see below)
- those travelling for less than one month to enzootic areas but who may be exposed to rabies because of their travel activities, or those who would have limited access to post-exposure medical care.

Further information is available from the National Travel Health Network and Centre (www.nathnac.org.uk) and, in Scotland, from Health Protection Scotland (www.hps.scot.nhs.uk). Country-by-country advice is also contained in *Health information for overseas travel* (Department of Health, 2001). All travellers to enzootic areas should also be informed by their medical advisers of the practical steps to be taken if they are bitten by an animal or have some other types of exposure which puts them at risk of rabies.

A risk assessment should be undertaken when considering immunisation for children less than one year of age.

Reinforcing doses

For those at regular and continuous risk, a single reinforcing dose of vaccine should be given one year after the primary course has been completed. Further doses should be given at three- to five-year intervals thereafter. For those at intermittent risk or who are travelling again to rabies-enzootic areas without ready access to safe, medical care, a booster dose should be given, from two years after the primary course has been completed.

Serological testing is advised only for those who work with the live viruses. Such individuals should have their antibodies tested every three to six months, and be given reinforcing doses of vaccine as necessary to maintain their immune status. The World Health Organization (WHO) currently considers a minimal acceptable antibody titre to be 0.5IU/ml.

Post-exposure management

Post-exposure management normally consists of wound treatment and risk assessment for appropriate immunisation. Treatment and immunisation after a possible rabies exposure will depend on the circumstances of the exposure, including the local incidence of rabies in the species involved and the immune status of the person.

Wound treatment

As soon as possible after the incident, the wound or site of exposure (e.g. mucous membrane) should be cleaned by thorough flushing under a running tap for several minutes and washing with soap or detergent and water. A suitable disinfectant should be applied and the wound covered with a simple dressing.

Suitable disinfectants include 40 to 70% alcohol, tincture or aqueous solution of povidone-iodine, or quaternary ammonium compounds, for example cetrimide solution 0.15%.

Primary suture could cause further damage to the wound and may increase the risk of introduction of rabies virus to the nerves. It should be avoided or postponed.

Risk assessment

Each case requires a full, expert risk assessment based on the information outlined below. Advice on the assessment of the risk and appropriate management should be obtained from the Health Protection Agency (HPA) Centre for Infection, Colindale, London (Tel: 020 8200 6868); in Scotland from Health Protection Scotland (Tel: 0141 300 1100); and in Northern Ireland from the Public Health Laboratory, Belfast City Hospital (Tel: 028 9032 9241).

As much as possible of the following information must be collected:

The site and severity of the wound

High-risk exposures are those with broken skin, including single or multiple transdermal bites or scratches, or where mucous membranes or an existing skin lesion have been contaminated by the animal's saliva or other body fluid. Intact skin is a barrier against infection. Bites represent a higher risk than scratches. Proximal bites (e.g. face, fingers) represent a higher risk than distal wounds. Bat bites and scratches may not be visible.

The circumstances of the bite (or other contact)

An unprovoked attack carries a higher risk than one that is provoked.

The species, behaviour and appearance of the animal

A frantic or paralysed dog or cat represents a high risk of infection. The name and address of the owner of the animal should be obtained, if possible. The dog or cat should be observed for 15 days to see if it begins to behave abnormally; the relevant period is not known for animals other than cats and dogs. If the dog or cat is feral or stray and observation is impossible, try to contact a local doctor or veterinarian who may know whether rabies occurs in the locality. Bat rabies may be suspected if the bat is sick or grounded without injury, or if an uninjured bat is found dead. Apparently healthy bats may have rabies.

The vaccination status of the animal

A regularly vaccinated animal is unlikely to be rabid but, rarely, vaccinated dogs have transmitted rabies.

The origin of the animal, the location of the incident and the incidence of rabies in that species

It is important to know whether the implicated animal is indigenous to that locality or originates elsewhere, and to ascertain the incidence of rabies in the originating area. If necessary, the assistance of local veterinary officials should be sought or advice should be taken from a local doctor.

Terrestrial animals (not bats)

The risk of rabies by country and territory, as of the time of writing, is provided below. This list covers all popular destinations but is not exhaustive and may become out of date. For updated information on rabies by country, see WHO's *Rabies Bulletin Europe* (www.who-rabies-bulletin.org), or the epidemiology website of the Centers for Disease Control and Prevention (CDC), USA (www.cdc.gov/ncidod/dvrd/rabies/epidemiology/epidemiology.htm).

- **No risk**: Animals originating from the following countries and territories are considered to pose 'no risk' of rabies (free of terrestrial rabies):
    - **Europe**: Belgium, Cyprus, Denmark, Faroe Islands, Finland, France, Gibraltar, Greece, Iceland, Ireland, Italy (except the northern and eastern border regions), Luxembourg, Malta, the Netherlands, Norway (mainland), Portugal, Spain (mainland, excluding North African coast territories) and the Canary Islands, Sweden and the UK.

  - **Americas**: Anguilla, Antigua and Barbuda, Bahamas, Barbados, Bermuda, the British Virgin Islands, the Cayman Islands, Dominica, the French Antilles, Guadaloupe, Jamaica, Martinique, Montserrat, Netherlands Antilles, St Christopher and Nevis, St Lucia, St Martin, St Pierre and Miquelon, St Vincent and the Grenadines, the Turks and Caicos Islands, the Virgin Islands and Uruguay
  - **Asia**: Bahrain, Brunei Darussalam, Hong Kong, Japan, Kuwait, the Maldives, Qatar, Singapore, Taiwan and the United Arab Emirates
  - **Oceania**: American Samoa, Australia, the Cook Islands, Federated States of Micronesia, Fiji, French Polynesia, Guam, Kiribati, the Marshall Islands, New Caledonia, New Zealand, Niue, the Northern Mariana Islands, Palau, Papua New Guinea, Samoa, Sao Tome and Principe, the Solomon Islands, Tonga, Vanuatu and Western Samoa.
- **Low risk**: Animals originating from the following countries and territories are considered to pose a 'low risk' of rabies:
  - **Europe**: Austria, Bulgaria, the Czech Republic, Germany and Switzerland
  - **Americas**: Canada, USA (CDC, Atlanta provides information on the risk of rabies in different parts of the USA).
- **High risk**: Animals originating from the following countries, where terrestrial rabies is enzootic, are considered 'high risk':
  - Colombia, Cuba, the Dominican Republic, Ecuador, El Salvador, Guatemala, India, parts of Mexico, Nepal, Pakistan, Peru, Philippines, Sri Lanka, Thailand, Turkey and Vietnam.

Countries in Asia, Africa and South America not otherwise mentioned as 'no risk' or 'low risk' should be considered as 'high risk'.

Bats

Both classical rabies virus and rabies-related lyssaviruses may be acquired from bats depending on the species and origin. Information on the local epidemiology of rabies in bats should be sought.

Following a case of EBLV infection in a bat handler in the UK, bat exposures are an increasing cause for concern. Assessment of the risk from a possible bat contact is more difficult than for a terrestrial animal. Transmission of EBLV can occur in the absence of a recognised contact (e.g. waking to find a bat in the room). Information that is required for an accurate risk assessment includes:

- the nature of the contact, e.g. a definite bite or scratch, handling or touching, or a possible unrecognised exposure
- origin and condition of the bat, e.g. species and behaviour of the bat. If the species of the bat is unknown, then size and location may help to determine the most likely type. If the bat is available, urgent testing can be arranged
- severity and site of the wound.

Advice should be sought from the HPA, Virus Reference Department, Colindale, London (Tel: 020 8200 4400) or Communicable Disease Surveillance Centre (Tel: 020 8200 6868) in England and Wales; Health Protection Scotland (Tel: 0141 300 1100) in Scotland; or the Public Health Laboratory, Belfast City Hospital (Tel: 028 9032 9241) in Northern Ireland.

Post-exposure immunisation and immunoglobulin

Treatment, including cleaning the wound as above, must not be delayed, and should be started as soon as possible while enquiries are made about the local epidemiology of rabies in the country concerned (see above) and, where possible, the ownership and condition of the biting animal.

As the incubation period for rabies can be prolonged, treatment should still be considered even if the interval from exposure is lengthy. Specialist advice should be sought (as above).

Contraindications

Pre-exposure rabies vaccine should not be given to those who have had:

- a confirmed anaphylactic reaction to a previous dose of rabies vaccine, or
- a confirmed anaphylactic reaction to any component of the vaccine.

There are no absolute contraindications to post-exposure rabies vaccine. In the event of a hypersensitivity reaction to a dose of a pre-exposure course, such individuals should still receive post-exposure vaccination if indicated, because the risks of rabies outweigh the risks of hypersensitivity. When a hypersensitivity reaction occurs during post-exposure immunisation, further doses should be given under close medical supervision.

Precautions

Minor illnesses without fever or systemic upset are not valid reasons to postpone pre-exposure immunisation.

Table 27.1 Guide to post-exposure prophylaxis following risk assessment

	Post-exposure prophylaxis	
Rabies risk	**Unimmunised /incompletely immunised individual***	**Fully immunised individual**
No risk	None	None
Low risk	Five doses (each 1ml) rabies vaccine on days 0, 3, 7, 14 and 30	Two doses (each 1ml) rabies vaccine on days 0 and 3
High risk	Five doses (each 1ml) rabies vaccine on days 0, 3, 7, 14 and 30, plus HRIG on day 0 only	Two doses (each 1ml) rabies vaccine on days 0 and 3

* Persons who have not received a full course of pre- or post-exposure tissue culture rabies vaccine.

If an individual is acutely unwell, pre-exposure immunisation should be postponed until they have recovered. This is to avoid confusing the differential diagnosis of any acute illness by wrongly attributing any signs or symptoms to the adverse effects of the vaccine.

Pregnant women and breast-feeding

Pregnant women and breast-feeding mothers should only be given pre-exposure vaccination if the risk of exposure to rabies is high and rapid access to post-exposure prophylaxis would be limited. Post-exposure treatment should be given to pregnant women when indicated.

The single site, intradermal 0.1ml pre-exposure vaccine regimen should not be used in those taking chloroquine for malaria prophylaxis, as this suppresses the antibody response.

Immunosuppression and HIV infection

Individuals with immunosuppression and HIV infection (regardless of CD4 count) should be given rabies vaccines in accordance with the recommendations above. These individuals may not make a full antibody response. Re-immunisation should be considered after treatment is finished and recovery has occurred.

Individuals who are immunosuppressed or with HIV who are exposed may require a different regime for post-exposure management. Specialist advice should be sought urgently.

Further guidance is provided by the Royal College of Paediatrics and Child Health (www.rcpch.ac.uk) the British HIV Association (BHIVA) *Immunisation guidelines for HIV-infected adults* (BHIVA, 2006) and the Children's HIV Association of UK and Ireland (CHIVA) immunisation guidelines (www.bhiva.org/chiva).

Adverse reactions

Rabies vaccine may cause local reactions such as redness, swelling or pain at the site of injection within 24 to 48 hours of administration. Systemic reactions such as headache, fever, muscle aches, vomiting and urticarial rashes are rare. Delayed hypersensitivity reactions have been reported from the US. Reactions may become more severe with repeated doses. Neurological conditions, such as Guillain-Barré syndrome, have been reported extremely rarely; a causal association with vaccination is not established.

HRIG may cause local pain and low-grade fever, but no serious adverse reactions have been reported.

All suspected adverse reactions to vaccines occurring in children, or in individuals of any age after vaccines labelled with a black triangle (▼), should be reported to the Commission on Human Medicines using the Yellow Card scheme. Serious suspected adverse reactions to vaccines in adults should also be reported through the Yellow Card scheme.

Management of cases

Human rabies is a notifiable disease. In the event of a case of human rabies, the Consultant in Communicable Disease Control (in England, Wales or Northern Ireland) or the Consultant in Public Health Medicine for Communicable Disease and Environmental Health (in Scotland) should be informed.

Supplies

- Rabies Vaccine BP is available from Sanofi Pasteur MSD (Tel: 0800 085 5511).
- Rabipur is available from Novartis Vaccines (Tel: 08457 451500) or MASTA (Tel: 0113 238 7500) .

Rabies vaccine for pre-exposure immunisation of those at occupational risk and bat handlers is supplied by the Department of Health and should be obtained from the HPA Virus Reference Department (Tel: 020 8200 4400). For others, it can be obtained through local pharmacies by private prescription. In Scotland, the vaccine is available through normal GP channels.

For post-exposure use, vaccine is supplied by centres listed in the HPA directory. Information may be obtained from the HPA Virus Reference Department (Tel: 020 8200 4400) or Communicable Disease Surveillance Centre (Tel: 020 8200 6868) in England; the National Public Health Service (Virology Cardiff) for Wales (Tel: 029 2074 7747); Health Protection Scotland (Tel: 0141 300 1100); and the Public Health Laboratory, Belfast City Hospital (Tel: 028 9032 9241) in Northern Ireland.

HRIG is manufactured by Bio Products Laboratory and supplied through the HPA for England. Supply centres for rabies vaccine and HRIG are listed in the Department of Health's *Memorandum on rabies: prevention and control* (www.dh.gov.uk – enter title in the search box).

Rabies vaccine and HRIG for use in post-exposure treatment are available free of charge to patients. If vaccine held for pre-exposure prophylaxis is used for post-exposure treatment, it will be replaced free of charge.

References

American Academy of Pediatrics (2003) Active immunization. In: Pickering LK (ed.) *Red Book: 2003 Report of the Committee on Infectious Diseases,* 26th edition. Elk Grove Village, IL: American Academy of Pediatrics, p 33.

Briggs DJ and Schwenke JR (1992) Longevity of rabies antibody titre in recipients of human diploid cell rabies vaccine. *Vaccine* **10**: 125–9.

British HIV Association (2006) *Immunisation guidelines for HIV-infected adults:* www.bhiva.org/pdf/2006/Immunisation506.pdf.

Cabasso VJ, Dobkin MB, Roby RE and Hammar AH (1974) Antibody response to human diploid cell rabies vaccine. *Appl Microbiol* **27**: 553–61.

Department of Health (2001) *Health information for overseas travel*, 2nd edition. London: TSO.

Fekadu M, Shaddock JH, Sanderlin DW and Smith JS (1988) Efficacy of rabies vaccines against Duvenhage virus isolated from the European house bats (*Eptesicus serotinus*), classic rabies and rabies-related viruses. *Vaccine* **6**: 533.

Fooks AR, Brookes SM, Johnson N *et al.* (2003) European bat lyssaviruses: an emerging zoonosis. *Epidemiol Infect* **131**(3): 1029–39.

Hossain J, Crowcroft NS, Lea G *et al.* (2004) Audit of rabies post-exposure prophylaxis in England and Wales in 1990 and 2000. *Commun Dis and Public Health* **7**(2): 105–11.

Nathwani D, McIntyre PG, White K *et al.* (2003) Fatal human rabies caused by European bat lyssavirus type 2a infection in Scotland. *Clin Infect Dis* **37**: 598–601.

Nicholson KG, Prestage H, Cole PJ *et al.* (1981) Multisite intradermal rabies vaccination. *Lancet* **ii**: 915–18.

Plotkin SA and Orenstein WA (eds) (2004) *Vaccines,* 4th edition. Philadelphia: WB Saunders Company.

Rupprecht CE, Hanlon CA and Hemachudha T (2002) Rabies re-examined. *Lancet Infect Dis* **2**: 327–43.

Strady A, Lang J, Lienard M *et al.* (1998) Antibody persistence following pre-exposure regimens of cell-culture rabies vaccines: 10-year follow-up and proposal for a new booster policy. *J Infect Dis* **177**(5): 1290–5.

Strady C, Jaussaud R, Bequinot I *et al.* (2000) Predictive factors for the neutralizing antibody response following pre-exposure rabies immunization: validation of a new booster dose strategy. *Vaccine* **18**(24): 2661–7.

Turner GS, Nicholson KG, Tyrrell DAJ and Aoki FY (1982) Evaluation of a human diploid cell strain rabies vaccine: final report of a three-year study of pre-exposure immunisation. *J Hyg* (Lond) **89**: 101–10.

World Health Organization (2006) Fact Sheet No 99: *Rabies.* www.who.int/rabies/en/WHO_guide_rabies_pre_post_exp_treat_humans.pdf.

Zuckerman JN (2000) The importance of injecting vaccines into muscle. *BMJ* **321**: 1237–8.

28

Rubella

NOTIFIABLE

The disease

Rubella is a mild disease caused by a togavirus. There may be a mild prodromal illness involving a low-grade fever, malaise, coryza and mild conjunctivitis. Lymphadenopathy involving post-auricular and sub-occipital glands may precede the rash. The rash is usually transitory, erythematous and mostly seen behind the ears and on the face and neck. Clinical diagnosis is unreliable as the rash may be fleeting and is not specific to rubella.

Rubella is spread by droplet transmission. The incubation period is 14 to 21 days, with the majority of individuals developing a rash 14 to 17 days after exposure. Individuals with rubella are infectious from one week before symptoms appear to four days after the onset of the rash.

Complications include thrombocytopaenia (the rate may be as high as one in 3000 infections) and post-infectious encephalitis (one in 6000 cases) (Lokletz and Reynolds, 1965; Plotkin and Orenstein, 2004). In adults, arthritis and arthralgia may occasionally be seen after rubella infection; chronic arthritis has rarely been reported (Plotkin and Orenstein, 2004).

Maternal rubella infection in pregnancy may result in fetal loss or in congenital rubella syndrome (CRS). CRS presents with one or more of the following:

- cataracts and other eye defects
- deafness
- cardiac abnormalities
- microcephaly
- retardation of intra-uterine growth
- inflammatory lesions of brain, liver, lungs and bone marrow.

Infection in the first eight to ten weeks of pregnancy results in damage in up to 90% of surviving infants; multiple defects are common. The risk of damage declines to about 10 to 20% with infection occurring between 11 and 16 weeks gestation (Miller *et al.*, 1982). Fetal damage is rare with infection after 16 weeks of pregnancy, with only deafness being reported following infections up to 20 weeks of pregnancy. Some infected infants may appear normal at birth but perceptive deafness may be detected later (Miller *et al.*, 1982; Plotkin and Orenstein, 2004).

History and epidemiology of the disease

Before the introduction of rubella immunisation, rubella occurred commonly in children, and more than 80% of adults had evidence of previous rubella infection (Morgan Capner *et al.*, 1988).

Rubella immunisation was introduced in the UK in 1970 for pre-pubertal girls and non-immune women of childbearing age to prevent rubella infection in pregnancy. Rather than interrupting the circulation of rubella, the aim of this strategy was to directly protect women of childbearing age by increasing the proportion with antibody to rubella; this increased from 85 to 90% before 1970 to 97 to 98% by 1987 (Vyse *et al.*, 2002). Surveillance for congenital rubella was established in 1971 to monitor the impact of the vaccination programme. During the period 1971–75 there were an average of 48 CRS births and 742 terminations annually in the UK (Tookey and Peckham, 1999) (see Figure 28.1).

Although the selective immunisation policy was effective in reducing the number of cases of CRS and terminations of pregnancy, cases of rubella in pregnancy continued to occur. This was mainly because the few women who remained susceptible to rubella could still acquire rubella infection from their own and/or their friends' children.

Universal immunisation against rubella, using the measles, mumps and rubella (MMR) vaccine, was introduced in October 1988. The aim of this policy was to interrupt circulation of rubella among young children, thereby protecting susceptible adult women from exposure. At the same time, rubella was made a notifiable disease. A considerable decline in rubella in young children followed the introduction of MMR, with a concomitant fall in rubella infections in pregnant women – from 167 in 1987 to one in 2003.

A seroprevalence study in 1989 showed a high rate of rubella susceptibility in school-age children, particularly in males (Miller *et al.*, 1991). In 1993, there was a large increase in both notifications and laboratory-confirmed cases of rubella. Many of the individuals affected would not have been eligible for MMR or for the rubella vaccine. For this reason, the combined measles-rubella (MR) vaccine was used for the schools campaign in November 1994 (see Chapter 21). At that time, insufficient stocks of MMR were available to vaccinate all of

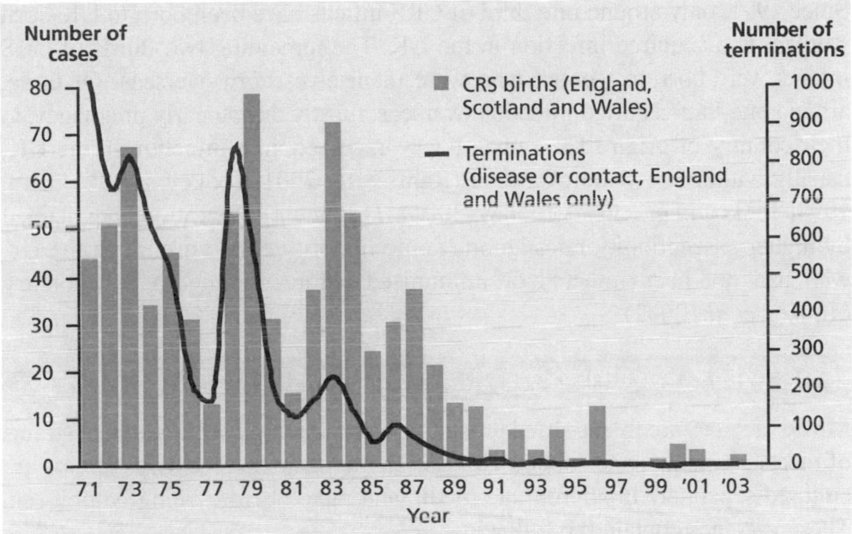

Figure 28.1 Congenital rubella syndrome births (source: National Congenital Rubella Surveillance Programme 1971–2004) and rubella-associated terminations (source: Office for National Statistics 1971–2003)

these children against mumps. Over 8 million children aged between 5 and 16 years were immunised with the MR vaccine.

In October 1996, a two-dose MMR schedule was introduced and the selective vaccination policy of teenage girls ceased. A single dose of rubella-containing vaccine as used in the UK confers around 95 to 100% protection against rubella (Plotkin and Orenstein, 2004).

In Finland, a two-dose MMR schedule was introduced in 1982; high coverage of each dose has been achieved consistently. Indigenous measles, mumps and rubella have been eliminated since 1994 (Peltola *et al.*, 1994). The United States introduced its two-dose schedule in 1989 and, in 2000, announced that it had interrupted endemic transmission (Plotkin and Orenstein, 2004, Chapter 20). MMR is now routinely given in over 100 countries, including those in the European Union, North America and Australasia.

A further resurgence of rubella was observed in the UK in 1996. Many of these cases occurred in colleges and universities in males who had already left school before the 1994 MR campaign (Vyse *et al.*, 2002). Sporadic rubella cases have been reported since then, mainly linked to imported cases (Health Protection Agency website).

Since 1991, only around one-third of CRS infants have been born to UK-born women who acquired infection in the UK. The remaining two-thirds of CRS infants were born to women who were themselves born overseas. Of these, around one-half acquired infection overseas, mostly during early pregnancy, in their country of origin. The remaining women acquired infection in the UK, usually within two years of arrival (Rahi *et al.*, 2001; Tookey and Peckham, 1999; Tookey *et al.*, 2002; Tookey, 2004). This latter observation is explained by higher susceptibility rates among some minority ethnic groups in the UK who had not been infected or immunised before coming to this country (Tookey *et al.*, 2002).

The MMR vaccination

MMR vaccines are freeze-dried preparations containing live, attenuated strains of measles, mumps and rubella viruses. The three attenuated virus strains are cultured separately in appropriate media and mixed before being lyophilised. These vaccines contain the following:

Priorix®

Each 0.5ml dose of reconstituted vaccine contains:

not less than $10^{3.0}$ cell culture infective dose$_{50}$ ($CCID_{50}$) of the Schwarz measles virus
not less than $10^{3.7}$ $CCID_{50}$ of the RIT 4385 mumps virus
not less than $10^{3.0}$ $CCID_{50}$ of the Wistar RA 27/3 rubella virus strains.

M-M-R™II

Each 0.5ml dose when reconstituted contains not less than the equivalent of:

1000 tissue culture infective dose$_{50}$ ($TCID_{50}$) of the more attenuated Enders line of the Edmonston strain of measles virus
20,000 $TCID_{50}$ of mumps virus (Jeryl Lynn® Level B strain)
1000 $TCID_{50}$ of rubella virus (Wistar RA 27/3 strain).

MMR vaccine does not contain thiomersal or any other preservatives. The vaccine contains live organisms that have been attenuated (modified). MMR is recommended when protection against measles, mumps and/or rubella is required.

Storage

The unreconstituted vaccine and its diluent should be stored in the original packaging at +2˚C to +8˚C and protected from light. All vaccines are sensitive to some extent to heat and cold. Heat speeds up the decline in potency of most vaccines, thus reducing their shelf life. Effectiveness cannot be guaranteed for vaccines unless they have been stored at the correct temperature. Freezing may cause increased reactogenicity and loss of potency for some vaccines. It can also cause hairline cracks in the container, leading to contamination of the contents.

The vaccines should be reconstituted with the diluent supplied by the manufacturer and either used within one hour or discarded.

Presentation

Rubella vaccine is only available as part of a combined product (MMR).

Priorix is supplied as a whitish to slightly pink pellet of lyophilised vaccine for reconstitution with the diluent supplied. The reconstituted vaccine must be shaken well until the pellet is completely dissolved in the diluent.

M-M-R II is supplied as a lyophilised powder for reconstitution with the diluent supplied. The reconstituted vaccine must be shaken gently to ensure thorough mixing. The reconstituted vaccine is yellow in colour and should only be used if clear and free from particulate matter.

Dosage and schedule

Two doses of 0.5ml at the recommended interval (see below).

Administration

Vaccines are routinely given intramuscularly into the upper arm or anterolateral thigh. However, for individuals with a bleeding disorder, vaccines should be given by deep subcutaneous injection to reduce the risk of bleeding.

MMR vaccine can be given at the same time as other vaccines such as DTaP/IPV, MenC and hepatitis B. The vaccine should be given at a separate site, preferably in a different limb. If given in the same limb, they should be given at least 2.5cm apart (American Academy of Pediatrics, 2003). If MMR cannot be given at the same time as an inactivated vaccine, it can be given at any interval before or after.

MMR should ideally be given at the same time as other live vaccines, such as BCG. If live vaccines are given simultaneously, then each vaccine virus will begin to replicate and an appropriate immune response is made to each vaccine. After a live vaccine is given, natural interferon is produced in response to that vaccine. If a second live vaccine is given during this response, the interferon may prevent replication of the second vaccine virus. This may attenuate the response to the second vaccine. Based on evidence that MMR vaccine can lead to an attenuation of the varicella vaccine response (Mullooly and Black, 2001), the recommended interval between live vaccines is currently four weeks. For this reason, if live vaccines cannot be administered simultaneously, a four-week interval is recommended.

Four weeks should be left between giving MMR vaccine and carrying out tuberculin testing. The measles vaccine component of MMR can reduce the delayed-type hypersensitivity response. As this is the basis of a positive tuberculin test, this could give a false negative response.

When MMR is given within three months of receiving blood products, such as immunoglobulin, the response to the measles component may be reduced. This is because such blood products may contain significant levels of measles-specific antibody, which could then prevent vaccine virus replication. Where possible, MMR should be deferred until three months after receipt of such products. If immediate measles protection is required in someone who has recently received a blood product, MMR vaccine should still be given. To confer longer-term protection, MMR should be repeated after three months.

Where rubella protection is required for post-partum women who have received anti-D immunoglobulin, no deferral is necessary as the response to the rubella component is normally adequate (Edgar and Hambling, 1977; Black *et al.*, 1983). Blood transfusion around the time of delivery may inhibit the rubella response and, therefore, a test for rubella antibody should be undertaken six to eight weeks after vaccination. The vaccination should be repeated if necessary.

Disposal

Equipment used for vaccination, including used vials or ampoules, should be disposed of at the end of a session by sealing in a proper, puncture-resistant 'sharps' box (UN-approved, BS 7320).

Recommendations for the use of the vaccine

The objective of the immunisation programme is to provide two doses of MMR vaccine at appropriate intervals for all eligible individuals.

Over 90% of individuals will seroconvert to measles, mumps and rubella antibodies after the first dose of the MMR vaccines currently used in the UK (Tischer and Gerike, 2000). Antibody responses from pre-licence studies may be higher, however, than clinical protection under routine use. Evidence shows that a single dose of measles-containing vaccine confers protection in around 90% of individuals for measles (Morse *et al.*, 1994; Medical Research Council, 1977). A single dose of a rubella-containing vaccine confers around 95 to 100% protection (Plotkin and Orenstein, 2004). A single dose of a mumps-containing vaccine used in the UK confers between 61% and 91% protection against mumps (Plotkin and Orenstein, 2004). A more recent study in the UK suggested that a single dose of MMR is around 64% effective against mumps (Harling *et al.*, 2005).

Therefore, two doses of MMR are required to produce satisfactory protection against measles, mumps and rubella.

MMR is recommended when protection against measles, mumps and/or rubella is required. MMR vaccine can be given irrespective of a history of measles, mumps or rubella infection. There are no ill effects from immunising such individuals because they have pre-existing immunity that inhibits replication of the vaccine viruses.

Children under ten years of age

The first dose of MMR should be given at any time after the first birthday, ideally at 13 months of age. Immunisation before 13 months of age provides earlier protection in localities where the risk of measles is higher, but residual maternal antibodies may reduce the response rate to the vaccine. The optimal age chosen for scheduling children is therefore a compromise between risk of disease and level of protection.

If a dose of MMR is given before the first birthday, either because of travel to an endemic country, or because of a local outbreak, then this dose should be ignored, and two further doses given at the recommended times after the first birthday and pre-school.

A second dose is normally given before school entry but can be given routinely at any time from three months after the first dose. Allowing three months between doses is likely to maximise the response rate, particularly in young children under the age of 18 months where maternal antibodies may reduce the response to vaccination (Orenstein *et al.*, 1986; Redd *et al.*, 2004; de Serres *et al.*, 1995). Where protection against measles is urgently required, the second dose can be given one month after the first (ACIP, 1998). If the child is given the second dose less than three months after the first dose and at less than 18 months of age, then the routine pre-school dose (a third dose) should be given in order to ensure full protection.

Children aged ten years or over and adults

All children should have received two doses of MMR vaccine before they leave school. The teenage (school-leaving) booster session or appointment is an opportunity to ensure that unimmunised or partially immunised children are given MMR. If two doses of MMR are required, then the second dose should be given one month after the first.

MMR vaccine can be given to individuals of any age. Entry into college, university or other higher education institutions, prison or military service provides an opportunity to check an individual's immunisation history. Those who have not received MMR should be offered appropriate MMR immunisation.

All seronegative women of childbearing age who need to be protected against rubella should be offered MMR vaccine. Satisfactory evidence of protection would include documentation of having received two doses of rubella-containing vaccine or a positive antibody test for rubella.

The decision on when to vaccinate other adults needs to take into consideration the past vaccination history, the likelihood of an individual remaining susceptible and the future risk of exposure and disease:

- individuals who were born between 1980 and 1990 may not be protected against mumps but are likely to be vaccinated against measles and rubella. They may never have received a mumps-containing vaccine or had only one dose of MMR, and had limited opportunity for exposure to natural mumps. They should be recalled and given MMR vaccine. If this is their first dose, a further dose of MMR should be given from one month later.
- individuals born between 1970 and 1979 may have been vaccinated against measles and many will have been exposed to mumps and rubella during childhood. However, this age group should be offered MMR wherever feasible, particularly if they are considered to be at high risk of exposure. Where such adults are being vaccinated because they have been demonstrated to be susceptible to at least one of the vaccine components, then either two doses should be given, or there should be evidence of seroconversion to the relevant antigen.

- individuals born before 1970 are likely to have had all three natural infections and are less likely to be susceptible. MMR vaccine should be offered to such individuals on request or if they are considered to be at high risk of exposure. Where such adults are being vaccinated because they have been demonstrated to be susceptible to at least one of the vaccine components, then either two doses should be given or there should be evidence of seroconversion to the relevant antigen.

Individuals with unknown or incomplete vaccination histories

Children coming from developing countries will probably have received a measles-containing vaccine in their country of origin but may not have received mumps or rubella vaccines (www-nt.who.int/immunization_monitoring/en/globalsummary/countryprofileselect.cfm). Unless there is a reliable history of appropriate immunisation, individuals should be assumed to be unimmunised and the recommendations above should be followed. Individuals aged 18 months and over who have not received MMR should receive two doses at least one month apart. An individual who has already received one dose of MMR should receive a second dose to ensure that they are protected.

Healthcare workers

Protection of healthcare workers is especially important in the context of their ability to transmit measles, mumps or rubella infections to vulnerable groups. While they may need MMR vaccination for their own benefit, on the grounds outlined above, they also should be immune to measles, mumps and rubella for the protection of their patients.

Satisfactory evidence of protection would include documentation of:

- having received two doses of MMR, or
- positive antibody tests for measles and rubella.

Individuals who are travelling or going to reside abroad

All travellers to epidemic or endemic areas should ensure that they are fully immunised according to the UK schedule (see above).

Contraindications

There are very few individuals who cannot receive MMR vaccine. When there is doubt, appropriate advice should be sought from a consultant paediatrician, immunisation co-ordinator or consultant in communicable disease control rather than withholding the vaccine.

The vaccine should not be given to:

- those who are immunosuppressed (see chapter 6 for more detail)
- those who have had a confirmed anaphylactic reaction to a previous dose of a measles-, mumps- or rubella-containing vaccine
- those who have had a confirmed anaphylactic reaction to neomycin or gelatin
- pregnant women.

Anaphylaxis after MMR is extremely rare (3.5 to 14.4 per million doses) (Bohlke *et al.*, 2003; Patja *et al.*, 2000; Pool *et al.*, 2002; D'Souza *et al.*, 2000). Minor allergic conditions may occur and are not contraindications to further immunisation with MMR or other vaccines. A careful history of that event will often distinguish between anaphylaxis and other events that are either not due to the vaccine or are not life-threatening. In the latter circumstances, it may be possible to continue the immunisation course. Specialist advice must be sought on the vaccines and circumstances in which they could be given. The lifelong risk to the individual of not being immunised must be taken into account.

Precautions

Minor illnesses without fever or systemic upset are not valid reasons to postpone immunisation. If an individual is acutely unwell, immunisation should be postponed until they have fully recovered. This is to avoid confusing the differential diagnosis of any acute illness by wrongly attributing any sign or symptoms to the adverse effects of the vaccine.

Idiopathic thrombocytopaenic purpura

Idiopathic thrombocytopaenic purpura (ITP) has occurred rarely following MMR vaccination, usually within six weeks of the first dose. The risk of developing ITP after MMR vaccine is much less than the risk of developing it after infection with wild measles or rubella virus.

If ITP has occurred within six weeks of the first dose of MMR, then blood should be taken and tested for measles, mumps and rubella antibodies before a second dose is given. Serum should be sent to the Health Protection Agency (HPA) Virus Reference Laboratory (Colindale), which offers free, specialised serological testing for such children. If the results suggest incomplete immunity against measles, mumps or rubella, then a second dose of MMR is recommended.

Allergy to egg

Children with egg allergy should have MMR vaccine. Recent data suggest that anaphylactic reactions to MMR vaccine are not associated with hypersensitivity to egg antigens but to other components of the vaccine (such as gelatin) (Fox and Lack, 2003). In three large studies with a combined total of over 1,000 patients with egg allergy, no severe cardiorespiratory reactions were reported after MMR vaccination (Fasano *et al.*, 1992; Freigang *et al.*, 1994; Aickin *et al.*, 1994; Khakoo and Lack, 2000).

If there is a history of confirmed anaphylactic reaction to egg-containing food, paediatric advice should be sought with a view to immunisation under controlled conditions, such as admission to hospital as a day case.

Pregnancy and breast-feeding

There is no evidence that rubella-containing vaccines are teratogenic. In the USA, UK and Germany, 661 women were followed through active surveillance, including 293 who were vaccinated (mainly with single rubella vaccine) in the high-risk period (i.e. the six weeks after the last menstrual period). Only 16 infants had evidence of infection and none had permanent abnormalities compatible with CRS (Best *et al.*, 2004). However, as a precaution, MMR vaccine should not be given to women known to be pregnant. If MMR vaccine is given to adult women, they should be advised to guard against pregnancy for one month.

Termination of pregnancy following inadvertent immunisation should not be recommended (Tookey *et al.*, 1991). The potential parents should be given information on the evidence of lack of risk from vaccination in pregnancy. Surveillance of inadvertent MMR administration in pregnancy is being conducted by the HPA Immunisation Department, to whom such cases should be reported (Tel: 020 8200 4400).

Pregnant women who are found to be susceptible to rubella should be immunised with MMR after delivery.

Breast-feeding is not a contraindication to MMR immunisation, and MMR vaccine can be given to breast-feeding mothers without any risk to their baby. Very occasionally, rubella vaccine virus has been found in breast milk, but this has not caused any symptoms in the baby (Buimovici-Klein *et al.*, 1997; Landes *et al.*, 1980; Losonsky *et al.*, 1982). The vaccine does not work when taken orally. There is no evidence of mumps and measles vaccine viruses being found in breast milk.

Premature infants

It is important that premature infants have their immunisations at the appropriate chronological age, according to the schedule (see chapter 11).

Immunosuppression and HIV

MMR vaccine is not recommended for patients with severe immunosuppression (see Chapter 6) (Angel *et al.*, 1996). MMR vaccine can be given to HIV-positive patients without or with moderate immunosuppression (as defined in Table 28.1).

Table 28.1 CD4 count/μl (% of total lymphocytes)

Age	<12 months	1–5 years	6–12 years	>12 years
No suppression	⩾1500 (⩾25%)	⩾1000 (15–24%)	⩾500 (⩾25%)	⩾500 (⩾25%)
Moderate suppression	750–1499 (15–24%)	500–999 (15–24%)	200–499 (15–24%)	200–499 (15–24%)
Severe suppression	<750 (<15%)	<500 (<15%)	<200 (<15%)	<200 (<15%)

Further guidance is provided by the Royal College of Paediatrics and Child Health (www.rcpch.ac.uk), the British HIV Association (BHIVA) *Immunisation guidelines for HIV-infected adults* (BHIVA, 2006) and the Children's HIV Association of UK and Ireland (CHIVA) immunisation guidelines (www.bhiva.org/chiva).

Neurological conditions

The presence of a neurological condition is not a contraindication to immunisation. If there is evidence of current neurological deterioration, including poorly controlled epilepsy, immunisation should be deferred until the condition has stabilised. Children with a personal or close family history of seizures should be given MMR vaccine. Advice about likely timing of any fever and management of a fever should be given. Doctors and nurses should seek specialist paediatric advice rather than refuse immunisation.

Adverse reactions

Adverse reactions following the MMR vaccine (except allergic reactions) are due to effective replication of the vaccine viruses with subsequent mild illness. Such events are to be expected in some individuals. Events due to the measles component occur six to 11 days after vaccination. Events due to the mumps and rubella components usually occur two to three weeks after vaccination but may occur up to six weeks after vaccination. These events only occur in individuals who are susceptible to that component, and are therefore less common after second and subsequent doses. Individuals with vaccine-associated symptoms are not infectious to others.

Common events

Following the first dose of MMR vaccine, malaise, fever and/or a rash may occur, most commonly about a week after immunisation, and last about two to three days. In a study of over 6000 children aged one to two years, the symptoms reported were similar in nature, frequency, time of onset and duration to those commonly reported after measles vaccine alone (Miller *et al.*, 1989). Parotid swelling occurred in about 1% of children of all ages up to four years, usually in the third week.

Adverse reactions are considerably less common after a second dose of MMR vaccine than after the first dose. One study showed no increase in fever or rash after re-immunisation of college students compared with unimmunised controls (Chen *et al.*, 1991). An analysis of allergic reactions reported through the US Vaccine Adverse Events Reporting System in 1991–93 showed fewer reactions among children aged six to 19 years, considered to be second-dose recipients, than among those aged one to four years, considered to be first-dose recipients (Chen *et al.*, 1991). In a study of over 8000 children there was no increased risk of convulsions, rash or joint pain in the months after the second dose of the MMR vaccination given between four and six years of age (Davis *et al.*, 1997).

Rare and more serious events

Febrile seizures are the most commonly reported neurological event following measles immunisation. Seizures occur during the sixth to eleventh day in one in 1000 children vaccinated with MMR – a rate similar to that reported in the same period after measles vaccine. The rate of febrile seizures following MMR is lower than that following infection with measles disease (Plotkin and Orenstein, 2004). There is good evidence that febrile seizures following MMR immunisation do not increase the risk of subsequent epilepsy compared with febrile seizures due to other causes (Vestergaard *et al.*, 2004).

One strain of mumps virus (Urabe) in an MMR vaccine previously used in the UK was associated with an increased risk of aseptic meningitis (Miller *et al.*, 1993). This vaccine was replaced in 1992 (Department of Health, 1992) and is no longer licensed in the UK. A study in Finland using MMR containing a different mumps strain (Jeryl Lynn), similar to those used currently in MMR in the UK, did not identify any association between MMR and aseptic meningitis (Makela *et al.*, 2002).

Because MMR vaccine contains live, attenuated viruses, it is biologically plausible that it may cause encephalitis. A recent large record linkage study in Finland looking at over half a million children aged between one and seven years did not identify any association between MMR and encephalitis (Makela *et al.*, 2002).

ITP is a condition that may occur following MMR and is most likely due to the rubella component. This usually occurs within six weeks and resolves spontaneously. ITP occurs in about one in 22,300 children given a first dose of MMR in the second year of life (Miller *et al.,* 2001). If ITP has occurred within six weeks of the first dose of MMR, then blood should be taken and tested for measles, mumps and rubella antibodies before a second dose is given (see above).

Arthropathy (arthralgia or arthritis) has also been reported to occur rarely after MMR immunisation, probably due to the rubella component. If it is caused by the vaccine, it should occur between 14 and 21 days after immunisation. Where it occurs at other times, it is highly unlikely to have been caused by vaccination. Several controlled epidemiological studies have shown no excess risk of chronic arthritis in women (Slater, 1997).

All suspected adverse reactions to vaccines occurring in children, or in individuals of any age after vaccines labelled with a black triangle (▼), should be reported to the Commission on Human Medicines using the Yellow Card scheme. Serious, suspected adverse reactions to vaccines in adults should be reported through the Yellow Card scheme.

Other conditions reported after vaccines containing measles, mumps and rubella

Following the November 1994 MR immunisation campaign, only three cases of Guillain-Barré syndrome (GBS) were reported. From the background rate, between one and eight cases would have been expected in this population over this period. Therefore, it is likely that these three cases were coincidental and not caused by the vaccine. Analysis of reporting rates of GBS from acute flaccid paralysis surveillance undertaken in the WHO Region of the Americas has shown no increase in rates of GBS following measles immunisation campaigns when 80 million children were immunised (da Silveira *et al.*, 1997). In a population that received 900,000 doses of MMR, there was no increased risk of GBS at any time after vaccinations (Patja *et al.*, 2001). This evidence refutes the suggestion that MMR causes GBS.

Although gait disturbance has been reported after MMR, a recent epidemiological study showed no evidence of a causal association between MMR and gait disturbance (Miller *et al.*, 2005).

In recent years, the postulated link between measles vaccine and bowel disease has been investigated. There was no increase in the incidence of inflammatory bowel disorders in those vaccinated with measles-containing vaccines compared with controls (Gilat *et al.*, 1987; Feeney *et al.*, 1997). No increase in the incidence of inflammatory bowel disease has been observed since the introduction of MMR vaccination in Finland (Pebody *et al.*, 1998) or in the UK (Seagroatt, 2005).

There is overwhelming evidence that MMR does not cause autism (www.iom.edu/report.asp?id=20155). Over the past seven years, a large number of studies have been published looking at this issue. Such studies have shown:

- no increased risk of autism in children vaccinated with MMR compared with unvaccinated children (Farrington *et al.*, 2001; Madsen and Vestergaard, 2004)
- no clustering of the onset of symptoms of autism in the period following MMR vaccination (Taylor *et al.*, 1999; De Wilde *et al.*, 2001; Makela *et al.*, 2002)
- that the increase in the reported incidence of autism preceded the use of MMR in the UK (Taylor *et al.*, 1999)
- that the incidence of autism continued to rise after 1993, despite the withdrawal of MMR in Japan (Honda *et al.*, 2005)
- that there is no correlation between the rate of autism and MMR vaccine coverage in either the UK or the USA (Kaye *et al.*, 2001; Dales *et al.*, 2001)
- no difference between the proportion of children developing autism after MMR who have a regressive form compared with those who develop autism without vaccination (Fombonne, 2001; Taylor *et al.*, 2002; Gillberg and Heijbel, 1998)
- no difference between the proportion of children developing autism after MMR who have associated bowel symptoms compared with those who develop autism without vaccination (Fombonne, 2001; Fombonne, 1998; Taylor *et al.*, 2002)
- that no vaccine virus can be detected in children with autism using the most sensitive methods available (Afzal *et al.*, 2006).

For the latest evidence, see the Department of Health's website: www.mmrthe facts.nhs.uk.

It has been suggested that combined MMR vaccine could potentially overload the immune system. From the moment of birth, humans are exposed to countless numbers of foreign antigens and infectious agents in their everyday environment. Responding to the three viruses in MMR would use only a tiny proportion of the total capacity of an infant's immune system (Offit *et al.*, 2002). The three viruses in MMR replicate at different rates from each other and would be expected to reach high levels at different times.

A study examining the issue of immunological overload found a lower rate of admission for serious bacterial infection in the period shortly after MMR vaccination compared with other time periods. This suggests that MMR does not cause any general suppression of the immune system (Miller *et al.*, 2003).

Management of cases, contacts and outbreaks

Diagnosis

Prompt notification of measles, mumps and rubella to the local health protection unit (HPU) is required to ensure public health action can be taken promptly. Notification should be based on clinical suspicion and should not await laboratory confirmation. Since 1994, few clinically diagnosed cases are subsequently confirmed to be true measles, mumps or rubella. Confirmation rates do increase, however, during outbreaks and epidemics.

The diagnosis of measles, mumps and rubella can be confirmed through non-invasive means. Detection of specific IgM in oral fluid (saliva) samples, ideally between one and six weeks after the onset of rash or parotid swelling, has been shown to be highly sensitive and specific for confirmation of these infections (Brown *et al.*, 1994; Ramsay *et al.*, 1991; Ramsay *et al.*, 1998). It is recommended that oral fluid samples should be obtained from all notified cases, other than during a large epidemic. Advice on this procedure can be obtained from the local HPU.

Infants with suspected congenital rubella infection should be reported to the National Congenital Rubella Surveillance Programme, either directly to the Institute of Child Health (Tel: 020 7905 2604) or via the British Paediatric Surveillance Unit (Tel: 020 7323 7911).

Protection of contacts with MMR

Antibody response to the rubella component of MMR vaccine does not develop soon enough to provide effective prophylaxis after exposure to suspected rubella. Even where it is too late to provide effective post-exposure prophylaxis with MMR, the vaccine can provide protection against future exposure to all three infections. Therefore, contact with suspected measles, mumps or rubella provides a good opportunity to offer MMR vaccine to previously unvaccinated individuals. If the individual is already incubating measles, mumps or rubella, MMR vaccination will not exacerbate the symptoms. In these circumstances, individuals should be advised that a rubella-like illness occurring shortly after vaccination is likely to be due to natural infection. If there is doubt about an individual's vaccination status, MMR should still be given as there are no ill effects from vaccinating those who are already immune.

Protection of contacts with immunoglobulin

Human normal immunoglobulin is not routinely used for post-exposure protection from rubella since there is no evidence that it is effective. It is **not** recommended for the protection of pregnant women exposed to rubella. It should only be considered when termination of pregnancy is unacceptable. Serological follow-up of recipients is essential.

To prevent or attenuate an attack:
Dose: 750mg

Supplies

- M-M-R™II – manufactured by Sanofi Pasteur MSD.
- Priorix® – manufactured by GlaxoSmithKline.

These vaccines are supplied by Healthcare Logistics (Tel: 0870 871 1890) as part of the national childhood immunisation programme.

In Scotland, supplies should be obtained from local childhood vaccine holding centres. Details of these are available from Scottish Healthcare Supplies (Tel: 0131 275 6154).

In Northern Ireland, supplies should be obtained from local childhood vaccine holding centres. Details of these are available from the regional pharmaceutical procurement service (Tel: 02890 552368).

Human normal immunoglobulin

England and Wales:
Health Protection Agency, Centre for Infections
(Tel: 020 8200 6868).

Scotland:
Blood Transfusion Service
(Tel: 0141 3577700).

Northern Ireland:
Public Health Laboratory, Belfast City Hospital
(Tel: 01232 329241).

References

ACIP (1998) Measles, mumps, and rubella – vaccine use and strategies for elimination of measles, rubella, and congenital rubella syndrome and control of mumps: recommendations of the Advisory Committee on Immunization Practices (ACIP). *MMWR* **47**(RR-8): 1–57. www.cdc.gov/mmwr/preview/mmwrhtml/00053391.htm.

Afzal MA, Ozoemena LC, O'Hare A *et al.* (2006) Absence of detectable measles virus genome sequence in blood of autistic children who have had their MMR vaccination during the routine childhood immunisation schedule of the UK. *J Med Virol* **78**: 623–30.

Aickin R, Hill D and Kemp A (1994) Measles immunisation in children with allergy to egg. *BMJ* **308**: 223–5.

American Academy of Pediatrics (2003) Active immunization. In: Pickering LK (ed.) *Red Book: 2003 Report of the Committee on Infectious Diseases*, 26th edition. Elk Grove Village, IL: American Academy of Pediatrics.

Angel JB, Udem SA, Snydman DR *et al.* (1996) Measles pneumonitis following measles-mumps-rubella vaccination of patients with HIV infection, 1993. *MMWR* **45**: 603–6.

Best JM, Cooray S and Banatvala JE (2004) Rubella. In: Mahy BMJ and ter Meulen V (eds) *Topley and Wilson's Virology*, 10th edition. London: Hodder Arnold.

Black NA, Parsons A, Kurtz JB *et al.* (1983) Post-partum rubella immunisation: a controlled trial of two vaccines. *Lancet* **2**(8357): 990–2.

Bohlke K, Davis RL, Moray SH *et al.* (2003) Risk of anaphylaxis after vaccination of children and adolescents. *Pediatrics* **112**: 815–20.

British HIV Association (2006) *Immunisation guidelines for HIV-infected adults*. BHIVA. www.bhiva.org/pdf/2006/Immunisation506.pdf

Brown DW, Ramsay ME, Richards AF and Miller E (1994) Salivary diagnosis of measles: a study of notified cases in the United Kingdom, 1991–3. *BMJ* **308**(6935): 1015–17.

Buimovici-Klein E, Hite RL, Byrne T and Cooper LR (1997) Isolation of rubella virus in milk after postpartum immunization. *J Pediatr* **91**: 939–43.

Chen RT, Moses JM, Markowitz LE and Orenstein WA (1991) Adverse events following measles-mumps-rubella and measles vaccinations in college students. *Vaccine* **9**: 297–9.

Dales L, Hammer SJ and Smith NJ (2001) Time trends in autism and in MMR immunization coverage in California. *JAMA* **285**(22): 2852–3.

da Silveira CM, Salisbury DM and de Quadros CA (1997) Measles vaccination and Guillain-Barré syndrome. *Lancet* **349**(9044): 14–16.

Davis RL, Marcuse E, Black S *et al.* (1997) MMR2 immunization at 4 to 5 years and 10 to 12 years of age: a comparison of adverse clinical events after immunization in the Vaccine Safety Datalink project. *Pediatrics* **100**: 767–71.

Department of Health (1992) *Changes in supply of vaccine.* Circular (PL/CMO(92)11).

de Serres G, Boulianne N, Meyer F and Ward BJ (1995) Measles vaccine efficacy during an outbreak in a highly vaccinated population: incremental increase in protection with age at vaccination up to 18 months. *Epidemiol Infect* **115**: 315–23.

De Wilde S, Carey IM, Richards N *et al.* (2001) Do children who become autistic consult more often after MMR vaccination? *Br J General Practice* **51**: 226–7.

D'Souza RM, Campbell-Lloyd S, Isaacs D *et al.* (2000) Adverse events following immunisation associated with the 1998 Australian Measles Control Campaign. *Commun Dis Intell* **24**: 27–33.

Edgar WM and Hambling MH (1977) Rubella vaccination and anti-D immunoglobulin administration in the puerperium. *Br J Obstet Gynaecol* **84**(10): 754–7.

Farrington CP, Miller E and Taylor B (2001) MMR and autism: further evidence against a causal association. *Vaccine* **19**: 3632–5.

Fasano MB, Wood RA, Cooke SK and Sampson HA (1992) Egg hypersensitivity and adverse reactions to measles, mumps and rubella vaccine. *J Pediatr* **120**: 878–81.

Feeney M, Gregg A, Winwood P and Snook J (1997) A case-control study of measles vaccination and inflammatory bowel disease. The East Dorset Gastroenterology Group. *Lancet* **350**: 764–6.

Fombonne E (1998) Inflammatory bowel disease and autism. *Lancet* **351**: 955.

Fombonne E (2001) Is there an epidemic of autism? *Pediatrics* **107**: 411–12.

Fox A and Lack G (2003) Egg allergy and MMR vaccination. *Br J Gen Pract* **53**(495): 801–2.

Freigang B, Jadavji TP and Freigang DW (1994) Lack of adverse reactions to measles, mumps and rubella vaccine in egg-allergic children. *Ann Allergy* **73**: 486–8.

Gilat T, Hacohen D, Lilos P and Langman MJ (1987) Childhood factors in ulcerative colitis and Crohn's disease. An international co-opreative study. *Scan J Gastroenterology* **22**: 1009–24.

Gillberg C and Heijbel H (1998) MMR and autism. *Autism* **2**: 423–4.

Harling R, White JM, Ramsay ME *et al.* (2005) The effectiveness of the mumps component of the MMR vaccine: a case control study. *Vaccine* **23**(31): 4070–4.

Health Protection Agency (2006) Measles deaths, England and Wales, by age group, 1980-2004. www.hpa.org.uk/infections/topics_az/measles/data_death_age.htm

Honda H, Shimizu J and Rutter M (2005) No effect of MMR withdrawal on the incidence of autism: a total population study. *J Child Psychol Psychiatry* **46**(6): 572–9.

Kaye JA, del Mar Melero-Montes M and Jick H (2001) Mumps, measles and rubella vaccine and the incidence of autism recorded by general practitioners: a time trend analysis. *BMJ* **322**(7284): 460–3.

Khakoo GA and Lack G (2000) Recommendations for using MMR vaccine in children allergic to eggs. *BMJ* **320**: 929–32.

Landes RD, Bass JW, Millunchick EW and Oetgen WJ (1980) Neonatal rubella following postpartum maternal immunisation. *J Pediatr* **97**: 465–7.

Lokletz H and Reynolds FA (1965) Post-rubella thrombocytopaenic purpura. Report of nine new cases and review of published cases. *Lancet* **85**: 226–30.

Losonsky GA, Fishaut JM, Strussenberg J and Ogra PL (1982) Effect of immunization against rubella on lactation products. Development and characterization of specific immunologic reactivity in breast milk. *J Infect Dis* **145**: 654–60.

Madsen KM and Vestergaard M (2004) MMR vaccination and autism: what is the evidence for a causal association? *Drug Saf* **27**: 831–40.

Makela A, Nuorti JP and Peltola H (2002) Neurologic disorders after measles-mumps-rubella vaccination. *Pediatrics* **110**: 957–63.

Medical Research Council (1977) Clinical trial of live measles vaccine given alone and live vaccine preceded by killed vaccine. Fourth report of the Medical Research Council by the measles sub-committee on development of vaccines and immunisation procedures. *Lancet* **ii**: 571–5.

Miller C, Miller E, Rowe K *et al.* (1989) Surveillance of symptoms following MMR vaccine in children. *Practitioner* **233**(1461): 69–73.

Miller E, Cradock-Watson JE and Pollock TM (1982) Consequences of confirmed maternal rubella at successive stages of pregnancy. *Lancet* **2**: 781–4.

Miller EM, Waight P, Vurdein JE *et al.* (1991) Rubella surveillance to December 1990: a joint report from the PHLS and National Congenital Rubella Surveillance Programme. *CDR Review* **1**(4): R33–37.

Miller E, Goldacre M, Pugh S *et al.* (1993) Risk of aseptic meningitis after measles, mumps, and rubella vaccine in UK children. *Lancet* **341**(8851): 979–82.

Miller E, Waight P, Farrington P *et al.* (2001) Idiopathic thrombocytopaenic purpura and MMR vaccine. *Arch Dis Child* **84**: 227–9.

Miller E, Andrews N, Waight P and Taylor B (2003) Bacterial infections, immune overload, and MMR vaccine. Measles, mumps, and rubella. *Arch Dis Child* **88**(3): 222–3.

Miller E, Andrews N, Grant A *et al.* (2005) No evidence of an association between MMR vaccine and gait disturbance. *Arch Dis Child* **90**(3): 292–6.

Morgan Capner P, Wright J, Miller CL and Miller E (1988) Surveillance of antibody to measles, mumps and rubella by age. *BMJ* **297**: 770–2.

Morse D, O'Shea M, Hamilton G *et al.* (1994) Outbreak of measles in a teenage school population: the need to immunize susceptible adolescents. *Epidemiol Infect* **113**: 355–65.

Mullooly J and Black S (2001) Simultaneous administration of varicella vaccine and other recommended childhood vaccines – United States, 1995–1999. *MMWR* **50**(47): 1058–61.

Offit PA, Quarles J, Gerber MA *et al.* (2002) Addressing parents' concerns: do multiple vaccines overwhelm or weaken the infant's immune system? *Pediatrics* **109**(1): 124–9.

Orenstein WA, Markowitz L, Preblud SR *et al.* (1986) Appropriate age for measles vaccination in the United States *Dev Biol Stand* **65**: 13–21.

Patja A, Davidkin I, Kurki T *et al.* (2000) Serious adverse events after measles-mumps-rubella vaccination during a fourteen-year prospective follow-up. *Pediatr Infect Dis J* **19**: 1127–34.

Patja A, Paunio M, Kinnunen E *et al.* (2001) Risk of Guillain-Barré syndrome after measles-mumps-rubella vaccination. *J Pediatr* **138**: 250–4.

Pebody RG, Paunio M and Ruutu P (1998) Measles, measles vaccination, and Crohn's disease has not increased in Finland. *BMJ* **316**(7146): 1745–6.

Peltola H, Heinonen OP and Valle M (1994) The elimination of indigenous measles, mumps and rubella from Finland by a 12-year two-dose vaccination program. *NEJM* **331**(21): 1397–402.

Plotkin SA and Orenstein (eds) (2004) *Vaccines,* 4th edition. Philadelphia: WB Saunders Company, Chapters 19, 20 and 26.

Pool V, Braun MM, Kelso JM *et al.* (2002) Prevalence of anti-gelatin IgE antibodies in people with anaphylaxis after measles-mumps-rubella vaccine in the United States. *Pediatrics* **110**(6):e71. www.pediatrics.org/cgi/content/full/110/6/e71

Rahi K, Adams G, Russell-Eggitt I and Tookey P (2001) Epidemiological surveillance of rubella must continue (letter). *BMJ* **323**: 112.

Ramsay ME, Brown DW, Eastcott HR and Begg NT (1991) Saliva antibody testing and vaccination in a mumps outbreak. *CDR (Lond Engl Rev)* **1**(9): R96–8).

Ramsay ME, Brugha R, Brown DW *et al.* (1998) Salivary diagnosis of rubella: a study of notified cases in the United Kingdom, 1991–4. *Epidemiol Infect* **120**(3): 315–19.

Redd SC, King GE, Heath JL *et al.* (2004) Comparison of vaccination with measles-mumps-rubella at 9, 12 and 15 months of age. *J Infect Dis* **189**: S116–22.

Seagroatt V (2005) MMR vaccine and Crohn's disease: ecological study of hospital admissions in England, 1991 to 2002. *BMJ* **330**: 1120–1.

Slater PE (1997) Chronic arthropathy after rubella vaccination in women. False alarm? *JAMA* **278**: 594–5.

Taylor B, Miller E, Farrington CP *et al.* (1999) Autism and measles, mumps and rubella: no epidemiological evidence for a causal association. *Lancet* **353**(9169): 2026–9.

Taylor B, Miller E, Langman R *et al.* (2002) Measles, mumps and rubella vaccination and bowel problems or developmental regression in children with autism; population study. *BMJ* **324**(7334): 393–6.

Tischer A and Gerike E (2000) Immune response after primary and re-vaccination with different combined vaccines against measles, mumps, rubella. *Vaccine* **18**(14): 1382–92.

Tookey PA, Jones G, Miller BH and Peckham CS (1991) Rubella vaccination in pregnancy. *CDR London Engl Rev* **1**(8): R86–8.

Tookey PA and Peckham CS (1999) Surveillance of congenital rubella in Great Britain, 1971–96. *BMJ* **318**: 769–70.

Tookey PA, Cortina-Borja M and Peckham CS (2002) Rubella susceptibility among pregnant women in North London, 1996–1999. *J Public Health Med* **24**(3): 211–16.

Tookey PA (2004) Rubella in England, Scotland and Wales. *Euro Surveill* **9**: 21–2.

Vestergaard M, Hviid A, Madsen KH *et al.* (2004) MMR vaccination and febrile seizures. Evaluation of susceptible subgroups and long-term prognosis. *JAMA* **292**: 351–7.

Vyse AJ, Gay NJ, White JM *et al.* (2002) Evolution of surveillance of measles, mumps, and rubella in England and Wales: Providing the platform for evidence based vaccination policy. *Epidemiologic Reviews* **24**(2): 125–36.

WHO (2005) Vaccine Preventable Diseases Monitoring System. Global summary. www-nt.who.int/immunization_monitoring/en/globalsummary/countryprofileselect.cfm

29

Smallpox and vaccinia NOTIFIABLE

Introduction

In December 1979, the Global Commission for the Certification of Smallpox Eradication declared the world free of smallpox and this declaration was ratified by the World Health Assembly in May 1980.

In response to the threat of a bioterrorist release of smallpox, in 2003 the Department of Health published *Guidelines for smallpox response and management in the post-eradication era (smallpox plan)* available at www.dh.gov.uk/PublicationsAndStatistics/Publications/PublicationsPolicyAndGuidance/PublicationsPolicyAndGuidanceArticle/fs/en?CONTENT_ID=4070830&chk=XRWF7m

This outlines the vaccination of response teams who could safely manage and diagnose suspected cases of smallpox. In 2003–04 more than 300 healthcare and ambulance workers were vaccinated, along with a small number of staff in laboratories designated to receive specimens from suspected cases.

An information pack entitled *Smallpox vaccination of Regional Response Groups: information for health care workers administering or receiving the smallpox vaccine* has been developed specifically for non-emergency vaccination of such first responders. It includes information on administration and types of vaccine. It also has guidance on pre-vaccination screening and exclusion criteria and on work restrictions following vaccination. It is available at www.dh.gov.uk/PublicationsAndStatistics/Publications/PublicationsPolicyAndGuidance/PublicationsPolicyAndGuidanceArticle/fs/en?CONTENT_ID=4009816&chk=InmH7S

Outside the context of this plan there is no indication for smallpox vaccination for any individual with the exception of some laboratory staff and specific workers at identifiable risk.

Recommendations

Workers in laboratories where pox viruses (such as monkeypox or genetically modified vaccinia) are handled, and others whose work involves an identifiable risk of exposure to pox virus, should be advised of the possible risk and vaccination should be considered. Detailed guidance for laboratory staff has been prepared (Advisory Committee on Dangerous Pathogens and the Advisory Committee on Genetic Modification, 1990). Further advice on the need for vaccination and on contraindications should be obtained from the Health Protection Agency (HPA) Virus Reference Department (Tel: 020 8200 4400); if vaccination is considered desirable, vaccine can be obtained through HPA on this number. In Scotland, advice can be obtained from Health Protection Scotland (Tel: 0141 300 1100).

Vaccination is not recommended for people exhuming bodies in crypts, since the theoretical risk involved poses less risk than the vaccination.

Reference

Advisory Committee on Dangerous Pathogens and Advisory Committee on Genetic Modification (1990) *Vaccination of laboratory workers handling vaccinia and related pox viruses in infectious situations for humans*. London: TSO.

30

Tetanus

NOTIFIABLE

The disease

Tetanus is an acute disease caused by the action of tetanus toxin, released following infection by the bacterium *Clostridium tetani.* Tetanus spores are present in soil or manure and may be introduced into the body through a puncture wound, burn or scratch – which may go unnoticed. Neonatal tetanus is due to infection of the baby's umbilical stump. The bacteria grow anaerobically at the site of the injury and have an incubation period of between four and 21 days (most commonly about ten days).

The disease is characterised by generalised rigidity and spasms of skeletal muscles. The muscle stiffness usually involves the jaw (lockjaw) and neck and then becomes generalised. The case–fatality ratio ranges from 10 to 90%; it is highest in infants and the elderly. It varies inversely with the length of the incubation period and the availability of intensive care.

Tetanus can never be eradicated because the spores are commonly present in the environment, including soil. Tetanus is not spread from person to person.

History and epidemiology of the disease

Tetanus immunisation was first provided in the UK to the Armed Forces in 1938. From the mid-1950s it was introduced in some localities as part of the primary immunisation of infants, then nationally in 1961. The disease had almost disappeared in children under 15 years of age by the 1970s (Galbraith *et al.*, 1981). In 1970, it was recommended that people with tetanus-prone wounds should routinely be offered passive immunisation and complete a primary immunisation course.

Between 1984 and 2004, there were 198 cases of tetanus (combined data from notifications, deaths and laboratory reports) in England and Wales (Rushdy *et al.*, 2003). Seventy-four per cent occurred in individuals aged 45 years or over, and 16% were in individuals aged from 25 to 44 years. The highest incidence of tetanus was in adults over 65 years of age, with no cases of tetanus reported in infants or children under five years of age. Three cases were notified in Northern Ireland between 1984 and 2002.

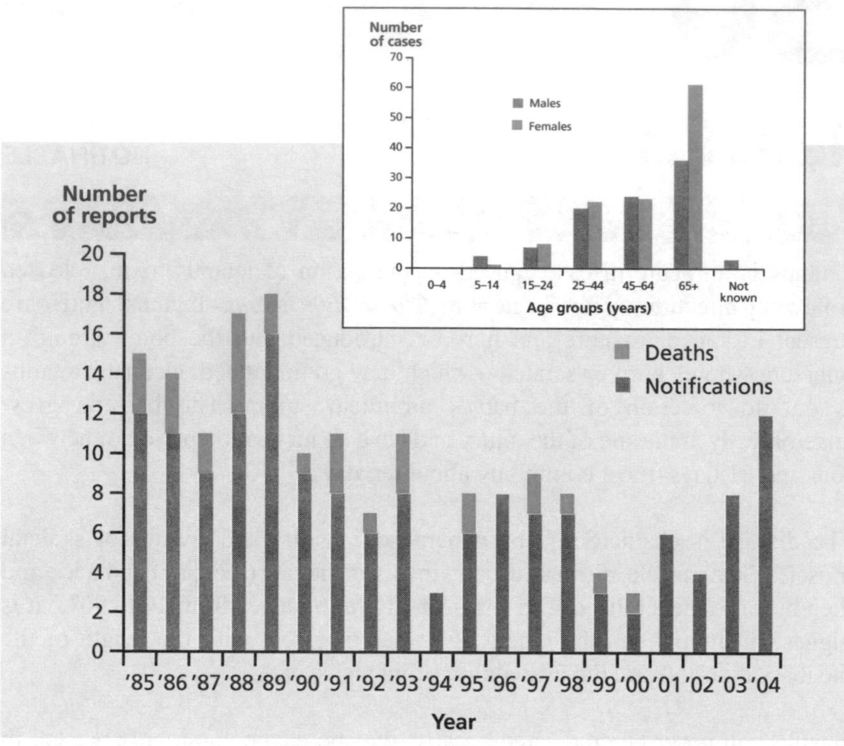

Figure 30.1 Tetanus cases and deaths in England and Wales (1984–2004)

Twenty cases of tetanus were reported in injecting drug users (IDUs) between July 2003 and February 2004 (Health Protection Agency (HPA), 2004). Seven were closely clustered in time and possibly caused by a contaminated batch of illicit drugs (HPA, 2003). Tetanus in IDUs had previously been reported rarely in the UK, in contrast to the US, where IDUs accounted for 15 to 18% of cases reported between 1995 and 2000 (Centers for Disease Control and Prevention (CDC), 2003).

Neonatal tetanus is an important cause of death in many countries in Asia and Africa due to infection of the baby's umbilical stump. Worldwide elimination of neonatal tetanus by 1995 was one of the targets of the World Health Organization (WHO), and the number of countries in which neonatal tetanus occurs is progressively decreasing. Turkey was the only country in the WHO European Region still reporting cases, with 32 cases in 2002 (www-nt.who.int/immunization_monitoring/en/globalsummary/countryprofileselect.cfm).

The tetanus vaccination

The vaccine is made from a cell-free purified toxin extracted from a strain of *C. tetani*. This is treated with formaldehyde that converts it into tetanus toxoid. This is adsorbed onto an adjuvant, either aluminium phosphate or aluminium hydroxide, to improve its immunogenicity.

Tetanus vaccines contain more than 20IU of tetanus toxoid.

The tetanus vaccine is only given as part of combined products:

- diphtheria/tetanus/acellular pertussis/inactivated polio vaccine/ *Haemophilus influenzae* type b (DTaP/IPV/Hib)
- diphtheria/tetanus/acellular pertussis/inactivated polio vaccine (DTaP/IPV or dTaP/IPV)
- tetanus/diphtheria/inactivated polio vaccine (Td/IPV).

The above vaccines are thiomersal-free. They are inactivated, do not contain live organisms and cannot cause the diseases against which they protect.

Td/IPV vaccine should be used where protection is required against tetanus, diphtheria or polio in order to provide comprehensive, long-term protection against all three diseases.

Storage

Vaccines should be stored in the original packaging at +2˚C to +8˚C and protected from light. All vaccines are sensitive to some extent to heat and cold. Heat speeds up the decline in potency of most vaccines, thus reducing their shelf life. Effectiveness cannot be guaranteed for vaccines unless they have been stored at the correct temperature. Freezing may cause increased reactogenicity and loss of potency for some vaccines. It can also cause hairline cracks in the container, leading to contamination of the contents.

Presentation

Tetanus vaccine should only be used as part of combined products. It is supplied as a cloudy white suspension either in a single dose ampoule or in a pre-filled syringe. The suspension may sediment during storage and should be shaken to distribute the suspension uniformly before administration.

Administration

Vaccines are routinely given intramuscularly into the upper arm or anterolateral thigh. This is to reduce the risk of localised reactions, which are more common when vaccines are given subcutaneously (Mark *et al.*, 1999; Diggle and Deeks, 2000; Zuckerman, 2000). However, for individuals with a bleeding disorder, vaccines should be given by deep subcutaneous injection to reduce the risk of bleeding.

Tetanus-containing vaccines can be given at the same time as other vaccines such as MMR, MenC and hepatitis B. The vaccines should be given at a separate site, preferably in a different limb. If given in the same limb, they should be given at least 2.5cm apart (American Academy of Pediatrics, 2003). The site at which each vaccine was given should be noted in the child's records.

Dosage and schedule

- First dose of 0.5ml of a tetanus-containing vaccine.
- Second dose of 0.5ml, one month after the first dose.
- Third dose of 0.5ml, one month after the second dose.
- Fourth and fifth doses of 0.5ml should be given at the recommended intervals (see below).

Disposal

Equipment used for vaccination, including used vials or ampoules, should be disposed of at the end of a session by sealing in a proper, puncture-resistant 'sharps' box (UN-approved, BS 7320).

Recommendations for the use of the vaccine

The objective of the immunisation programme is to provide a minimum of five doses of tetanus-containing vaccine at appropriate intervals for all individuals. In most circumstances, a total of five doses of vaccine at the appropriate intervals are considered to give satisfactory long-term protection.

To fulfil this objective, the appropriate vaccine for each age group is determined also by the need to protect individuals against diphtheria, pertussis, Hib and polio.

Primary immunisation

Infants and children under ten years of age

The primary course of tetanus vaccination consists of three doses of a tetanus-containing vaccine with an interval of one month between each dose. DTaP/IPV/Hib is recommended to be given at two, three and four months of age but can be given at any stage from two months up to ten years of age. If the primary course is interrupted it should be resumed but not repeated, allowing an interval of one month between the remaining doses.

Children aged ten years or over, and adults

The primary course of tetanus vaccination consists of three doses of a tetanus-containing vaccine with an interval of one month between each dose. Td/IPV is recommended for all individuals aged ten years or over. If the primary course is interrupted it should be resumed but not repeated, allowing an interval of one month between the remaining doses.

Reinforcing immunisation

Children under ten years should receive the first tetanus booster combined with diphtheria, pertussis and polio vaccines. The first booster of a tetanus-containing vaccine should ideally be given three years after completion of the primary course, normally between three and a half years and five years of age. When primary vaccination has been delayed, this first booster dose may be given at the scheduled visit provided it is one year since the third primary dose. This will re-establish the child on the routine schedule. DTaP/IPV or dTaP/IPV should be used in this age group. Td/IPV should not be used routinely for this purpose in this age group because it has been shown not to give equivalent diphtheria antitoxin response when compared with other recommended preparations.

Individuals aged ten years or over who have only had three doses of a tetanus-containing vaccine, with the last dose at least five years ago, should receive the first tetanus booster combined with diphtheria and polio vaccines (Td/IPV).

The second booster dose of Td/IPV should be given to all individuals ideally ten years after the first booster dose. When the previous doses have been delayed, the second booster should be given at the school session or scheduled appointment provided a minimum of five years have lapsed between the first and second boosters. This will be the last scheduled opportunity to ensure long-term protection.

If a person attends for a routine booster dose and has a history of receiving a vaccine following a tetanus-prone wound, attempts should be made to identify which vaccine was given. If the vaccine given at the time of the injury was the same as that due at the current visit and was given after an appropriate interval, then the routine booster dose is not required. Otherwise, the dose given at the time of injury should be discounted as it may not provide long-term protection against all antigens, and the scheduled immunisation should be given. Such additional doses are unlikely to produce an unacceptable rate of reactions (Ramsay *et al.*, 1997).

Intravenous drug users are at greater risk of tetanus. Every opportunity should be taken to ensure that they are fully protected against tetanus. Booster doses should be given if there is any doubt about their immunisation status.

Vaccination of children with unknown or incomplete immunisation status

Where a child born in the UK presents with an inadequate immunisation history, every effort should be made to clarify what immunisations they may have had (see Chapter 11 on vaccination schedules). A child who has not completed the primary course should have the outstanding doses at monthly intervals. Children may receive the first booster dose as early as one year after the third primary dose to re-establish them on the routine schedule. The second booster should be given at the time of leaving school to ensure long-term protection by this time, provided a minimum of five years is left between the first and second boosters.

Children coming to the UK who have a history of completing immunisation in their country of origin may not have been offered protection against all the antigens currently used in the UK. They will probably have received tetanus-containing vaccines in their country of origin (www-nt.who.int/immunization_monitoring/en/globalsummary/countryprofileselect.cfm)

Children coming from developing countries, from areas of conflict or from hard-to-reach population groups may not have been fully immunised. Where there is no reliable history of previous immunisation, it should be assumed that they are unimmunised, and the full UK recommendations should be followed (see Chapter 11).

Children coming to the UK may have had a fourth dose of a tetanus-containing vaccine that is given at around 18 months in some countries. This dose should be discounted as it may not provide satisfactory protection until the time of the teenage booster. The routine pre-school and subsequent boosters should be given according to the UK schedule.

Travellers and those going to reside abroad

All travellers should ensure that they are fully immunised according to the UK schedule (see above). Additional doses of vaccines may be required according to the destination and the nature of travel intended (see Departments of Health, 2001 (the Yellow Book) for more information).

For travellers to areas where medical attention may not be accessible and whose last dose of a tetanus-containing vaccine was more than ten years previously, a booster dose should be given prior to travelling, even if the individual has received five doses of vaccine previously. This is a precautionary measure in case immunoglobulin is not available to the individual should a tetanus-prone injury occur.

Where tetanus, diphtheria or polio protection is required and the final dose of the relevant antigen was received more than ten years ago, Td/IPV should be given.

Tetanus vaccination in laboratory workers

Individuals who may be exposed to tetanus in the course of their work, in microbiology laboratories, are at risk and must be protected (see Chapter 12).

Contraindications

There are very few individuals who cannot receive tetanus-containing vaccines. When there is doubt, appropriate advice should be sought from a consultant paediatrician, immunisation co-ordinator or consultant in communicable disease control rather than withholding the vaccine.

The vaccines should not be given to those who have had:

- a confirmed anaphylactic reaction to a previous dose of a tetanus-containing vaccine, or
- a confirmed anaphylactic reaction to neomycin, streptomycin or polymyxin B (which may be present in trace amounts).

Confirmed anaphylaxis occurs extremely rarely. Data from the UK, Canada and the US point to rates of 0.65 to 3 anaphylaxis events per million doses of vaccine given (Bohlke *et al.,* 2003; Canadian Medical Association, 2002). Other allergic conditions may occur more commonly and are not contraindications to further immunisation. A careful history of the event will often distinguish between anaphylaxis and other events that either are not due to the vaccine or are not life-threatening. In the latter circumstance, it may be possible to continue the immunisation course. Specialist advice must be sought on the vaccines and circumstances in which they could be given. The risk to the individual of not being immunised must be taken into account.

Precautions

Minor illnesses without fever or systemic upset are not valid reasons to postpone immunisation.

If an individual is acutely unwell, immunisation should be postponed until they have fully recovered. This is to avoid wrongly attributing any new symptom or the progression of symptoms to the vaccine.

Systemic and local reactions following a previous immunisation

This section gives advice on the immunisation of children with a history of a severe or mild systemic or local reaction within 72 hours of a preceding vaccine. Immunisation with tetanus-containing vaccine **should** continue following a history of:

- fever, irrespective of its severity
- hypotonic-hyporesponsive episodes (HHE)
- persistent crying or screaming for more than three hours
- severe local reaction, irrespective of extent.

Children who have had severe reactions, as above, have continued and completed immunisation with tetanus-containing vaccines without recurrence (Vermeer-de Bondt *et al.*, 1998; Gold *et al.*, 2000).

In Canada, a severe general or local reaction to DTaP/IPV/Hib is not a contraindication to further doses of the vaccine (Canadian Medical Association, 2002). Adverse events after childhood immunisation are carefully monitored in Canada (Le Saux *et al.*, 2003), and experience there suggests that further doses were not associated with recurrence or worsening of the preceding events (S Halperin and R Pless, pers. comm., 2003).

Pregnancy and breast-feeding

Tetanus-containing vaccines may be given to pregnant women when protection is required without delay. There is no evidence of risk from vaccinating pregnant women or those who are breast-feeding with inactivated virus, bacterial vaccines or toxoids (Plotkin and Orenstein, 2004).

Premature infants

It is important that premature infants have their immunisations at the appropriate chronological age, according to the schedule. There is no evidence that premature babies are at an increased risk of adverse reactions from vaccines (Slack *et al.*, 2001).

Immunosuppression and HIV infection

Individuals with immunosuppression or HIV infection (regardless of CD4 count) should be given tetanus-containing vaccines in accordance with the recommendations above. These individuals may not make a full antibody response. Re-immunisation should be considered after treatment is finished and recovery has occurred. Specialist advice may be required.

Further guidance is provided by the Royal College of Paediatrics and Child Health (www.rcpch.ac.uk), the British HIV Association (BHIVA) *Immunisation guidelines for HIV-infected adults* (BHIVA, 2006) and the Children's HIV Association of UK and Ireland (CHIVA) Immunisation guidelines (www.bhiva.org/chiva).

Neurological conditions

Pre-existing neurological conditions

The presence of a neurological condition is not a contraindication to immunisation. Where there is evidence of a neurological condition in a child, the advice given in the flow chart in Figure 30.2 should be followed.

If a child has a stable, pre-existing neurological abnormality such as spina bifida, congenital abnormality of the brain or perinatal hypoxic ischaemic encephalopathy, they should be immunised according to the recommended schedule. When there has been a documented history of cerebral damage in the neonatal period, immunisation should be carried out unless there is evidence of an evolving neurological abnormality.

If there is evidence of current neurological deterioration, including poorly controlled epilepsy, immunisation should be deferred and the child should be referred to a child specialist for investigation to see if an underlying cause can be identified. If a cause is not identified, immunisation should be deferred until the condition has stabilised. If a cause is identified, immunisation should proceed as normal.

A family history of seizures is not a contraindication to immunisation. When there is a personal or family history of febrile seizures, there is an increased

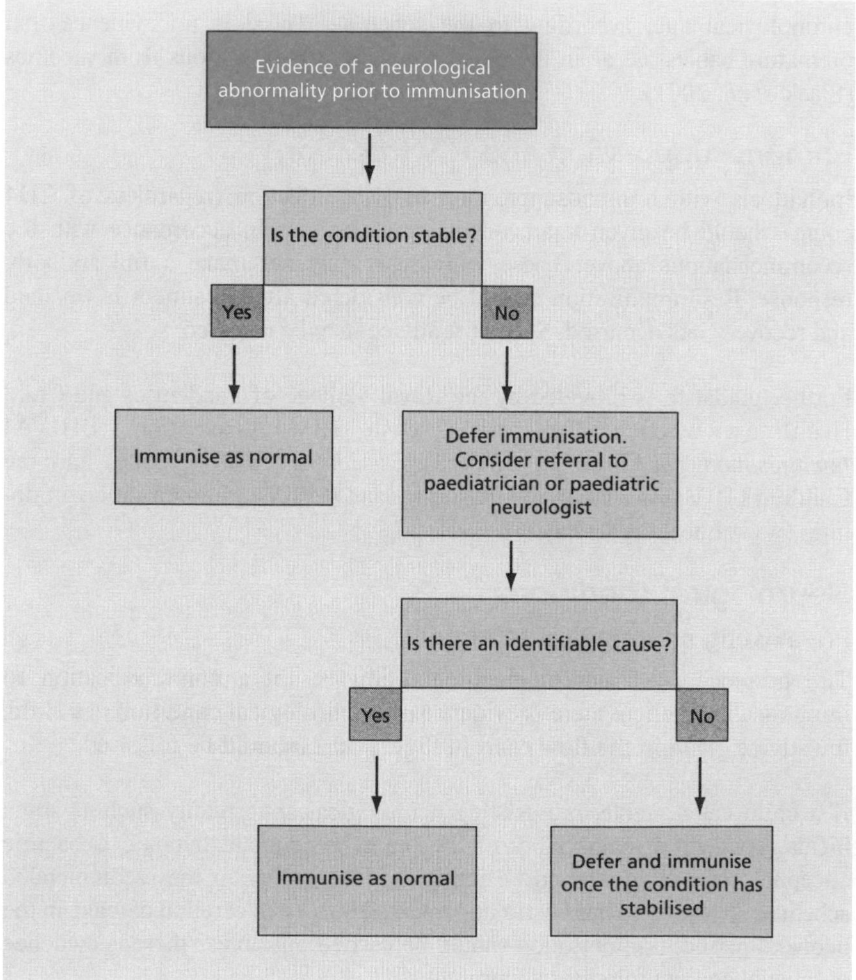

Figure 30.2 Flow chart for evidence of a neurological condition before immunisation

risk of these occurring after any fever, including that caused by immunisation. Seizures associated with fever are rare in the first six months of life and most common in the second year of life. After this age, the frequency falls and they are rare after five years of age.

When a child has had a seizure associated with fever in the past, with no evidence of neurological deterioration, immunisation should proceed as recommended. Advice on the prevention and management of fever should be given before immunisation.

When a child has had a seizure that is not associated with fever, and there is no evidence of neurological deterioration, immunisation should proceed as recommended. When immunised with DTP vaccine, children with a family or personal history of seizures had no significant adverse events and their developmental progress was normal (Ramsay *et al.*, 1994).

Neurological abnormalities following immunisation

If a child experiences encephalopathy or encephalitis within seven days of immunisation, the advice in the flow chart in Figure 30.3 should be followed. It is unlikely that these conditions will have been caused by the vaccine and they should be investigated by a specialist. Immunisation should be deferred in children where no underlying cause is found, and the child has not recovered completely within seven days, until the condition has stabilised. If a cause is identified or the child recovers within seven days, immunisation should proceed as recommended.

If a seizure associated with a fever occurs within 72 hours of an immunisation, further immunisation should be deferred if no underlying cause has been found and the child did not recover completely within 24 hours, until the condition is stable. If a cause is identified or the child recovers within 24 hours, immunisation should continue as recommended.

Deferral of immunisation

There will be very few occasions when deferral of immunisation is required (see p 45). Deferral leaves the child unprotected; the period of deferral should be minimised so that immunisation can commence as soon as possible. If a specialist recommends deferral, this should be clearly communicated to the general practitioner, who must be informed as soon as the child is fit for immunisation.

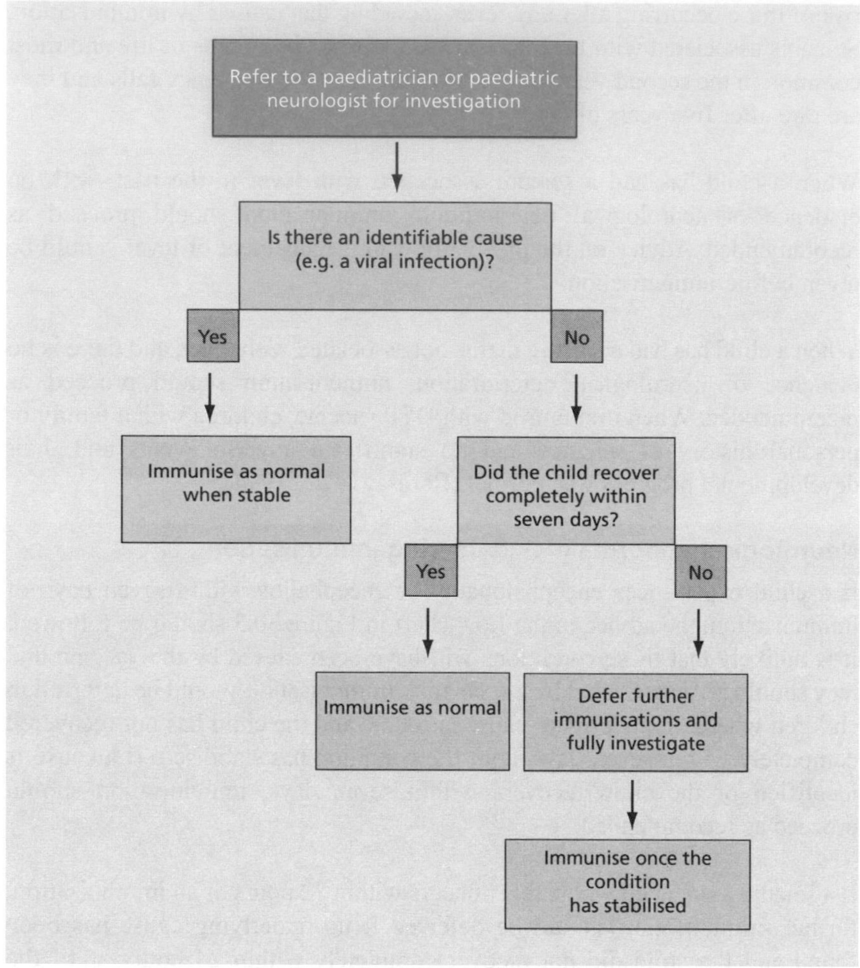

Figure 30.3 Flow chart for encephalitis or encephalopathy occurring within seven days of immunisation

Adverse reactions

Pain, swelling or redness at the injection site are common and may occur more frequently following subsequent doses. A small painless nodule may form at the injection site; this usually disappears and is of no consequence. The incidence of local reactions is lower with tetanus vaccines combined with acellular pertussis vaccines than with whole-cell pertussis vaccines and is similar to that after DT vaccine (Miller, 1999; Tozzi and Olin, 1997).

Fever, convulsions, high-pitched screaming and episodes of pallor, cyanosis and limpness (HHE) occur with equal frequency after both DTaP and DT vaccines (Tozzi and Olin, 1997).

Confirmed anaphylaxis occurs extremely rarely. Data from the UK, Canada and the US point to rates of 0.65 to 3 anaphylaxis events per million doses of vaccine given (Bohlke *et al.*, 2003; Canadian Medical Association, 2002). Other allergic conditions may occur more commonly and are not contraindications to further immunisation.

All suspected adverse reactions to vaccines occurring in children, or in individuals of any age to vaccines labelled with a black triangle (▼), should be reported to the Commission on Human Medicines through the Yellow Card scheme. Serious suspected adverse reactions to vaccines in adults should be reported through the Yellow Card scheme.

Management of patients with tetanus-prone wounds

Tetanus-prone wounds include:

- wounds or burns that require surgical intervention that is delayed for more than six hours
- wounds or burns that show a significant degree of devitalised tissue or a puncture-type injury, particularly where there has been contact with soil or manure
- wounds containing foreign bodies
- compound fractures
- wounds or burns in patients who have systemic sepsis.

Thorough cleaning of wounds is essential. If the wound, burn or injury fulfils the above criteria and is considered to be high risk, human tetanus immunoglobulin should be given for immediate protection, irrespective of the tetanus immunisation history of the patient. This is a precautionary recommendation since there is insufficient current evidence to support other alternatives. High risk is regarded as heavy contamination with material likely to contain tetanus spores and/or extensive devitalised tissue.

Injecting drug users may be at risk from tetanus-contaminated illicit drugs, especially when they have sites of focal infection such as skin abscesses that may promote growth of anaerobic organisms (Health Protection Agency, 2003).

Although any wound can give rise to tetanus, clean wounds are considered to have a low likelihood of harbouring tetanus spores and of developing the anaerobic and acidic conditions that promote spore germination (Wassilak *et al.*, 2004). Therefore, in the case of wounds such as clean cuts, human tetanus immunoglobulin need not be given.

Tetanus vaccine given at the time of a tetanus-prone injury may not boost immunity early enough to give additional protection within the incubation period of tetanus (Porter *et al.*, 1992). Therefore, tetanus vaccine is not considered adequate for treating a tetanus-prone wound. However, this provides an opportunity to ensure that the individual is protected against future exposure (see Table 30.1).

Patients who are immunosuppressed may not be adequately protected against tetanus, despite having been fully immunised. They should be managed as if they were incompletely immunised.

For those whose immunisation status is uncertain, and individuals born before 1961 who may not have been immunised in infancy, a full course of immunisation is likely to be required.

Dosage of human tetanus immunoglobulin

For prevention: 250IU by intramuscular injection, or 500IU if more than 24 hours have elapsed since injury or there is a risk of heavy contamination or following burns. This preparation is available in 1ml ampoules containing 250IU.

Management of cases

Early recognition and treatment may be life saving but few clinicians in the UK now have experience of managing tetanus. Recent experience has pointed to injecting drug users as being at significant risk of tetanus. But injecting drug users are often reluctant to present to health services. Awareness of the risk and value of vaccination in this group, and awareness among those working with them, is extremely important.

For **treatment**: The dose of tetanus immunoglobulin for intravenous use is 5000–10,000IU by infusion. If intravenous administration is not possible, 150IU/kg of the intramuscular preparation may be given in multiple sites.

IMMUNISATION STATUS	CLEAN WOUND	TETANUS-PRONE WOUND	
	Vaccine	Vaccine	Human tetanus immunoglobulin
Fully immunised, i.e. has received a total of five doses of vaccine at appropriate intervals	None required	None required	Only if high risk (see p 379)
Primary immunisation complete, boosters incomplete but up to date	None required (unless next dose due soon and convenient to give now)	None required (unless next dose due soon and convenient to give now)	Only if high risk (see p 379)
Primary immunisation incomplete or boosters not up to date	A reinforcing dose of vaccine and further doses as required to complete the recommended schedule (to ensure future immunity)	A reinforcing dose of vaccine and further doses as required to complete the recommended schedule (to ensure future immunity)	Yes: one dose of human tetanus immunoglobulin in a different site
Not immunised or immunisation status not known or uncertain	An immediate dose of vaccine followed, if records confirm the need, by completion of a full five-dose course to ensure future immunity	An immediate dose of vaccine followed, if records confirm the need, by completion of a full five-dose course to ensure future immunity	Yes: one dose of human tetanus immunoglobulin in a different site

Table 30.1 Immunisation recommendations for clean and tetanus-prone wounds

Supplies

Vaccines

- Pediacel (diphtheria/tetanus/5-component acellular pertussis/ inactivated polio vaccine/*Haemophilus influenzae* type b (DTaP/IPV/Hib)) – manufactured by Sanofi Pasteur MSD.
- Repevax (diphtheria/tetanus/5-component acellular pertussis/ inactivated polio vaccine (dTaP/IPV)) – manufactured by Sanofi Pasteur MSD.
- Infanrix IPV (diphtheria/tetanus/3-component acellular pertussis/ inactivated polio vaccine (DTaP/IPV)) – manufactured by GlaxoSmithKline.
- Revaxis (diphtheria/tetanus/inactivated polio vaccine (Td/IPV)) – manufactured by Sanofi Pasteur MSD.

These vaccines are supplied by Healthcare Logistics (Tel: 0870 871 1890) as part of the national childhood immunisation programme.

In Scotland, supplies should be obtained from local childhood vaccine-holding centres. Details of these are available from Scottish Healthcare Supplies (Tel: 0141 282 2240).

In Northern Ireland, supplies should be obtained from local childhood vaccine-holding centres. Details of these are available from the regional pharmaceutical procurement service (Tel: 028 90 552368).

Human tetanus immunoglobulin

Intravenous product

Human tetanus immunoglobulin for intravenous use is available on a named-patient basis from the Scottish National Blood Transfusion Service (Tel: 0131 536 5300, Fax: 0131 536 5781).

In England and Wales it is available from Bio Products Laboratory (Tel: 020 8258 2342).

In Northern Ireland, the source of anti-tetanus immunoglobulin is the Northern Ireland Blood Transfusion Services (Tel: 028 90 439017) (issued via hospital pharmacies).

Intramuscular products

Human tetanus immunoglobulin for intramuscular use is available from Bio Products Laboratory (Tel: 020 8258 2342) and as Liberim T from the Scottish National Blood Transfusion Service (Tel: 0131 536 5300, Fax: 0131 536 5781).

References

American Academy of Pediatrics (2003) Active immunization. In: Pickering LK (ed) *Red Book: 2003 Report of the Committee on Infectious Diseases*, 26th edition. Elk Grove Village, IL: American Academy of Pediatrics, p 33.

Bohlke K, Davis RL, Marcy SH *et al.* (2003) Risk of anaphylaxis after vaccination of children and adolescents. *Pediatrics* **112**: 815–20.

British HIV Association (2006) *Immunisation guidelines for HIV-infected adults:* www.bhiva.org/pdf/2006/Immunisation506.pdf.

Canadian Medical Association (2002) *Canadian Immunisation Guide*, 6th edition. Canadian Medical Association.

Centers for Disease Control and Prevention (2003) Tetanus surveillance – United States, 1998–2000. *Morbid Mortal Wkly Rep Surveill Summ* **52** (SS03): 1–12.

Department of Health (2001) *Health information for overseas travel* 2nd edition. London: TSO.

Diggle L and Deeks J (2000) Effect of needle length on incidence of local reactions to routine immunisation in infants aged 4 months: randomised controlled trial. *BMJ* **321**: 931–3.

Galbraith NS, Forbes P and Tillett H (1981) National surveillance of tetanus in England and Wales 1930–79. *J Infect* **3**: 181–91.

Gold M, Goodwin H, Botham S *et al.* (2000) Re-vaccination of 421 children with a past history of an adverse reaction in a specialised service. *Arch Dis Child* **83**: 128–31.

Health Protection Agency (2003) Cluster of cases of tetanus in injecting drug users in England. *CDR Wkly* **13**: 47.

Health Protection Agency (2004) Ongoing outbreak of tetanus in injecting drug users. *CDR Wkly* **14**: 2–4.

Le Saux N, Barrowman NJ, Moore D *et al.* (2003) Canadian Paediatric Society/Health Canada Immunization Monitoring Program–Active (IMPACT). Decrease in hospital admissions for febrile seizures and reports of hypotonic-hyporesponsive episodes presenting to hospital emergency departments since switching to acellular pertussis vaccine in Canada: a report from IMPACT. *Pediatrics* **112**(5): e348.

Mark A, Carlsson RM and Granstrom M (1999) Subcutaneous versus intramuscular injection for booster DT vaccination in adolescents. *Vaccine* **17**: 2067–72.

Miller E (1999) Overview of recent clinical trials of acellular pertussis vaccines. *Biologicals* **27**: 79–86.

Plotkin SA and Orenstein WA (eds) (2004) *Vaccines,* 4th edition. Philadelphia: WB Saunders Company, Chapter 8.

Porter JDH, Perkin MA, Corbel MJ *et al.* (1992) Lack of early antitoxin response to tetanus booster. *Vaccine* **10**: 334– 6.

Ramsay M, Begg N, Holland B and Dalphinis J (1994) Pertussis immunisation in children with a family or personal history of convulsions: a review of children referred for specialist advice. *Health Trends* **26**: 23–4.

Ramsay M, Joce R and Whalley J (1997) Adverse events after school leavers received combined tetanus and low dose diphtheria vaccine. *CDR Review* **5**: R65–7.

Rushdy AA, White JM, Ramsay ME and Crowcroft NS (2003) Tetanus in England and Wales 1984–2000. *Epidemiol Infect* **130**: 71–7.

Slack MH, Schapira D, Thwaites RJ *et al.* (2001) Immune response of premature infants to meningococcal serogroup C and combined diphtheria-tetanus toxoids-acellular pertussis-*Haemophilus influenzae* type b conjugate vaccines. *J Infect Dis* **184**(12): 1617–20.

Tozzi AE and Olin P (1997) Common side effects in the Italian and Stockholm 1 Trials. *Dev Biol Stand* **89**: 105–8.

Vermeer-de Bondt PE, Labadie J and Rümke HC (1998) Rate of recurrent collapse after vaccination with whole cell pertussis vaccine: follow up study. *BMJ* **316**: 902.

Wassilak SG, Roper MH, Murphy TV and Orenstein WA (2004) Tetanus toxoid. In: Plotkin SA and Orenstein WA (eds). *Vaccines*, 4th edition. Philadelphia: WB Saunders Company, p 766.

Zuckerman JN (2000) The importance of injecting vaccines into muscle. *BMJ* **321**: 1237–8.

31

Tick-borne encephalitis

NOT NOTIFIABLE

The disease

Tick-borne encephalitis (TBE) is caused by members of the flavivirus family that can affect the central nervous system. Although TBE is most commonly recognised as a meningo-encephalitis, mild febrile illnesses can also occur.

There are three forms of the disease related to the virus subtypes, namely European, Far Eastern and Siberian (Hayasaka, 2001).

The incubation period is from two to 28 days (Dumpis *et al.*, 1999). The European form of the disease is biphasic with an initial viraemic phase of fever and influenza-like symptoms followed in some cases (after an afebrile period of one to 20 days) by central nervous system involvement. The case fatality rate of the European form is 1%. Long-lasting or permanent neuropsychiatric sequelae are observed in 10–20% of affected patients. The Far Eastern version is more gradual in onset and normally takes a more severe and longer course with a reported mortality of 5–20%.

TBE is transmitted to humans by the bite of an infected tick or, less commonly, by ingestion of unpasteurised milk from infected animals, especially goats. The virus is maintained in nature by small mammals, domestic livestock and certain species of birds.

More men tend to be infected than women and most of these infections are caused by leisure activity such as hiking (Kaiser, 1995). The incidence peaks in spring and early summer, but can occur throughout the year (Lindgren and Gustafson, 2001).

TBE occurs in most or parts of Austria, Germany, southern and central Sweden, France (Alsace region), Switzerland, Norway, Denmark, Poland, Croatia, Albania, the Baltic states (Estonia, Latvia and Lithuania), the Czech and Slovak Republics, Hungary, Russia (including Siberia), Ukraine, some other countries of the former Soviet Union, and northern and eastern regions of China (Hayasaka, 2001).

History and epidemiology of the disease

The TBE virus is almost exclusively restricted to areas of Europe and Asia. The disease has never been endemic in the UK. Since the 1930s, TBE has been a major public health problem in central Russia.

Austria has had a universal, annual, national vaccination campaign since 1980. There is widespread use of TBE vaccine in other central European countries.

The TBE vaccination

One licensed vaccine (FSME-IMMUN) is available currently. It is produced from virus grown in chick fibroblasts and then inactivated by formaldehyde; it is supplied as a suspension of 0.5ml for injection in a pre-filled syringe.

The vaccine contains the Neudörfl virus strain, has been shown to be effective against the European subtype of TBE, and is probably effective against the more aggressive Far Eastern subtype.

The vaccine contains aluminium hydroxide and trace quantities of neomycin and gentamicin, and is thiomersal-free. It is inactivated, does not contain live organisms and cannot cause the disease against which it protects.

Dosage and schedule

- First dose of 0.5ml (0.25ml FSME-IMMUN Junior for children aged one year and below 16 years of age) at day 0.
- Second dose of 0.5ml (0.25ml of FSME-IMMUN Junior for children aged one year and below 16 years of age) one to three months after the first dose.
- Third dose of 0.5ml (0.25ml FSME-IMMUN Junior for children aged one year and below 16 years of age) five to 12 months after the second dose.

For rapid short-term protection of children and adults the second dose may be given two weeks after the first dose and gives at least 90% protection (Plotkin and Orenstein, 2004)

Storage

Vaccines should be stored in the original packaging at +2˚C to +8˚C and protected from light. All vaccines are sensitive to some extent to heat and cold.

Heat speeds up the decline in potency of most vaccines, thus reducing their shelf life. Effectiveness cannot be guaranteed for vaccines unless they have been stored at the correct temperature. Freezing may cause increased reactogenicity and loss of potency for some vaccines. It can also cause hairline cracks in the container, leading to contamination of the contents.

Administration

Vaccines are routinely given intramuscularly into the upper arm or anterolateral thigh. However, for individuals with a bleeding disorder, vaccines should be given by deep subcutaneous injection to reduce the risk of bleeding.

TBE vaccine can be given at the same time as other travel and routine vaccines. The vaccines should be given at separate sites, preferably in different limbs. If given in the same limb, they should be given at least 2.5cm apart (American Academy of Pediatrics, 2003).

Disposal

Equipment used for vaccination, including used vials or ampoules, should be disposed of at the end of a session by sealing in a proper, puncture-resistant 'sharps' box (UN-approved, BS 7320).

Recommendations for the use of the vaccine

TBE vaccine is used for the protection of individuals at high risk of exposure to the virus through travel or employment.

Awareness of risk areas is essential. The following measures are advised whether or not vaccine is given. Some protection against TBE is provided by covering arms, legs and ankles, and using insect repellents on socks and outer clothes (Dumpis *et al.*, 1999). Any ticks attaching to the skin should be removed completely as soon as possible. Evidence suggests that the best method is slow, straight removal with tweezers (Teece and Crawford, 2002). Unvaccinated individuals bitten by ticks in endemic areas should seek local medical advice.

Unpasteurised milk should not be drunk.

The vaccine is recommended particularly for spring and summer travel in warm, forested parts of the endemic areas, where ticks are most prevalent. Individuals who hike, camp, hunt and undertake fieldwork in endemic forested areas should be vaccinated.

TBE vaccine is recommended for those who will be going to reside in an area where TBE is endemic or epidemic, and particularly for those working in forestry, woodcutting, farming and the military (WHO, 1995).

More detailed country-by-country information is contained in *Health information for overseas travel* (Department of Health, 2001).

Laboratory workers who may be exposed to TBE should be vaccinated.

Infants and children under 36 months of age

Although the vaccine is not licensed in the UK for use on patients below 36 months of age, it is used routinely in Austria from 18 months of age. Use of the vaccine should be considered in young children if they are going to be at high risk.

The manufacturer notes that the product available in Austria for those under 36 months, FSME-IMMUN Junior, may be available on a named-patient basis via MASTA until the UK licence for it is granted.

Reinforcing immunisation

A booster dose is recommended every three years (Dumpis *et al.*,1999) after an initial three-dose schedule, if the individual continues to be at risk.

Contraindications

There are few individuals who cannot receive TBE vaccine.

The vaccine should not be given to those who have had:

- a confirmed anaphylactic reaction to a previous dose of TBE vaccine
- a confirmed anaphylactic reaction to one of the vaccine components
- a confirmed anaphylactic reaction to egg ingestion.

Precautions

Pregnancy and breast-feeding

TBE vaccine has not been associated directly with adverse outcomes of pregnancy. There is no evidence of risk from vaccinating pregnant women, or those who are breast-feeding, with inactivated virus or bacterial vaccines or toxoids (Hayasaka *et al.*, 2001).

Adverse reactions

Reported reactions to TBE vaccine are rare. Local reactions such as swelling, pain and redness at the injection site may occur.

Pyrexia, particularly after the first dose, can occur in children and adults, usually occurring within 12 hours of immunisation and settling within 24–48 hours (Dumpis *et al*., 1999; Kunz *et al*., 1980). Febrile convulsions have rarely occurred, and antipyretic treatment and cooling should be initiated in good time.

All suspected adverse reactions to vaccines occurring in children, or in individuals of any age after vaccines labelled with a black triangle (▼), should be reported to the Commission on Human Medicines using the Yellow Card scheme. Serious suspected adverse reactions to all vaccines in adults should also be reported through the Yellow Card scheme.

Management of cases

No specific therapy is available for TBE. FSME Bulin (TBE immunoglobulin) has been discontinued (Kluger, 1995) and is no longer available either in the UK or in Europe.

Supportive treatment can significantly reduce morbidity and mortality.

Supplies

FSME-IMMUN® and FSME-IMMUN Junior are both currently available from MASTA (Tel: 0113 238 7555) and Baxter Healthcare Ltd (Tel: 01635 206140).

References

American Academy of Pediatrics (2003). Active immunization. In: Pickering LK (ed.) *Red Book: 2003 Report of the Committee on Infectious Diseases*, 26th edition. Elk Grove Village, IL: American Academy of Pediatrics, p 33.

Department of Health (2001) *Health information for overseas travel*, 2nd edition. London: TSO.

Dumpis U, Crook D and Oksi J (1999) Tick-borne encephalitis. *Clinical Infect Dis* **28**: 882–90.

Hayasaka D, Goto A, Yoshii K *et al*. (2001) Evaluation of European tick-borne encephalitis virus vaccine against recent Siberian and far-eastern subtype strains. *Vaccine* **19**(32): 4774–9.

Kaiser R (1995) Tick-borne encephalitis in southern Germany. *Lancet* **345**(8947): 463.

Kluger G, Schottler A, Waldvogel K *et al.* (1995) Tick-borne encephalitis despite specific immunoglobulin prophylaxis. *Lancet* **346**: 1502.

Kunz C, Heinz FX and Hofmann H (1980) Immunogenicity and reactogenicity of a highly purified vaccine against tick-borne encephalitis. *J Med Virol* **6**: 103–9.

Lindgren E and Gustafson R (2001) Tick-borne encephalitis in Sweden and climate change. *Lancet* **358**: 16–18.

Plotkin SA and Orenstein WA (eds) (2004) *Vaccines,* 4th edition, Philadelphia: WB Saunders Company, p 1039–57.

Teece S and Crawford I (2002) Towards evidence based emergency medicine: best BETs from the Manchester Royal Infirmary. How to remove a tick. *Emerg Med J* **19**(4): 323–4.

WHO (1995) Tick-borne encephalitis. *WHO Wkly Epidemiol Rec* **70**: 120–2.

32

Tuberculosis

NOTIFIABLE

The disease

Human tuberculosis (TB) is caused by infection with bacteria of the *Mycobacterium tuberculosis* complex (*M. tuberculosis*, *M. bovis* or *M. africanum*) and may affect almost any part of the body. The most common form is pulmonary TB, which accounts for almost 60% of all cases in the UK (Table 32.1). Non-respiratory forms of TB are more common in young children in communities with connections to areas of the world with high prevalence, and in those with impaired immunity.

The symptoms of TB are varied and depend on the site of infection. General symptoms may include fever, loss of appetite, weight loss, night sweats and lassitude. Pulmonary TB typically causes a persistent productive cough, which may be accompanied by blood-streaked sputum or, more rarely, frank haemoptysis. Untreated, TB in most otherwise healthy adults is a slowly progressive disease that may eventually be fatal.

Almost all cases of TB in the UK are acquired through the respiratory route, by breathing in infected respiratory droplets from a person with infectious respiratory TB. Transmission is most likely when the index case has sputum that is smear positive for the bacillus on microscopy, and often after prolonged close contact such as living in the same household.

The initial infection may:

- be eliminated
- remain latent – where the individual has no symptoms but the TB bacteria remain in the body, or
- progress to active TB over the following weeks or months.

Latent TB infection may reactivate in later life, particularly if an individual's immune system has become weakened, for example by disease (e.g. HIV), certain medical treatments (e.g. cancer chemotherapy, corticosteroids) or in old age.

Table 32.1 Site of disease in cases of TB occurring in England, Wales and Northern Ireland in order of frequency (Health Protection Agency, Enhanced Tuberculosis Surveillance, data for 2001)

Site of disease	Number of cases	% of total cases
Pulmonary	3907	59.4
Extra-thoracic lymph nodes	1066	16.2
Pleural	484	7.4
Intra-thoracic lymph nodes	475	7.2
Bone/joint	310	4.7
Gastro-intestinal	227	3.5
Genito-urinary	115	1.7
Miliary	106	1.6
Meninges	99	1.5
CNS (other than meningitis)	52	0.8
Cryptic	49	0.7
Laryngeal	12	0.2
Other	452	6.9

History and epidemiology of the disease

Notifications of TB declined in the UK over most of the last century (Figure 32.1). In 1913, the first year of statutory notification, 117,139 new TB cases were recorded in England and Wales; the lowest number of reported cases (5086) was in 1987. Since then, new reported cases rose by nearly 40% to around 7000 in 2004 in England and Wales. In London, the numbers doubled, accounting for almost 3000 (40%) of the national total in 2004. In Scotland, the number of new cases remains relatively constant at around 400 each year.

The epidemiological changes in the UK have occurred against a background of deteriorating TB control in many parts of the world such that the World Health Organization (WHO) declared TB a global public health emergency in 1993.

The resurgence of TB in some parts of the UK has been associated with changing patterns in its epidemiology. Over the last 50 years, it has moved from a disease that occurred across all parts of the population to one occurring predominantly in specific population subgroups. Rates are higher in certain communities, mainly by virtue of their connections to higher-prevalence areas of the world. In other communities, endemic factors such as homelessness and alcohol misuse are important factors. In 2003, two-thirds of

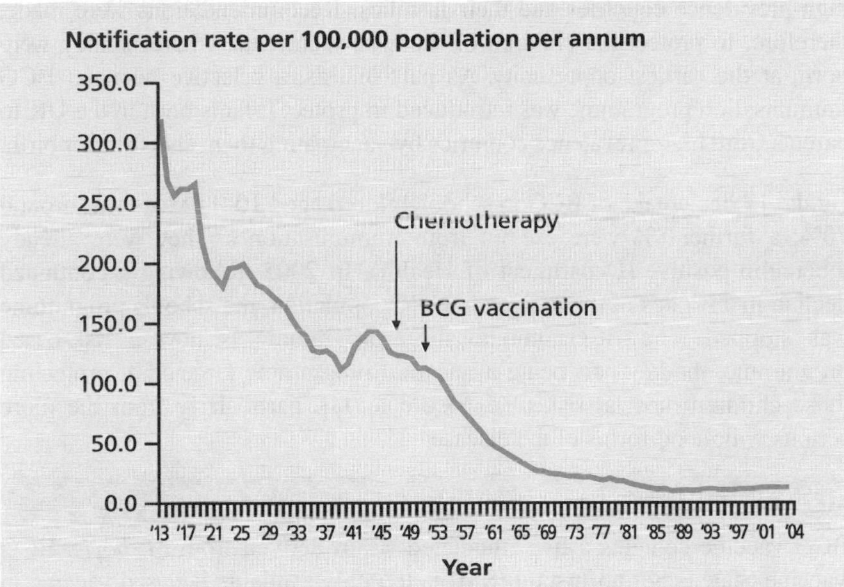

Figure 32.1 Notifications of TB in England and Wales 1913–2004

patients with TB were born abroad (Health Protection Agency, 2003); the proportion is reversed in Scotland. TB is also concentrated in certain areas of the UK, mainly inner city areas.

In the UK, mortality from TB decreased rapidly after the introduction of effective chemotherapy in the 1940s and the introduction of routine adolescent BCG (Bacillus Calmette-Guérin vaccine) programmes in 1953. However, there are still around 350 deaths each year either directly due to or associated with TB (Health Protection Agency, 2005). Although levels of drug-resistant and multidrug-resistant TB remain low in the UK, they increased slightly between 1998 and 2003 (Health Protection Agency, 2004).

The BCG immunisation programme

The BCG immunisation programme was introduced in the UK in 1953 and has undergone several changes since, in response to changing trends in the epidemiology of TB. The programme was initially targeted at children of school-leaving age (then 14 years), as the peak incidence of TB was in young, working-age adults.

In the 1960s, when TB rates in the indigenous population were continuing to decline, rates were shown to be much higher in new immigrants from high-prevalence countries and their families. Recommendations were made, therefore, to protect the children of these new entrants, wherever they were born, at the earliest opportunity. As part of this, a selective neonatal BCG immunisation programme was introduced to protect infants born in the UK to parents from high-prevalence countries by vaccinating them shortly after birth.

By the 1990s, uptake of BCG in schoolchildren aged 10–14 years was around 70%; a further 8% were exempt from immunisation as they were already tuberculin-positive (Department of Health). In 2005, following a continued decline in TB rates in the indigenous UK population, the schools programme was stopped. The BCG immunisation programme is now a risk-based programme, the key part being a neonatal programme targeted at protecting those children most at risk of exposure to TB, particularly from the more serious childhood forms of the disease.

The Bacillus Calmette-Guérin (BCG) vaccine

BCG vaccine contains a live attenuated strain derived from *M. bovis*. BCG Vaccine Statens Serum Institut (SSI) is the only available licensed vaccine in the UK. It contains the Danish strain 1331. BCG vaccine does not contain thiomersal or any other preservatives. It contains live organisms that have been attenuated (modified).

Studies of the effectiveness of BCG vaccine have given widely varying results, between countries and between studies, ranging from no protection to 70 to 80% protection in UK schoolchildren (Sutherland and Springett, 1987, Rodrigues *et al.*, 1991). However, meta-analyses have shown the vaccine to be 70 to 80% effective against the most severe forms of the disease, such as TB meningitis in children (Rodrigues *et al.*, 1993). It is less effective in preventing respiratory disease, which is the more common form in adults. Protection has been shown to last for 10 to 15 years (WHO, 1999). Data on duration of protection after this time are limited, but protection may wane with time.

There are few data on the protection afforded by BCG vaccine when it is given to adults (aged 16 years or over), and virtually no data for persons aged 35 years or over. BCG is not usually recommended for people aged over 16 years, unless the risk of exposure is great (e.g. healthcare or laboratory workers at occupational risk or where vaccination is indicated for travel).

Storage

The unreconstituted vaccine and its diluent should be stored in the original packaging at +2°C to +8°C and protected from light. All vaccines are sensitive to some extent to heat and cold. Effectiveness of vaccines cannot be guaranteed unless they have been stored at the correct temperature. Heat speeds up the decline in potency of most vaccines, thus reducing their shelf life. Freezing may cause increased reactogenicity and loss of potency in some vaccines. It can also cause hairline cracks in the container, leading to contamination of the contents. If the vaccine and/or diluent has been frozen, it must not be used.

The vaccine should be reconstituted with the diluent supplied by the manufacturer and used immediately. Unused reconstituted vaccine should be discarded after four hours. The vaccine is usable for up to four hours at room temperature after reconstitution.

Presentation

The vaccine is a freeze-dried powder for suspension for injection. BCG Vaccine SSI is supplied in a glass vial containing the equivalent of 10 adult or 20 infant doses, fitted with a bromobutyl rubber stopper which does not contain latex. The powder must be reconstituted with 1ml of the diluted Sauton SSI diluent which is supplied separately.

Administration of BCG vaccination

In all cases, BCG vaccine must be administered strictly intradermally, normally into the lateral aspect of the left upper arm at the level of the insertion of the deltoid muscle (just above the middle of the left upper arm – the left arm is recommended by WHO). Sites higher on the arm, and particularly the tip of the shoulder, are more likely to lead to keloid formation and should be avoided. Jet injectors and multiple puncture devices should not be used.

The upper arm should be positioned approximately 45° to the body. This can be achieved in older children and adults if the hand is placed on the hip with the arm abducted from the body, but in infants and younger children this will not be possible. For this age group, the arm must be held firmly in an extended position (see Chapter 4).

If the skin is visibly dirty it should be washed with soap and water. The vaccine is administered through either a specific tuberculin syringe or, alternatively, a 1ml graduated syringe fitted with a 26G 10mm (0.45mm × 10mm) needle for each individual. The correct dose (see below) of BCG vaccine should be drawn into the tuberculin syringe and the 26G short bevelled needle attached to give the injection. The needle must be attached firmly and the intradermal injection administered with the bevel uppermost.

The operator stretches the skin between the thumb and forefinger of one hand and with the other slowly inserts the needle, with the bevel upwards, about 3mm into the superficial layers of the dermis almost parallel with the surface. The needle can usually be seen through the epidermis. A correctly given intradermal injection results in a tense, blanched, raised bleb, and considerable resistance is felt when the fluid is being injected. A bleb is typically of 7mm diameter following a 0.1ml intradermal injection, and 3mm following a 0.05ml intradermal injection. If little resistance is felt when injecting and a diffuse swelling occurs as opposed to a tense blanched bleb, the needle is too deep. The needle should be withdrawn and reinserted intradermally before more vaccine is given.

No further immunisation should be given in the arm used for BCG immunisation for at least three months because of the risk of regional lymphadenitis. The subject must always be advised of the normal reaction to the injection and about caring for the vaccination site (see below).

BCG should ideally be given at the same time as other live vaccines such as MMR. If live vaccines cannot be administered simultaneously, a four-week interval is recommended.

Dosage and schedule

A single dose of:

- 0.05ml for infants under 12 months
- 0.1ml for children aged 12 months or older and adults.

Disposal

Equipment used for vaccination, including used vials or ampoules, should be disposed of at the end of a session by sealing in a proper, puncture-resistant 'sharps' box (UN-approved, BS-7320).

Recommendations for the use of the vaccine

The aim of the UK BCG immunisation programme is to immunise those at increased risk of developing severe disease and/or of exposure to TB infection.

BCG immunisation should be offered to:

- all infants (aged 0 to 12 months) living in areas of the UK where the annual incidence of TB is 40/100,000 or greater

- all infants (aged 0 to 12 months) with a parent or grandparent who was born in a country where the annual incidence of TB is 40/100,000 or greater
- previously unvaccinated children aged one to five years with a parent or grandparent who was born in a country where the annual incidence of TB is 40/100,000 or greater. These children should be identified at suitable opportunities, and can normally be vaccinated without tuberculin testing
- previously unvaccinated, tuberculin-negative children aged from six to under 16 years of age with a parent or grandparent who was born in a country where the annual incidence of TB is 40/100,000 or greater. These children should be identified at suitable opportunities, tuberculin tested and vaccinated if negative (see section on tuberculin testing prior to BCG vaccination)
- previously unvaccinated tuberculin-negative contacts of cases of respiratory TB (following recommended contact management advice – see National Institute for Health and Clinical Excellence (NICE), 2006)
- previously unvaccinated, tuberculin-negative new entrants under 16 years of age who were born in or who have lived for a prolonged period (at least three months) in a country with an annual TB incidence of 40/100,000 or greater.

Individuals at occupational risk

People in the following occupational groups are more likely than the general population to come into contact with someone with TB:

- healthcare workers who will have contact with patients or clinical materials
- laboratory staff who will have contact with patients, clinical materials or derived isolates
- veterinary and staff such as abattoir workers who handle animal species known to be susceptible to TB, e.g. simians
- prison staff working directly with prisoners
- staff of care homes for the elderly
- staff of hostels for homeless people and facilities accommodating refugees and asylum seekers.

Unvaccinated, tuberculin-negative individuals aged under 35 years in these occupations are recommended to receive BCG. There are no data on the protection afforded by BCG vaccine when it is given to adults aged 35 years or over.

Not all healthcare workers are at an equal risk of TB. There are likely to be categories of healthcare workers who are at particular risk of TB, and should be part of the clinical risk assessment when the use of BCG is being considered for a healthcare worker over 35 years of age.

Travellers and those going to reside abroad

BCG may be required for previously unvaccinated, tuberculin-negative individuals according to the destination and the nature of travel (Cobelens *et al.*, 2000). The vaccine is recommended for those under 35 years who are going to live or work with local people for more than three months in a country where the annual incidence of TB is 40/100,000 or greater (see Department of Health, 2001, *Health information for overseas travel*, for more information).

Individual requests for BCG vaccination

People seeking vaccination for themselves or their children should be assessed for specific risk factors for TB. Those without risk factors should not be offered BCG vaccination but should be advised of the current policy and given written information. Further information is available at www.immunisation.nhs.uk. People with risk factors should be tuberculin tested and offered BCG vaccination according to local service arrangements.

Repeat BCG vaccination

Although the protection afforded by BCG vaccine may wane with time, there is no evidence that repeat vaccination offers significant additional protection and repeat BCG vaccination is not recommended.

Contraindications

The vaccine should not be given to:

- those who have already had a BCG vaccination
- those with a past history of TB
- those with an induration of 6mm or more following Mantoux (SSI) tuberculin skin testing
- those who have had a confirmed anaphylactic reaction to a component of the vaccine
- neonates in a household where an active TB case is suspected or confirmed
- people who are immunocompromised by virtue of disease or treatment, e.g.:

- patients receiving corticosteroid or other immunosuppressive treatment, including general radiation. Inhaled steroids are not a contraindication
- those suffering from a malignant condition such as lymphoma, leukaemia, Hodgkin's disease or other tumour of the reticuloendothelial system.

BCG is contraindicated in symptomatic HIV-positive individuals. In countries such as the UK where the risk of TB is low, it is recommended that BCG is also withheld from all those known to be or suspected to be HIV positive, regardless of clinical status. Where vaccination is indicated, for example infants born to HIV-positive mothers, this can be administered after two appropriately timed negative postnatal PCR tests for HIV infection (see Chapter 6 Contraindications and special considerations).

Precautions

Minor illnesses without fever or systemic upset are not valid reasons to postpone immunisation.

If an individual is acutely unwell, immunisation should be postponed until they have fully recovered. This is to avoid confusing the differential diagnosis of any acute illness by wrongly attributing any sign or symptoms to the adverse effects of the vaccine.

Individuals with generalised septic skin conditions should not be vaccinated. If eczema exists, an immunisation site should be chosen that is free from skin lesions.

Pregnancy and breast-feeding

Although no harmful effects on the fetus have been observed from BCG during pregnancy, it is wise to avoid vaccination, particularly in the first trimester, and wherever possible to delay until after delivery. A further tuberculin test may be required if more than three months has elapsed since the test on which a recommendation for BCG was based. Breast-feeding is not a contraindication to BCG.

Premature infants

It is important that premature infants have their immunisations at the appropriate chronological age, according to recommendations. There is no evidence that premature babies are at an increased risk of adverse reactions from vaccines.

Previous BCG vaccination

BCG should not be administered to previously vaccinated individuals as there is an increased risk of adverse reactions and no evidence of additional protection. Evidence of a previous BCG vaccination includes: documentary evidence; a clear, reliable history of vaccination; or evidence of a characteristic scar.

Determining a reliable history of BCG vaccination may be complicated by:

- absent or limited documentary evidence
- unreliable recall of vaccination
- absence of a characteristic scar in some individuals vaccinated intradermally
- absence of a scar in a high proportion of individuals vaccinated percutaneously
- use of non-standard vaccination sites.

Individuals with an uncertain history of prior BCG vaccination should be tuberculin tested before being given BCG. The final decision whether to offer BCG, where there is a possible history of previous vaccination but no proof, must balance the risk of possible revaccination against the potential benefit of vaccination and the individual's risk of exposure to TB, particularly in an occupational setting.

Immunisation reaction and care of the immunisation site

The expected reaction to successful BCG vaccination, seen in 90 to 95% of recipients, is induration at the injection site followed by a local lesion which starts as a papule two or more weeks after vaccination. It may ulcerate and then slowly subside over several weeks or months to heal, leaving a small, flat scar. It may also include enlargement of a regional lymph node to less than 1cm.

It is not necessary to protect the site from becoming wet during washing and bathing. The ulcer should be encouraged to dry, and abrasion (by tight clothes, for example) should be avoided. Should any oozing occur, a temporary dry dressing may be used until a scab forms. It is essential that air is not excluded. If absolutely essential (e.g. to permit swimming), an impervious dressing may be used but it should be applied only for a short period as it may delay healing and cause a larger scar.

Further observation after routine vaccination with BCG is not necessary, other than as part of monitoring of the quality of the programme, nor is further tuberculin testing recommended.

Adverse reactions

Severe injection site reactions, large, local discharging ulcers, abscesses and keloid scarring are most commonly caused by faulty injection technique, excessive dosage or vaccinating individuals who are tuberculin positive. It is essential that all health professionals are properly trained in all aspects of the process involved in tuberculin skin tests and BCG vaccination. Training materials for health professionals are available from Department of Health Publications (e-mail: dh@prolog.uk.com). For further information, see www.immunisation.nhs.uk.

Other adverse reactions

Adverse reactions to the vaccine include headache, fever and enlargement of a regional lymph node to greater than 1cm and which may ulcerate.

Allergic reactions (including anaphylactic reactions), more severe local reactions such as abscess formation, and disseminated BCG complications (such as osteitis or osteomyelitis) are rare.

All serious or unusual adverse reactions possibly associated with BCG vaccination (including abscess and keloid scarring) should be recorded and reported to the Commission on Human Medicines through the Yellow Card system, and vaccination protocols and techniques should be reviewed. Every effort should be made to recover and identify the causative organism from any lesion constituting a serious complication.

Management of adverse reactions

Individuals with severe local reactions (ulceration greater than 1cm, caseous lesions, abscesses or drainage at the injection site) or with regional suppurative lymphadenitis with draining sinuses following BCG vaccination should be referred to a chest physician or paediatrician for investigation and management.

An adherent, suppurating or fistulated lymph node may be incised and drained, and left to heal. There is little evidence to support the use of either locally instilled anti-mycobacterial agents or systemic treatment of patients with severe persistent lesions.

Disseminated BCG infection should be referred to a chest physician or paediatrician for specialist advice and will normally require systemic anti-TB treatment following current guidance for managing *M. bovis* infection (currently Joint Tuberculosis Committee of the British Thoracic Society, 2000, and NICE, 2006).

In vitro testing has shown that, for treatment purposes, BCG SSI is susceptible to both isoniazid and rifampicin.

Overdose

Overdose increases the risk of a severe local reaction and suppurative lymphadenitis, and may lead to excessive scar formation. The extent of the reaction is likely to depend on whether any – and how much – of the vaccine was injected subcutaneously or intramuscularly instead of intradermally.

Any incident resulting in administration of an overdose of BCG vaccine should be documented according to local policy. The vaccine recipient or their carer and the local chest physician should be informed. The clinician should decide whether preventive chemotherapy is indicated and ensure arrangements are made for appropriate monitoring for early signs of an adverse reaction.

Tuberculin skin testing prior to BCG immunisation – the Mantoux test

BCG should not be administered to an individual with a positive tuberculin test – it is unnecessary and may cause a more severe local reaction. Those with *strongly* positive tests should be referred to a chest clinic for assessment of the need for further investigation and treatment.

A tuberculin skin test is necessary prior to BCG vaccination for:

- all individuals aged six years or over
- infants and children under six years of age with a history of residence or prolonged stay (more than three months) in a country with an annual TB incidence of 40/100,000 or greater
- those who have had close contact with a person with known TB
- those who have a family history of TB within the last five years.

BCG can be given up to three months following a negative tuberculin test.

The Mantoux test is used as a screening test for tuberculosis infection or disease and as an aid to diagnosis. The local skin reaction to tuberculin purified protein derivative (PPD) injected into the skin is used to assess an individual's sensitivity to tuberculin protein. The greater the reaction, the more likely it is that an individual is infected or has active TB disease.

The standard test for use in the UK is the Mantoux test using 2TU/0.1ml tuberculin PPD.

Purified protein derivative

Storage

Tuberculin PPD SSI should be stored in the original packaging at +2°C to +8°C and protected from light. Freezing may cause loss of activity.

Presentation

Tuberculin PPD SSI is a sterile preparation made from a culture of seven selected strains of *M. tuberculosis*. It is available as a clear colourless to light yellow solution for injection. It is available as 2TU/0.1ml (for routine screening) and 10TU/0.1ml (for clinical diagnostic purposes) and is supplied in glass vials with a chlorobutyl rubber stopper that does not contain latex.

Dosage

0.1ml of the appropriate tuberculin PPD preparation.

The preparation for routine use and in patients in whom TB is suspected contains 2TU/0.1ml.

A 10TU/0.1ml preparation may be used if a second Mantoux test is required for clinical diagnostic purposes.

Administration of the Mantoux test

In all cases, the Mantoux test should be administered intradermally (sometimes referred to as intracutaneous administration) normally on the flexor surface of the left forearm at the junction of the upper third with the lower two-thirds.

If the skin is visibly dirty it should be washed with soap and water. The Mantoux test is performed using the 0.1ml tuberculin syringe or, alternatively, a 1ml graduated syringe fitted with a short bevel 26G (0.45mm × 10mm) needle. A separate syringe and needle must be used for each subject to prevent cross-infection. 0.1ml of PPD should be drawn into the tuberculin syringe and the 25G or 26G short bevelled needle attached to give the injection. The needle must be attached firmly and the intradermal injection administered with the bevel uppermost.

The operator stretches the skin between the thumb and forefinger of one hand and with the other slowly inserts the needle, with the bevel upwards, about

3mm into the superficial layers of the dermis almost parallel with the surface. The needle can usually be seen through the epidermis. A correctly given intradermal injection results in a tense, blanched, raised bleb, and considerable resistance is felt when the fluid is being injected. A bleb is typically of 7mm diameter following 0.1ml intradermal injection. If little resistance is felt when injecting and a diffuse swelling occurs as opposed to a tense, blanched bleb, the needle is too deep. The needle should be withdrawn and reinserted intradermally.

Mantoux tests can be undertaken at the same time as inactivated vaccines are administered. Live viral vaccines can suppress the tuberculin response, and therefore testing should not be carried out within four weeks of having received a live viral vaccine such as MMR. Where MMR is not required urgently it should be delayed until the Mantoux has been read (see below).

Disposal

Equipment used for Mantoux testing, including used vials or ampoules, should be disposed of at the end of a session by sealing in a proper, puncture-resistant 'sharps' box (UN-approved, BS 7320).

Reading the Mantoux test

The results should be read 48 to 72 hours after the test is taken, but a valid reading can usually be obtained up to 96 hours later. The transverse diameter of the area of induration at the injection site is measured with a ruler and the result recorded in millimetres. **As several factors affect interpretation of the test, the size of the induration should be recorded and NOT just as a negative or positive result.** The area of erythema is irrelevant.

There is some variability in the time at which the test develops its maximum response. The majority of tuberculin-sensitive subjects will be positive at the recommended time of reading. A few, however, may have their maximum response just before or after the standard time.

Interpretation of the Mantoux test

For convenience, responses to the Mantoux test are considered in three categories of diameter, divided as follows:

Diameter of induration	Positivity	Interpretation
Less than 6mm	Negative – no significant hypersensitivity to tuberculin protein	Previously unvaccinated individuals may be given BCG provided there are no contraindications
6mm or greater, but less than 15mm	Positive – hypersensitive to tuberculin protein	Should not be given BCG.* May be due to previous TB infection or BCG or exposure to non-tuberculous mycobacteria
15mm and above	Strongly positive – strongly hypersensitive to tuberculin protein	Suggests tuberculosis infection or disease. Should be referred for further investigation and supervision (which may include preventive chemotherapy)

* When Mantoux tests are being performed as part of an immunisation programme, no further action is required for people with a reaction in this range. In other contexts (e.g. new immigrant screening, contact-tracing programmes), where the subject has not previously been vaccinated with BCG, and taking account of the precise size of the reaction and the circumstances of the case, referral to a chest clinic may be indicated for further investigation.

Factors affecting the result of the tuberculin test

The reaction to tuberculin protein may be suppressed by the following:

- glandular fever
- viral infections in general, including those of the upper respiratory tract
- live viral vaccines (tuberculin testing should not be carried out within four weeks of having received a live viral vaccine)
- sarcoidosis
- corticosteroid therapy
- immunosuppression due to disease or treatment, including HIV infection.

Subjects who have a negative test but who may have had an upper respiratory tract or other viral infection at the time of testing or at the time of reading should be re-tested two to three weeks after clinical recovery before being given BCG. If a second tuberculin test is necessary it should be carried out on the other arm: repeat testing at one site may alter the reactivity either by hypo- or more often hyper-sensitising the skin, and a changed response may reflect local changes in skin sensitivity only.

For further information and training materials on the administration, reading and interpretation of the Mantoux test, please see www.immunisation.nhs.uk.

Management of suspected cases, contacts and outbreaks

Contacts of cases known to be suffering from active pulmonary TB should be managed according to current guidance (Joint Tuberculosis Committee of the British Thoracic Society, 2000). Contacts of a sputum smear-positive index case should have a tuberculin test and, if positive or strongly positive (depending on prior vaccination status), be referred for assessment. Contacts with a negative tuberculin skin test when first seen may still be in the early stages of infection before tuberculin sensitivity has developed. A further skin test should therefore be performed six weeks after the last period of possible exposure. If the second skin test is positive, the patient has converted and must be referred for assessment and treatment. If the second test is negative, unvaccinated contacts under 16 years of age should be given BCG.

Exceptions to this advice include:

- newly born babies who are contacts of a smear-positive case, who should not be tested immediately but should be given prophylactic isoniazid chemotherapy and tuberculin tested after three to six months. If the skin test is positive, chemotherapy is continued; if negative, BCG vaccine is given provided the infant is no longer in contact with infectious TB. It is not necessary to use isoniazid-resistant BCG
- children under two years of age who have contact with a smear-positive case and have not received BCG. They should be given chemoprophylaxis even if the skin test is negative and then tuberculin tested after six weeks. If the skin test is positive, refer for assessment; if negative, BCG vaccine is given
- children under two years of age who have received BCG and who have contact with a smear-positive case. They should be skin tested and managed as for older children

- all HIV-positive contacts of a smear-positive case. They should be referred for consideration of chemoprophylaxis.

Newly born babies who are contacts of a TB case that is not smear positive should be immunised with BCG immediately.

Supplies

- BCG vaccine is manufactured by Statens Serum Institut (SSI).

- Tuberculin PPD is manufactured by Statens Serum Institut (SSI). Tuberculin PPD from SSI is not licensed medicine in the UK (although it has a marketing authorisation for use in other European countries).

References

Cobelens FG, van Deutekom H, Draayer-Jansen IW *et al.* (2000) Risk of infection with *Mycobacterium tuberculosis* in travellers to areas of high tuberculosis endemicity. *Lancet* **356**: 461–5.

Department of Health (2001) *Health information for overseas travel*, 2nd edition. London: TSO.

Department of Health, *Annual National Statistics: NHS Immunisation Statistics.*

Joint Tuberculosis Committee of the British Thoracic Society (2000) Control and prevention of tuberculosis in the United Kingdom: Code of Practice 2000. *Thorax* **55**: 887–901.

Health Protection Agency (2003) *Annual Report 2003.* www.hpa.org.uk/infections/topics_az/tb/menu.htm#menu_updates

Health Protection Agency (2004) Surveillance data.www.hpa.org.uk/infections/topics_az/tb/data_menu.htm

Health Protection Agency (2005) Tuberculosis mortality and mortality rate (per 100,000 population), England and Wales, 1982–2004). www.hpa.org.uk/infections/topics_az/tb/epidemiology/table11.htm

National Institute for Health and Clinical Excellence (2006) *Tuberculosis: Clinical diagnosis and management of tuberculosis, and measures for its prevention and control* (CG33). www.nice.org.uk/page.aspx?o=CG033.

Rodrigues LC, Gill ON and Smith PG (1991) BCG vaccination in the first year of life protects children of Indian subcontinent ethnic origin against tuberculosis in England. *Epidemiol Community Health* **45**: 78–80.

Rodrigues LC, Diwan VK and Wheeler JG (1993) Protective effect of BCG against tuberculous meningitis and military tuberculosis: a meta-analysis. *Int J Epidemiol* **22**: 1154–8.

Sutherland I and Springett VH (1987) Effectiveness of BCG vaccination in England and Wales in 1983. *Tubercle* **68**: 81–92.

World Health Organization (1999) Issues relating to the use of BCG in immunization programmes. A discussion document by Paul EM Fine, Ilona AM Carneiro, Julie B Milstien and C John Clements. www.who.int/entity/vaccine_research/documents/en/bcg_vaccines.pdf

33

Typhoid

NOTIFIABLE

The disease

Typhoid fever is a systemic infection caused by the gram-negative bacterium *Salmonella enterica,* subspecies *enterica,* serotype *typhi*. Paratyphoid fever is an illness clinically similar but usually less severe than typhoid and is caused by *S. paratyphi* A, B and C.

Following ingestion of contaminated food or water, *S. typhi* penetrates the intestinal mucosa, replicates and enters the bloodstream. The severity of symptoms varies. Clinical features range from mild fever, diarrhoea, myalgia and headache to severe disseminated disease with multi-organ involvement in 10 to 15% of cases. The case–fatality rate (CFR) is less than 1% with prompt antibiotic therapy, but may be as high as 20% in untreated cases. Typhoid has previously been thought to be a milder disease in children. Recent information, however, indicates that typhoid can cause significant morbidity in children aged one to five years who reside in endemic countries (Sinha *et al*., 1999).

Unlike other *Salmonella* species, both *S. typhi* and *S. paratyphi* only colonise humans. Most of the more than 2000 other serotypes of *Salmonella* cause only local infection of the gastro-intestinal tract (gastroenteritis or 'food poisoning') and are commonly found in many mammalian hosts.

Transmission is primarily via the oral route following ingestion of food or water contaminated by faeces and occasionally the urine of persons acutely ill with typhoid or those who are chronic carriers. Direct faecal–oral transmission can also occur. In healthy individuals, one million or more organisms may be required to cause illness; however, ingestion of fewer organisms may still result in illness, especially in susceptible individuals. The incubation period varies from one to three weeks, depending on host factors and the size of the infecting dose (Glynn and Bradley, 1992).

The risk of contracting typhoid fever is highest for travellers to areas of high endemicity. In the Indian subcontinent, a region of high incidence of typhoid fever (more than 100 cases per 100,000 people per year (Crump *et al*., 2004)), the attack rate for travellers has been estimated at 1 to 10 per

100,000 journeys (Mermin *et al.*, 1998; Steinberg *et al.*, 2004; Connor and Schwartz, 2005).

All patients with typhoid and paratyphoid excrete the organisms at some stage during their illness. About 10% of patients with typhoid excrete *S. typhi* for at least three months following the acute illness, and 2 to 5% become long-term carriers (more than one year). The likelihood of becoming a chronic carrier increases with age, especially in females and those with a biliary tract abnormality.

Typhoid can be successfully treated with antibiotic therapy and general medical support. Strains of *S. typhi* have become increasingly resistant to antibiotics, particularly in South Asia (Threlfall and Ward, 2001). This has implications for the treatment of typhoid fever as traditional antibiotic therapy (chloramphenicol, co-trimoxazole and amoxycillin) may not be effective. Treatment is usually with fluoroquinolones; third-generation cephalosporins or azithromycin may need to be given in resistant cases.

Following natural infection with typhoid, an immune response develops that may partially protect against reinfection and severity of disease (WHO, 2000).

History and epidemiology of the disease

Typhoid is predominantly a disease of countries with inadequate sanitation and poor standards of personal and food hygiene. The disease is endemic in South Asia and parts of South-East Asia, the Middle East, Central and South America, and Africa. Outbreaks of typhoid have been reported from countries in Eastern Europe (Kyrgyzstan, Tajikistan, Ukraine and Russia). In 2000, the global annual incidence of typhoid fever was estimated to be around 21.7 million cases with 216,510 deaths per year (CFR 1%) (Crump, Luby and Mintz, 2004).

Typhoid is rare in resource-rich countries where standards of sanitation are high. Typhoid and paratyphoid in England and Wales are usually imported diseases associated with foreign travel or contact with somebody who has travelled. Between 1990 and 2004, there were an average of 374 laboratory reports of typhoid and paratyphoid each year in England and Wales, nearly 70% of which reported recent foreign travel (HPA, 2005). Annually, cases of *S. typhi* have traditionally exceeded cases of *S. paratyphi* A and B. However, beginning in 1997, more cases of *S. paratyphi* A and B have occurred in each year except 2000.

The most frequently reported region of foreign travel for typhoid and paratyphoid A was South Asia; the Mediterranean and the Middle East were the most frequently reported regions for paratyphoid B (HPA, 2004). Occasional outbreaks of indigenous typhoid occur in the UK; the last community outbreak was in 2001 in Newport, Wales and involved five cases (Public Health Laboratory Services, 2001).

Prevention of typhoid and paratyphoid depends primarily on improving sanitation and water supplies in endemic areas and on scrupulous personal, food and water hygiene. Immunisation may be considered for individuals at risk from typhoid fever. There is no vaccine available to prevent paratyphoid infection.

The typhoid vaccination

Worldwide, three types of typhoid vaccine are available: a polysaccharide vaccine; an oral, live, attenuated vaccine; and a whole-cell inactivated vaccine.

Vi polysaccharide vaccine

One of the typhoid vaccines available in the UK is composed of purified Vi capsular polysaccharide from *S. typhi.* Each 0.5ml dose contains 25µg of antigen. A four-fold rise in antibody against Vi antigen has been detected seven days following primary immunisation with Vi vaccine. Maximum antibody response is achieved one month following vaccination and persists for about three years (Keitel *et al.*, 1994; Tacket *et al.*, 1998).

The efficacy of the Vi vaccine was evaluated in field trials in Nepal (Acharya *et al.*, 1987) and in Eastern Transvaal, South Africa (Klugman *et al.*, 1987; Klugman *et al.*, 1996). In the Nepalese study, vaccine efficacy at 20 months against culture-positive typhoid was 75% (95% CI = 49 to 87%) in adults and children aged five to 44 years. The South African study found the cumulative three-year efficacy of vaccine against culture-positive typhoid to be 55% (95% CI = 30 to 71%) in children aged six to 15 years.

Protective antibody titres to Vi antigen fall over time. Re-vaccination is necessary when continuing protection is required. Additional doses of Vi vaccine do not boost serum antibody levels; re-vaccination returns antibody levels to those achieved after the primary immunisation (Keitel *et al.*, 1994).

Non-conjugated polysaccharide vaccines are poorly immunogenic in infants and young children. There is little definitive data on the efficacy of Vi vaccine in children aged less than 18 months (Cadoz, 1998).

Protection by vaccination may be less if a large number of infective organisms are ingested. Because of the limited protection offered by the vaccine, the importance of scrupulous attention to personal, food and water hygiene must still be emphasised for those travelling to endemic areas.

Oral typhoid vaccine (Ty21a)

Oral typhoid vaccine contains a live, attenuated strain of *S. typhi* (Ty21a) in an enteric-coated capsule. A three-dose regimen gives a cumulative three-year efficacy of about 50 to 60% (Engels *et al.*, 1998). The vaccine is indicated for persons from six years of age.

Whole-cell typhoid vaccine

The injectable, killed, whole-cell typhoid vaccine contains heat-inactivated, phenol-preserved *S. typhi* organisms. A two-dose regimen gives a cumulative three-year efficacy of about 70%, and provides protection for up to five years (Engels *et al.*, 1998). This vaccine is highly reactogenic and is no longer used in the UK.

Storage

Both Vi polysaccharide and oral typhoid (Ty21a) vaccines should be stored in the original packaging at +2˚C to +8˚C and protected from light. All vaccines are sensitive to some extent to heat and cold. Heat speeds up the decline in potency of most vaccines, thus reducing their shelf life. Effectiveness cannot be guaranteed for vaccines unless they have been stored at the correct temperature. If Vi vaccines have been frozen they should not be used as this can reduce their potency and increase local reactions. If a blister containing Ty21a vaccine capsules is not intact, it should not be used.

Presentation

Vi vaccines are supplied in pre-filled syringes, each containing a single dose of 0.5ml. Vaccines are available as a single antigen product or combined with hepatitis A vaccine.

Ty21a vaccines are supplied in blister packs containing three capsules.

Dosage and schedule

A single dose of 0.5ml of Vi vaccine is recommended for adults and children over the age of 18 months. Reinforcing doses of 0.5ml should given as recommended.

The first Ty21a capsule is taken on day 0, the second capsule on day 2 and the third on day 4. The vaccine is recommended for children over the age of six years and adults. Reinforcing doses of three capsules should be given as recommended.

Dosage of monovalent typhoid vaccines

Vaccine product	Ages	Dose	Volume
Typhim Vi	18 months and older	25µg	0.5ml
Typherix	Two years and older	25µg	0.5ml

Dosage of combined typhoid and hepatitis A vaccines*

Vaccine product	Ages	Dose typhoid	Dose HAV†	Volume
Hepatyrix	15 years and older	25µg	1440 ELISA units	1ml
ViATIM	16 years and older	25µg	160 antigen units	1ml

* For booster doses of either typhoid or HAV, single antigen vaccines can be used
† HAV – hepatitis A vaccine

Administration

Vi vaccines are routinely given intramuscularly into the upper arm or anterolateral thigh. Intradermal injection may cause a severe local reaction and should be avoided. Vaccines should be given by deep subcutaneous injection to individuals with a bleeding disorder. Vaccines must not be given intravenously. Ty21a vaccine capsules are taken orally.

Both types of vaccine can be given at the same time as other vaccines, such as travel vaccines. Injectable vaccines should be given at separate sites, preferably in different limbs. If given in the same limb, they should be given at least 2.5cm apart (American Academy of Pediatrics, 2003). The site at which each vaccine was given should be noted in the individual's records.

Disposal

Equipment used for vaccination, including used vials or ampoules, should be disposed of at the end of a session by sealing in a proper, puncture-resistant 'sharps' box (UN-approved, BS 7320).

Recommendations for use of the vaccine

Typhoid vaccine is indicated for active immunisation against typhoid fever and is recommended for:

- travellers to countries where typhoid is endemic (e.g. South Asia, parts of South-East Asia, the Middle East, Central and South America, and Africa), especially if staying with or visiting the local population
- travellers to endemic areas (see above) with frequent and/or prolonged exposure to conditions where sanitation and food hygiene are likely to be poor
- laboratory personnel who may handle *S. typhi* in the course of their work.

Further information on vaccine use in travellers can be found in *Health information for overseas travel* (Department of Health, 2001).

Primary immunisation

The immunisation schedule of Vi vaccine consists of a single dose; for Ty21a vaccine, a three-dose course.

Vi vaccine

Children aged from 18 months and adults

A single dose of Vi vaccine is recommended for children and adults.

Ty21a vaccine

Children aged from six years and adults

One capsule on day 0, the second capsule on day 2 and the third on day 4. Capsules should be taken about one hour before a meal with a cold or lukewarm drink (temperature not to exceed 37˚C). The vaccine capsule should not be chewed, and should be swallowed as soon as possible after placing in the mouth.

Unless the immunisation schedule of three vaccine capsules is completed, an optimal immune response may not be achieved. Protection commences about seven to ten days after completion of the third dose.

Not all recipients of typhoid vaccines will be protected against typhoid fever, and travellers should be advised to take all necessary precautions to avoid contact with or ingestion of potentially contaminated food or water.

Reinforcing immunisation

Vi vaccine

A single dose of Vi vaccine should be administered at three-year intervals in adults and children over 18 months of age who remain at risk from typhoid fever.

Individuals who have received other non-Vi typhoid vaccines may receive reinforcing doses of Vi vaccine at three-year intervals.

Ty21a

In the case of travel from a non-endemic area to an area where typhoid is endemic, an annual booster consisting of three doses is recommended.

Children under 18 months of age

Young children may show a sub-optimal response to polysaccharide antigen vaccines. Children between the ages of 12 and 18 months should be immunised if the risk of typhoid fever is considered high. Immunisation is not recommended for children under one year of age. When children are too young to benefit fully from typhoid vaccination, scrupulous attention to personal, food and water hygiene measures should be exercised by the caregiver.

Contraindications

There are very few individuals who cannot receive typhoid vaccine. When there is doubt, appropriate advice should be sought from a travel health specialist. Severe reactions to a previous dose of non-Vi typhoid vaccine do not contraindicate the subsequent use of a Vi-containing vaccine. Most severe reactions to typhoid vaccines will have been associated with the inactivated whole-cell vaccine. Typhoid Vi vaccine should not be given to those who have had:

- a confirmed anaphylaxis to a Vi antigen-containing vaccine.

Ty21a vaccine should not be given to those who are:

- immunosuppressed (see Chapter 6 for more detail), or those who have had:

- confirmed anaphylaxis to any component of the Ty21a vaccine or enteric-coated capsule, including gelatin.

Precautions

Minor illnesses without fever or systemic upset are not valid reasons to postpone immunisation. If an individual is acutely unwell, immunisation should be postponed until they have fully recovered. This is to avoid confusing the differential diagnosis of any acute illness by wrongly attributing any sign or symptoms to the adverse effects of the vaccine.

In the event of a gastrointestinal illness, vaccination with the Ty21a vaccine should be postponed until after recovery. Ty21a vaccine should not be commenced within three days of completing any antibacterial agents, and similarly, antibacterial therapy should not commence within three days after the last dose of vaccine.

If malaria prophylaxis is also required, the fixed combination of atovaquone and proguanil can be given concomitantly with Ty21a. Doses of mefloquine and Ty21a should be separated by at least 12 hours. For other anti-malarials, there should be an interval of at least three days between the last dose of Ty21a and the first dose of malaria prophylaxis.

Pregnancy and breast-feeding

No data are available on the safety of Vi polysaccharide and Ty21a typhoid vaccines in pregnancy or during lactation. There is no evidence of risk from vaccinating pregnant women or those who are breast-feeding with inactivated viral or bacterial vaccines or toxoids (Plotkin and Orenstein, 2004). It is not known if Ty21a vaccine can cause fetal harm when administered to pregnant women or affect reproductive ability. If the risk of typhoid is high, vaccination should be considered.

Immunosuppression and HIV infection

Vi vaccine does not contain live organisms and may be given to HIV-positive individuals and those considered immunosuppressed, in the absence of contraindications.

Immunosuppressed individuals may have a sub-optimal immune response to Vi vaccine. The importance of scrupulous attention to personal, food and water hygiene must be emphasised for immunosuppressed persons travelling to endemic areas.

Ty21a vaccine should be avoided in immunosuppressed and HIV-infected individuals.

Further guidance is provided by the Royal College of Paediatrics and Child Health (www.rcpch.ac.uk), the British HIV Association (BHIVA) *Immunisation guidelines for HIV-infected adults* (BHIVA, 2006) and the Children's HIV Association of UK and Ireland (CHIVA) immunisation guidelines (www.bhiva.org/chiva).

Adverse reactions

Based on pooled estimates from clinical trials and post-marketing surveillance data, local reactions (pain, swelling, erythema and induration at injection site) are the most commonly reported symptoms following Vi vaccine (Engels *et al.*, 1998; Tacket *et al.*, 1986; Begier *et al.*, 2004). These symptoms are usually mild and transient. Systemic reactions following the vaccine are infrequent. Fever occurs in about 1% of vaccine recipients. Headache, nausea, diarrhoea and abdominal pain have been reported but are uncommon.

There have been rare reports of anaphylaxis following administration of Vi vaccine (Begier *et al.*, 2004).

Following Ty21a vaccine, the most commonly reported adverse events are gastro-intestinal symptoms, fever, influenza-like symptoms and headache.

All severe reactions should be reported to the Commission on Human Medicines using the Yellow Card scheme.

Management of cases, carriers, contacts and outbreaks

The local health protection unit (HPU) should be informed immediately whenever a patient is suspected of having typhoid fever. Reporting should not wait until there is laboratory confirmation. Early identification of the source of infection is vital in containing this disease. Reports should contain a travel history, including country of travel.

Cases, carriers and their close contacts in the following groups may pose an increased risk of spreading infection and may be considered for exclusion from work or school (Working Party of the PHLS *Salmonella* Committee, 1995):

- food handlers
- staff of healthcare facilities
- children aged less than five years of age who attend nurseries or other similar groups

- older children or adults who cannot maintain good standards of personal hygiene.

Advice on exclusion from work or school must be sought from the local HPU.

Both cases and carriers of *S. typhi* should be advised to be scrupulous in their hygiene practices. Carriers should be referred for specialist clinical management.

Typhoid vaccine is not recommended for close contacts of either cases or carriers, or during an outbreak of typhoid fever in the UK.

Supplies

Vi-containing vaccines

- Typhim Vi (typhoid vaccine)
- ViATIM (combined hepatitis A/typhoid vaccine)

These vaccines are available from
Sanofi Pasteur MSD
(Tel: 01628 785 291)
(Fax: 01628 671 722)
Customer care direct line: 01628 733 737.

- Typherix (typhoid vaccine)
- Hepatyrix (combined hepatitis A/typhoid vaccine)

These vaccines are available from
GlaxoSmithKline UK
(Tel: 0800 221 441)
(Fax: 0208 990 4321)
Medical information e-mail: customercontactuk@gsk.com and
MASTA
(Tel: 0113 238 7500)
(Fax: 0113 238 7541).

References

Acharya IL, Lowe CU, Thapa R *et al.* (1987) Prevention of typhoid fever in Nepal with the Vi capsular polysaccharide of *Salmonella typhi*. A preliminary report. *N Engl J Med* **317**: 1101–4.

American Academy of Pediatrics (2003) Active immunization. In: Pickering LK (ed.) *Red Book: 2003 Report of the Committee on Infectious Diseases*, 26th edition. Elk Grove Village, IL: American Academy of Pediatrics, p 33.

Begier EM, Burwen DR, Haber P and Ball R (2004) Post-marketing safety surveillance for typhoid fever vaccines from the Vaccine Adverse Event Reporting System, July 1990 through June 2002. *Clin Infect Dis* **38**: 771–9.

British HIV Association (2006) *Immunisation guidelines for HIV-infected adults:* www.bhiva.org/pdf/2006/Immunisation506.pdf.

Cadoz M (1998) Potential and limitations of polysaccharide vaccines in infancy. *Vaccine* **16**: 1391–5.

Connor BA and Schwartz E (2005) Typhoid and paratyphoid fever in travellers. *Lancet Infect Dis* **5**: 623–8.

Crump JA, Luby SP and Mintz ED (2004) The global burden of typhoid fever. *Bull World Health Organ* **82**: 346–53.

Department of Health (2001) *Health information for overseas travel.* London: The Stationery Office.

Engels EA, Falagas ME, Lau J and Bennish ML (1998) Typhoid fever vaccines: a meta-analysis of studies on efficacy and toxicity. *BMJ* **316**: 110–15.

Glynn JR and Bradley DJ (1992) The relationship between infecting dose and severity of disease in reported outbreaks of *Salmonella* infections. *Epidemiol Infect* **109**: 371–88.

Health Protection Agency (2004) *Illness in England, Wales, and Northern Ireland associated with foreign travel.* London: HPA.

HPA (2005) Laboratory reports of cases of typhoid and paratyphoid, England and Wales: 1990 to 2004. *CDR Wkly* 10 February 2005. www.hpa.org.uk/cdr/pages/enteric.htm#lab_typh

Keitel WA, Bond NL, Zahradnik JM *et al.* (1994) Clinical and serological responses following primary and booster immunization with *Salmonella typhi* Vi capsular polysaccharide vaccines. *Vaccine* **12**: 195–9.

Klugman KP, Gilbertson IT, Koornhof HJ *et al.* (1987) Protective effect of Vi capsular polysaccharide vaccine against typhoid fever. *Lancet* **ii**: 1165–9.

Klugman KP, Koornhof HJ, Robbins JB and Le Cam NN (1996) Immunogenicity, efficacy and serological correlate of protection of *Salmonella typhi* Vi capsular polysaccharide vaccine three years after immunization. *Vaccine* **14**: 435–8.

Mermin JH, Townes JM, Gerber M *et al.* (1998) Typhoid fever in the United States, 1985–1994. Changing risks of international travel and increasing antimicrobial resistance. *Arch Intern Med* **158**: 633–8.

Plotkin SA and Orenstein WA (eds) (2004) *Vaccines.* 4th edition. Philadelphia: WB Saunders Company p109–11.

Public Health Laboratory Services (2001) Typhoid in Newport, Wales – update. *Commun Dis Rep CDR Wkly* **11**:1.

Sinha A, Sazawal S, Kumar R *et al.* (1999) Typhoid fever in children aged less than 5 years. *Lancet* **354**: 734–7.

Steinberg EB, Bishop R, Haber P *et al.* (2004) Typhoid fever in travellers: who should be targeted for prevention? *Clin Infect Dis* **39**: 186–91.

Tacket CO, Ferreccio C, Robbins JB *et al.* (1986) Safety and immunogenicity of two *Salmonella typhi* Vi capsular polysaccharide vaccine candidates. *J Infect Dis* **154**: 342–5.

Tacket CO, Levine MM and Robbins JB (1998) Persistence of Vi antibody titers three years after vaccination with Vi polysaccharide against typhoid fever. *Vaccine* **6**: 307–8.

Threlfall EJ and Ward LR (2001) Decreased susceptibility to ciprofloxacin in *Salmonella enterica* serotype *typhi*, United Kingdom. *Emerg Infect Dis* **7**: 448–50.

Working Party of the PHLS *Salmonella* Committee (1995) The prevention of human transmission of gastrointestinal infections, infestations, and bacterial infestations. *Commun Dis Rep CDR Rev* **5**:1–16.

World Health Organization (2000) Typhoid vaccines. WHO position paper. *Wkly Epidemiol Rec* **75**: 257–64.

34

Varicella

NOTIFIABLE IN SCOTLAND AND NORTHERN IRELAND

The disease

Varicella (chickenpox) is an acute, highly infectious disease caused by the varicella zoster (VZ) virus.

The illness usually starts with one to two days of fever and malaise although this may be absent, particularly in young children. Vesicles begin to appear on the face and scalp, spreading to the trunk and abdomen and eventually to the limbs. After three or four days, the vesicles dry with a granular scab and are usually followed by further crops. Vesicles may be so few as to be missed or so numerous that they become confluent, covering most of the body. Virus is plentiful in the nasopharynx in the first few days and in the vesicles before they dry up; the infectious period is from one to two days before the rash appears until the vesicles are dry. This may be prolonged in immunosuppressed patients. Early treatment with high-dose oral aciclovir and analogues or systemic aciclovir shortens the duration and number of vesicles (Balfour *et al.*, 1992; Dunkle *et al.*, 1991).

Herpes zoster (shingles) is caused by the reactivation of the patient's varicella virus. Virus from lesions can be transmitted to susceptible individuals to cause chickenpox but there is no evidence that herpes zoster can be acquired from another individual with chickenpox. Although more common in the elderly, it can occur in children and is especially common in immunosuppressed individuals of any age. Vesicles appear in the dermatome, representing cranial or spinal ganglia where the virus has been dormant. The affected area may be intensely painful with associated paraesthesia.

Varicella is transmitted directly by personal contact or droplet spread. The incubation period is between one and three weeks. The secondary infection rate from household contact with a case of chickenpox can be as high as 90%. The infection is most common in children below the age of ten, in whom it usually causes mild disease.

The disease can be more serious in adults, particularly pregnant women and those who smoke, as they are at greater risk of fulminating varicella pneumonia. Pregnant women appear to be at greatest risk late in the second or early in the third trimester; of the nine deaths due to varicella in pregnancy in England and Wales between 1985 and 1998, seven occurred between 27 and 32 weeks' gestation (Enders and Miller, 2000). For neonates and immunosuppressed individuals, the risk of disseminated or haemorrhagic varicella is greatly increased.

Risks to the fetus and neonate from maternal chickenpox are related to the time of infection in the mother (Enders *et al.*, 1994; Miller *et al.*, 1990):

- **in the first 20 weeks of pregnancy** – congenital (fetal) varicella syndrome, which includes limb hypoplasia, microcephaly, cataracts, growth retardation and skin scarring. The mortality rate is high. From the largest available prospective study, the incidence has been estimated to be less than 1% in the first 12 weeks and around 2% between 13 and 20 weeks of pregnancy (Enders *et al.*, 1994). In this study, no cases of congenital varicella syndrome occurred among the 477 pregnancies in which maternal varicella occurred after 20 weeks' gestation.
- **in the second and third trimesters of pregnancy** – herpes zoster in an otherwise healthy infant. Occasional cases of fetal damage comprising chorioretinal damage, microcephaly and skin scarring following maternal varicella between 20 and 28 weeks' gestation have been reported (Tan and Koren, 2005), but the risk is likely to be substantially lower than that of the typical congenital varicella syndrome which occurs after maternal varicella in the first 20 weeks' gestation.
- **a week before, to a week after delivery** – severe and even fatal disease in the neonate. Before the introduction of human varicella zoster immunoglobulin (VZIG) in the UK, half the deaths in infants under one year old occurred in those aged less than three weeks in whom infection would have been contracted either before or during birth or in the first week of life.

History and epidemiology of the disease

The incidence of varicella is seasonal and classically reaches a peak from March to May, although in recent years seasonality has been less marked. Since chickenpox is so common in childhood, 90% of adults raised in the UK are immune.

Herpes zoster is less common than chickenpox and the incidence is highest in older people. The incidence of shingles increases with age and around one in four adults will experience an attack in their lifetime (Miller *et al.*, 1993).

The varicella vaccination

Varicella vaccines are lyophilised preparations containing live, attenuated virus derived from the Oka strain of varicella zoster virus. Two vaccines are currently available: Varilrix® (Oka-RIT) and Varivax® (Oka/Merck). On reconstitution, both preparations should be given as a 0.5ml dose. Although there are no data on interchangeability, it is likely that a course can be completed effectively with a different vaccine.

Varicella vaccines do not contain thiomersal. They contain live organisms which have been attenuated.

Transmission of vaccine virus from immunocompetent vaccinees to susceptible close contacts has occasionally been documented but the risk is very low. Transmission in the absence of a post-vaccination rash has not been documented (Annunziato and Gershon, 2000).

The two-dose vaccination schedule in adolescents and adults provides about 75% protection, and the single-dose schedule in children about 90% protection against clinical chickenpox (Annunziato and Gershon, 2000). In both age groups, most of the breakthrough infections are modified and vaccinated individuals who contract varicella have fewer lesions and less systemic upset than unvaccinated individuals.

Human varicella zoster immunoglobulin

Two licensed VZIG preparations are available in the UK: VZIG distributed in England and Wales is made by the Bio Products Laboratory (BPL), Elstree; and in Scotland and Northern Ireland, it is provided by the Protein Fractionation Centre (PFC), Edinburgh.

VZIG is prepared from pooled plasma of non-UK donors with suitably high titres of VZ antibody. The supply of VZIG is limited by the availability of suitable donors and its use is restricted to those at greatest risk and for whom there is evidence that it is likely to be effective.

Because of a theoretical risk of transmission of vCJD from plasma products, VZIG used in the UK is now prepared from plasma sourced from outside the UK, and supplies are scarce. All donors are screened for HIV, hepatitis B and C, and all plasma pools are tested for the presence of RNA from these viruses. A solvent detergent inactivation step for envelope viruses is included in the production process.

Storage

The unreconstituted vaccine and its diluent should be stored in the original packaging at +2˚C to +8˚C and protected from light. All vaccines are sensitive to some extent to heat and cold. Heat speeds up the decline in potency of most vaccines, thus reducing their shelf life. Effectiveness cannot be guaranteed for vaccines unless they have been stored at the correct temperature. Freezing may cause increased reactogenicity and loss of potency for some vaccines. It can also cause hairline cracks in the container, leading to contamination of the contents.

VZIG should be stored in a refrigerator between +2˚C and +8˚C. These products are tolerant to ambient temperatures for up to one week. They can be distributed in sturdy packaging outside the cold chain if needed.

Presentation

Varicella vaccines are available as lyophilised preparations for reconstitution with a diluent.

- Varilrix is a pink-coloured pellet, which on reconstitution may vary from a pink to a red solution.
- Varivax is an off-white powder, which on reconstitution produces a clear, colourless to pale yellow liquid.

After reconstitution of the lyophilised suspension, the vaccines must be used within one hour. Discard any unused vaccine one hour following reconstitution.

VZIG is a clear, pale yellow or light brown solution dispensed in vials containing 250mg protein in approximately 2–3ml of fluid (minimum potency 100IU of VZ antibody per ml) with added sodium chloride.

Dosage and schedules

Varicella vaccination

Children from one year to under 13 years of age

Children from one year to under 13 years of age should receive a single dose of varicella vaccine.

Children aged 13 years or older and adults

Children aged 13 years or older and adults should receive two doses of varicella vaccine, four to eight weeks apart.

Varicella zoster immunoglobulin

The dosage for both the BPL and PFC products are:

- 0–5 years, 250mg (one vial)
- 6–10 years, 500mg (two vials)
- 11–14 years, 750mg (three vials)
- 15 years or over, 1000mg (four vials).

If a second exposure occurs after three weeks, a further dose is required.

Contacts with bleeding disorders who cannot be given an intramuscular injection should be given intravenous normal immunoglobulin at a dose of 0.2g per kg body weight (i.e. 4ml/kg for a 5% solution) instead. This will produce serum VZ antibody levels equivalent to those achieved with VZIG (Paryani *et al.*, 1984).

Administration

Varicella vaccine should only be administered by deep subcutaneous injection.

Varicella vaccine can, and ideally should (see below), be given at the same time as other live vaccines such as MMR. The vaccines should be given at a separate site, preferably in a different limb. If given in the same limb, they should be given at least 2.5cm apart (American Academy of Pediatrics, 2003). The site at which each vaccine was given should be noted in the individual's records.

If live vaccines are given simultaneously, then each vaccine virus will begin to replicate and an appropriate immune response is made to each vaccine. After a live vaccine is given, natural interferon is produced in response to that vaccine. If a second live vaccine is given during this response, the interferon may prevent replication of the second vaccine virus. This may attenuate the response to the second vaccine. Based on evidence that MMR vaccine can lead to an attenuation of the varicella vaccine response (Mullooly and Black, 2001), the recommended interval between live vaccines is currently four weeks. For this reason, if live vaccines cannot be administered simultaneously, a four-week interval is recommended.

VZIG is given by intramuscular injection in the upper outer quadrant of the buttock or the anterolateral thigh.

When VZIG is being used for prevention of varicella, it must be remembered that it may interfere with the subsequent development of active immunity from live virus vaccines. If immunoglobulin has been administered first, then an interval of three months should be observed before administering a live virus vaccine. If immunoglobulin has been given within three weeks of administering a live vaccine, then the vaccine should be repeated three months later. This does not apply to yellow fever vaccine since VZIG does not contain significant amounts of antibody to this virus.

Disposal

Equipment used for vaccination, including used vials or ampoules, should be disposed of at the end of a session by sealing in a puncture-resistant 'sharps' box (UN-approved, BS 7320).

Recommendations for the use of the vaccine

Pre-exposure vaccination

The aim of varicella immunisation is to protect from exposure those who are at most risk of serious illness. This is done by immunising specific individuals who are in regular or close contact with those at risk. Since 2003, this recommendation includes vaccinating non-immune healthcare workers who themselves will derive benefit as they will be protected from contact with infectious patients. Varicella vaccine is also recommended for healthy susceptible close household contacts of immunocompromised patients.

Non-immune groups recommended to receive pre-exposure vaccination

Healthcare workers (see Figure 34.1)

The definition of a healthcare worker includes those working in general practice and hospitals who have patient contact, e.g. cleaners on wards, catering staff, ambulance staff, receptionists in general practice, as well as medical and nursing staff, whether employed directly or through contract.

Those with a definite history of chickenpox or herpes zoster can be considered protected. Healthcare workers with a negative or uncertain history of chickenpox or herpes zoster should be serologically tested and vaccine offered only to those without VZ antibody. A recent survey showed that a history of chickenpox is a less reliable predictor of immunity in individuals born and raised overseas (MacMahon *et al.*, 2004) and routine testing should be considered.

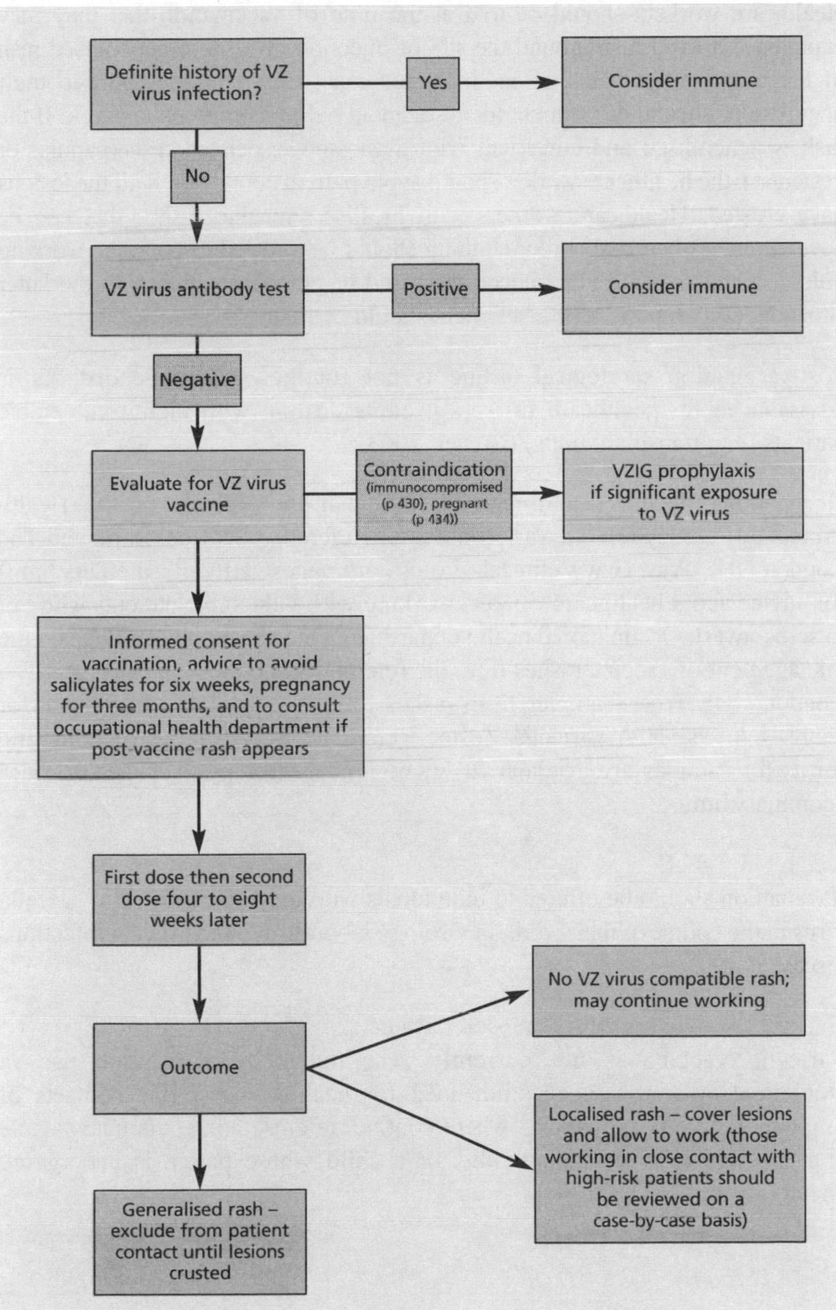

Figure 34.1 Procedure for vaccinating healthcare workers

Healthcare workers should be told at the time of vaccination that they may experience a local rash around the site of injection or a more generalised rash in the month after vaccination. In either case, they should report to their occupational health department for assessment before commencing work. If the rash is generalised and consistent with a vaccine-associated rash (papular or vesicular), the healthcare worker should avoid patient contact until all the lesions have crusted. Healthcare workers with localised vaccine rashes that can be covered with a bandage and/or clothing should be allowed to continue working unless in contact with immunocompromised or pregnant patients. In the latter situation, an individual risk assessment should be made.

Post-vaccination serological testing is not routinely recommended but is advisable in for healthcare workers in units dealing with highly vulnerable patients (e.g. transplant units) (Breuer, 2003).

Occupational health departments should visit the website of the Health Protection Agency (HPA), Varicella Zoster Reference Service, Barts and The London NHS Trust (www.clinical-virology.org/pages/vzrl/vzrl_summary.html) for advice about healthcare workers working with vulnerable patients who fail to seroconvert. Occupational health departments may also obtain advice on the management of vaccine rashes from the reference laboratory at Barts and The London NHS Trust (samples from rashes following vaccine can be sent for analysis to the HPA,Varicella Zoster Reference Service). Instructions and forms for samples are available at www.clinical-virology.org/pages/vzrl/vzrl _summary.html

Laboratory staff

Vaccination should be offered to individuals who may be exposed to varicella virus in the course of their work, in virology laboratories and clinical infectious disease units.

Contacts of immunocompromised patients

Varicella vaccine is not currently recommended for routine use in children. However, it is recommended for healthy susceptible contacts of immunocompromised patients where continuing close contact is unavoidable (e.g. siblings of a leukaemic child, or a child whose parent is undergoing chemotherapy).

Management of at-risk individuals following significant exposure to chickenpox or herpes zoster

The aim of post-exposure management is to protect individuals at high risk of suffering from severe varicella (see below) and those who may transmit infection to those at high risk (e.g. healthcare workers).

VZIG prophylaxis is recommended for individuals who fulfil all of the following three criteria:

- significant exposure to chickenpox or herpes zoster
- a clinical condition that increases the risk of severe varicella; this includes immunosuppressed patients, neonates and pregnant women (see below)
- no antibodies to VZ virus (see below).

The post-exposure management algorithms for immunosuppressed patients, neonates and pregnant women, and advice on antibody testing, are summarised below and in Figures 34.2, 34.3 and 34.4.

Definition of a significant exposure to VZ virus

Three aspects of the exposure are relevant:

- **type of VZ infection in the index case:** the risk of acquiring infection from an immunocompetent individual with non-exposed zoster lesions (e.g. thoracolumbar (the trunk)) is remote. The issue of VZIG should be restricted to those in contact with chickenpox, or those in contact with the following:
  - disseminated zoster
  - immunocompetent individuals with exposed lesions (e.g. ophthalmic zoster)
  - immunosuppressed patients with localised zoster on any part of the body (in whom viral shedding may be greater).
- **the timing of the exposure in relation to onset of rash in the index case:** VZIG should normally be restricted to patients exposed to a case of chickenpox or disseminated zoster between 48 hours before onset of rash until crusting of lesions, or day of onset of rash until crusting for those exposed to localised zoster.
- **closeness and duration of contact:** the following should be used as a guide to the type of exposure, other than maternal/neonatal and continuous home contact, that requires VZIG prophylaxis:

Varicella

- contact in the same room (e.g. in a house or classroom or a two- to four-bed hospital bay) for a significant period of time (15 minutes or more).
- face-to-face contact, e.g. while having a conversation
- in the case of large open wards, airborne transmission at a distance has occasionally been reported and giving VZIG to all susceptible high-risk contacts should be considered (particularly in paediatric wards where the degree of contact may be difficult to define).

Management of immunosuppressed patients

Immunosuppressed patients are described in detail in Chapter 6. They include:

- patients with evidence of severe primary immunodeficiency, for example, severe combined immunodeficiency (SCID), Wiskott-Aldrich syndrome and other combined immunodeficiency syndromes
- all patients currently being treated for malignant disease with immunosuppressive chemotherapy or radiotherapy, and for at least six months after terminating such treatment
- all patients who have received a solid organ transplant and are currently on immunosuppressive treatment
- patients who have received a bone marrow transplant until at least 12 months after finishing all immunosuppressive treatment, or longer where the patient has developed graft-versus-host disease. The decision to vaccinate should depend upon the type of transplant and immune status of the patient. Further advice can be found in current guidance produced by the European Group for Blood and Marrow Transplantation (www.ebmt.org) and the Royal College of Paediatrics and Child Health (www.rcpch.ac.uk)
- all patients receiving systemic high-dose steroids until at least three months after treatment has stopped. This would include children who receive prednisolone, orally or rectally, at a daily dose (or its equivalent) of 2mg/kg/day for at least one week, or 1mg/kg/day for one month. For adults, an equivalent dose is harder to define but immunosuppression should be considered in those who receive 40mg of prednisolone per day for more than one week. Occasionally, there may be individuals on lower doses of steroids who may be immunosuppressed, and are at increased risk from infections. Therefore, live vaccines should be considered with caution in discussion with a relevant specialist physician
- patients receiving other types of immunosuppressive drugs (e.g. azathioprine, ciclosporin, methotrexate, cyclophosphamide, leflunomide and the newer cytokine inhibitors) alone or in combination with lower

doses of steroids. The advice of the physician or immunologist in charge should be sought for at least six months after treatment

- patients with immunosuppression due to HIV infection (see section below).

Note: Patients with gammaglobulin deficiencies who are receiving replacement therapy with intravenous normal immunoglobulin do not require VZIG (see below).

Determination of VZ immune status

Whenever possible, immunosuppressed contacts should be tested irrespective of their history of chickenpox. However, VZIG administration should not be delayed past seven days after initial contact while an antibody test is done. Under these circumstances, VZIG should be given on the basis of a negative history of chickenpox. If the patient has a positive history of chickenpox, wait for the antibody results. Those with a positive history in whom VZ antibody is not detected by a sensitive assay should be given VZIG.

VZIG is not indicated in immunosuppressed contacts with detectable antibody as the amount of antibody provided by VZIG will not significantly increase VZ antibody titres in those who are already positive. Second attacks of chickenpox can occasionally occur in immunosuppressed VZ antibody positive patients, but these are likely to be related to defects in cell-mediated immunity.

Management of neonates

VZIG is recommended for infants whose mothers develop chickenpox (but not herpes zoster) in the period seven days before to seven days after delivery. VZIG can be given without antibody testing of the infant.

VZIG is not usually required for infants born more than seven days after the onset of maternal chickenpox or whose mothers develop zoster before or after delivery, as these infants will have maternal antibody.

VZIG is also recommended for:

- VZ antibody-negative infants exposed to chickenpox or herpes zoster (other than in the mother) in the first seven days of life
- VZ antibody-negative infants of any age, exposed to chickenpox or herpes zoster while still requiring intensive or prolonged special care nursing.

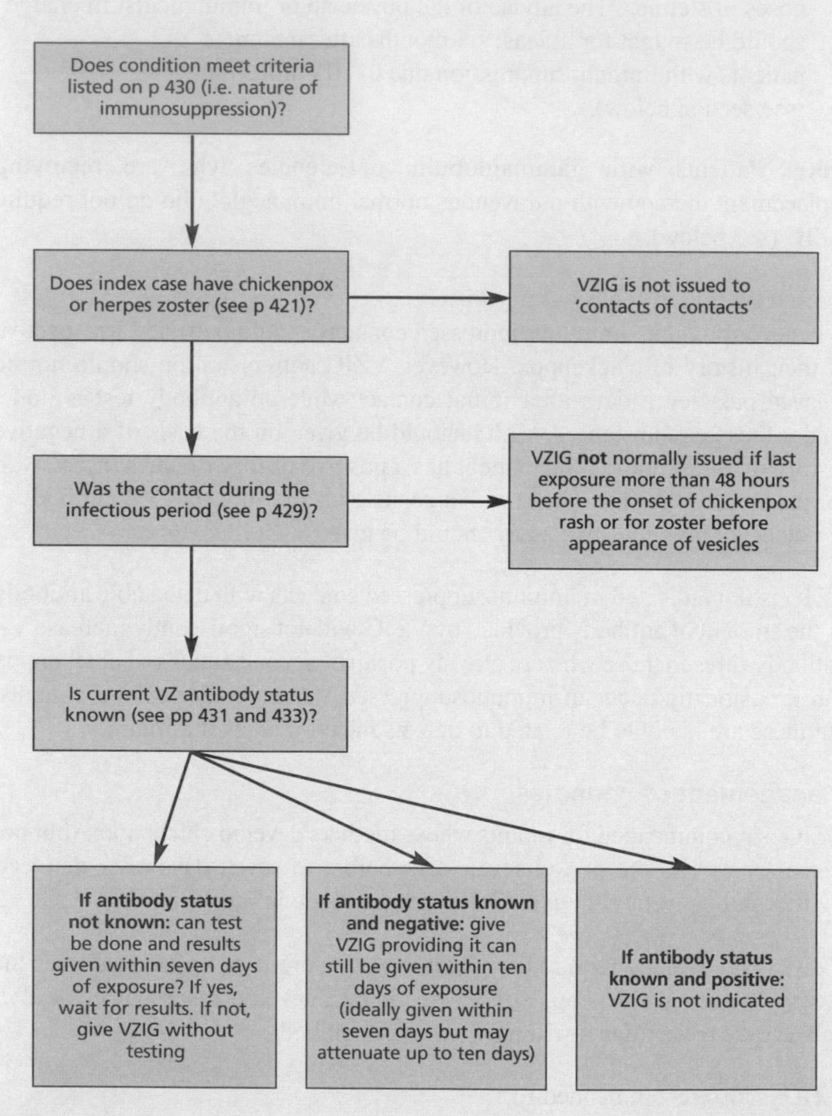

Figure 34.2 VZIG algorithm for immunocompromised patients who have been exposed to varicella zoster

For infants in these two exposure groups who were born before 28 weeks' gestation, or weighed less than 1000g at birth, or are more than 60 days old, or have had repeated blood sampling with replacement by packed red cell infusion, maternal antibodies may not be present despite a positive maternal history of chickenpox (Patou *et al.*, 1990; Gold *et al.*, 1993). It is recommended that, where possible, such infants are tested to determine their VZ antibody status in the event of a contact. Other infants whose mothers have a positive history of chickenpox and/or a positive VZ antibody result will usually have maternal antibody and do not require VZIG.

Management of pregnant women

VZIG is recommended for VZ antibody-negative pregnant contacts exposed at any stage of pregnancy, providing VZIG can be given within ten days of contact. However, when supplies of VZIG are short, issues to pregnant women may be restricted. Clinicians are advised to check availability of VZIG (see 'Supplies' below) before offering it to pregnant women.

Pregnant contacts with a positive history of chickenpox do not require VZIG. Those with a negative history must be tested for VZ antibody before VZIG is given (see below). The outcome in pregnant women is not adversely affected if administration of VZIG is delayed up to ten days after initial contact (Enders and Miller, 2000; Miller *et al.*, 1993). There is still time to test for VZ antibody even when the woman presents relatively late after contact.

Determination of VZ immune status

The majority of adults and a substantial proportion of children without a definite history of chickenpox will be VZ antibody positive. One UK study found that 11% of children aged 1 to 5 years, 37% aged 6 to 16 years and 89% of adults given VZIG on the basis of a negative history of chickenpox were VZ antibody positive (Evans *et al.*, 1980). To prevent wastage of VZIG, all individuals being considered for VZIG should have a serum sample tested for VZ antibody; only those without antibody require VZIG. If urgent VZ antibody testing is required for patients presenting late, VZIG can be ordered (see 'Supplies' below) at the same time that the blood is sent for testing and can be returned if the result is positive. VZ antibody testing should be available within 24 to 48 hours – seek advice from the local HPA or NHS laboratory.

VZ antibody detected in patients who have been transfused or who have received intravenous immunoglobulin in the previous three months may have been passively acquired. Although VZIG is not indicated if antibody from other blood products is detectable, re-testing in the event of a subsequent exposure will be required, as the patient may have become antibody negative.

About 15% of patients given VZIG who remain symptom-free after a home contact will have had a sub-clinical infection and will seroconvert asymptomatically (Evans *et al.*, 1980; Miller *et al.*, 1993). Patients who have received VZIG in the past following a close exposure should be re-tested for VZ antibody in the event of another exposure.

Effectiveness of VZIG prophylaxis

Immunosuppressed patients

About half of susceptible immunosuppressed home contacts will develop clinical chickenpox despite VZIG prophylaxis, and a further 15% will be infected sub-clinically (Evans *et al.*, 1980). Severe or fatal varicella can occur despite VZIG prophylaxis. Immunocompromised contacts given VZIG should still be monitored and aciclovir should be used at the first signs of illness.

Neonates

About half of neonates exposed to maternal varicella will become infected despite VZIG prophylaxis (Miller *et al.*, 1990). In up to two-thirds of these infants, infections are mild or asymptomatic but rare fatal cases have been reported despite VZIG prophylaxis in those with onset of maternal chickenpox in the period four days before to two days after delivery. Early treatment with intravenous aciclovir is recommended for infants in this exposure category who develop varicella despite VZIG prophylaxis.

Pregnant women

The rationale for the use of VZIG prophylaxis in pregnant women is twofold: reduction in severity of maternal disease and reduction of risk of fetal infection for women contracting varicella in the first 20 weeks of pregnancy. The risk of fatal varicella is estimated to be about five times higher in pregnant than non-pregnant adults with fatal cases concentrated late in the second or early in the third trimester (Enders and Miller, 2000).

One study showed a significant reduction in the risk of congenital VZ virus infection in women who developed varicella after VZIG prophylaxis compared with women who developed varicella without VZIG prophylaxis; however, the study was too small to assess whether the risk of congenital varicella syndrome was reduced (Enders *et al.*,1994). A case of congenital varicella syndrome has been reported in the infant of a woman exposed at the eleventh week of

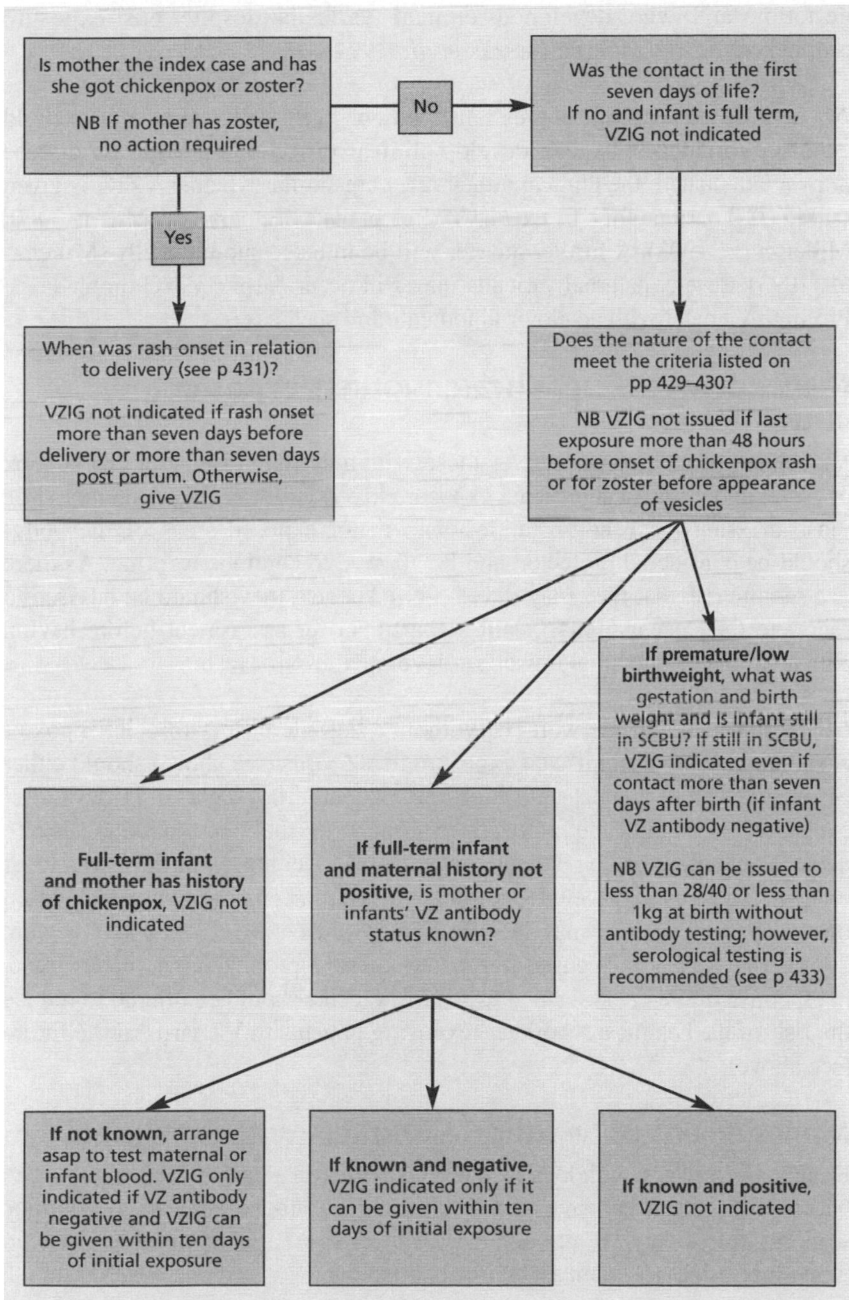

Figure 34.3 VZIG algorithm for neonates

gestation and who developed clinical varicella despite post-exposure prophylaxis with VZIG (Pasturszak *et al*., 1994).

About 50% of susceptible pregnant women given VZIG after a household exposure to chickenpox will develop clinical varicella, although the disease may be attenuated; the clinical attack rates are similar whether VZIG is given within 72 hours or four to ten days after contact (Enders and Miller, 2000; Miller *et al*., 1993). A further quarter will be infected sub-clinically (Miller *et al*., 1993). Severe maternal varicella may still occur despite VZIG prophylaxis. Prompt treatment with aciclovir is indicated in such cases.

Management of healthcare workers exposed to VZ virus infection

Vaccinated healthcare workers or those with a definite history of chickenpox or zoster and having a significant exposure to VZ virus (as above and including those dressing localised zoster lesions on non-exposed areas of the body) should be considered protected and be allowed to continue working. As there is a remote risk that they may develop chickenpox, they should be advised to report to their occupational health department for assessment before having patient contact if they feel unwell or develop a fever or rash.

Unvaccinated healthcare workers without a definite history of chickenpox or zoster and having a significant exposure to VZ virus (see above) should either be excluded from contact with high-risk patients from eight to 21 days after exposure, or should be advised to report to their occupational health department before having patient contact if they feel unwell or develop a fever or rash. There is some evidence that varicella vaccine administered within three days of exposure may be effective in preventing chickenpox (Ferson, 2001). (Varivax® is licensed for post-exposure prophylaxis.) In any case, irrespective of the interval since exposure, vaccine should be offered to reduce the risk of the healthcare workers exposing patients to VZ virus in the future (see above).

Management of healthcare workers with herpes zoster

Healthcare workers with localised herpes zoster on a part of the body that can be covered with a bandage and/or clothing should be allowed to continue working unless they are in contact with high-risk patients, in which case an individual risk assessment should be carried out.

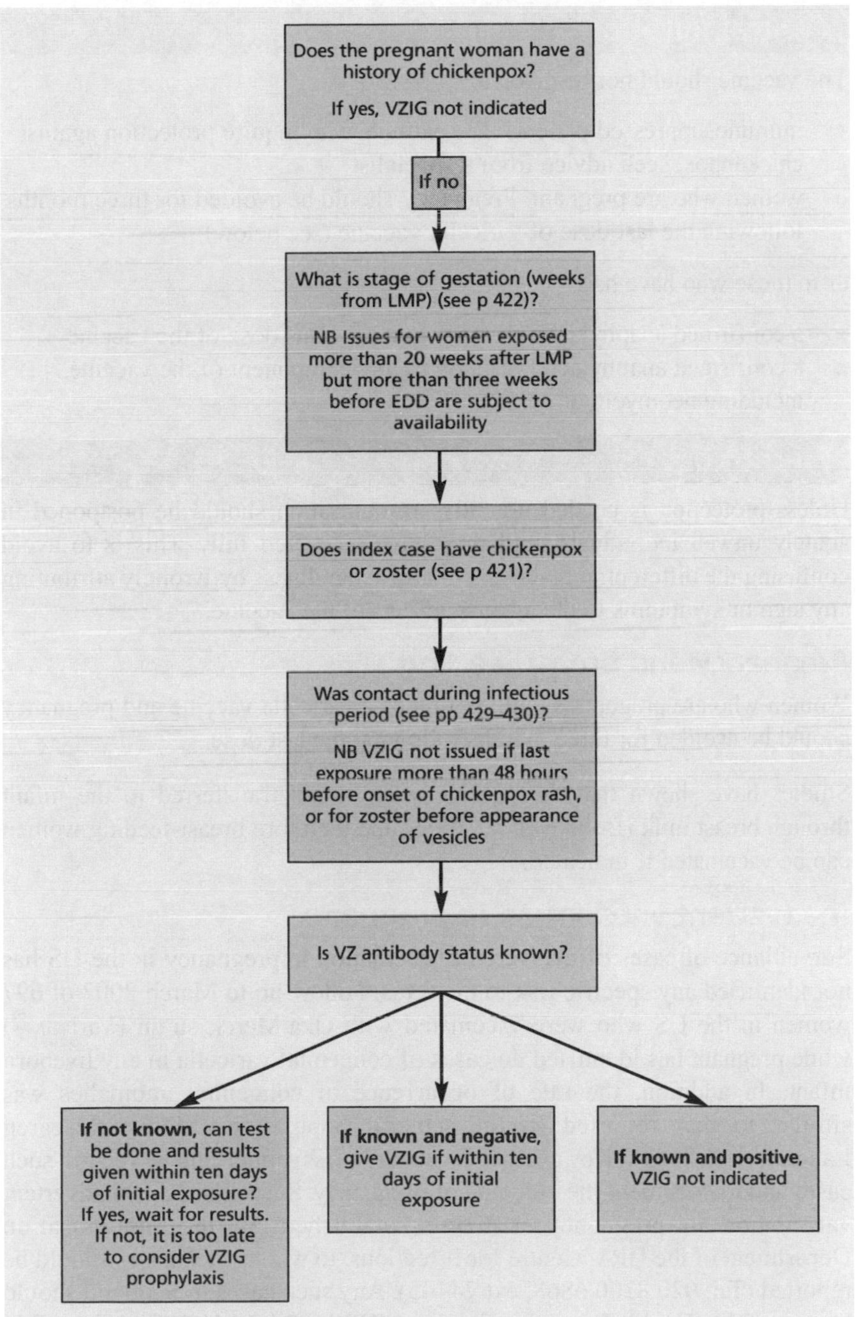

Figure 34.4 VZIG algorithm for pregnant women

Contraindications

The vaccine should not be given to:

- immunosuppressed patients. For patients who require protection against chickenpox, seek advice from a specialist
- women who are pregnant. Pregnancy should be avoided for three months following the last dose of varicella vaccine (see below)

or to those who have had:

- a confirmed anaphylactic reaction to a previous dose of the vaccine
- a confirmed anaphylactic reaction to any component of the vaccine, including neomycin or gelatin.

Precautions

Unless protection is needed urgently, immunisation should be postponed in acutely unwell individuals until they have recovered fully. This is to avoid confusing the differential diagnosis of any acute illness by wrongly attributing any sign or symptoms to the adverse effects of the vaccine.

Pregnancy and breast-feeding

Women who are pregnant should not receive varicella vaccine and pregnancy should be avoided for three months following the last dose.

Studies have shown that the vaccine virus is not transferred to the infant through breast milk (Bohlke *et al.*, 2003) and therefore breast-feeding women can be vaccinated if indicated.

Inadvertent vaccination in pregnancy

Surveillance of cases of inadvertent vaccination in pregnancy in the US has not identified any specific risk to the fetus. Follow-up to March 2002 of 697 women in the US who were vaccinated with Oka/Merck strain (Varivax®) while pregnant has identified no cases of congenital varicella in any liveborn infant. In addition, the rate of occurrence of congenital anomalies was similar to that reported in the general population (Merck Research Laboratories, 2003). However, it is nevertheless important to record such cases and to document the outcome of pregnancy. Surveillance of inadvertent vaccination in pregnancy is being established by the Immunisation Department of the HPA, Centre for Infections, to whom such cases should be reported (Tel: 020 8200 6868, ext 74405). Any such cases in Scotland should be reported to Health Protection Scotland (HPS) (Tel: 0141 300 1191) and in Wales, cases should be reported to the National Public Health Service for

Wales (Tel: 01352 700227 ext 4055). These will, in turn, contribute to the UK figures via the Immunisation Department of the HPA.

Immunosuppression and HIV infection

Varicella vaccine is contraindicated in immunosuppressed patients. For patients who require protection against chickenpox, seek advice from a specialist.

Further guidance is provided by the Royal College of Paediatrics and Child Health (www.rcpch.ac.uk), the British HIV Association (BHIVA) *Immunisation guidelines for HIV-infected adults* (BHIVA, 2006) and the Children's HIV Association of UK and Ireland (CHIVA) immunisation guidelines (www.bhiva.org/chiva).

Use of salicylates

Aspirin and systemic salicylates should not be given to children under 16 years of age, except under medical supervision. Vaccination with varicella vaccine is not contraindicated in individuals aged 16 years or over who need to take aspirin.

Adverse reactions

Varicella vaccines are well tolerated. Extensive clinical and post-marketing safety surveillance data from the US (for the Oka/Merck strain, Varivax®) shows the most commonly reported reactions are at the injection site (pain, redness and rash). Generalised symptoms, such as fever and rash, can also occur but less frequently. Management of these reactions in healthcare workers is detailed below.

Up to 10% of adults and 5% of children develop a vaccine-associated rash, either localised at the injection site or generalised, within one month of immunisation (Annunziato and Gershon, 2000). Varicella vaccine rashes may be papular or vesicular. Illness associated with the vaccine can be treated with aciclovir. It is important to determine whether the rash is due to the vaccine virus or to coincidental wild-type chickenpox. Samples from rashes following vaccine should be sent for analysis to the HPA Varicella Zoster Reference Service at Barts and The London NHS Trust (www.clinical-virology.org/pages/vzrl/vzrl_summary.html).

The vaccine virus strain can establish latent infection and reactivate to cause herpes zoster in immunocompetent individuals, but the risk is substantially lower than with wild varicella infection. Cases of zoster occurring in a vaccinee should be investigated and samples should be sent to the HPA Varicella Zoster Reference Service, as above.

Transmission of vaccine virus from immunocompetent vaccinees to susceptible close contacts has occasionally been documented but the risk is very low. Transmission in the absence of a post-vaccination rash has not been documented (Annunziato and Gershon, 2000).

All suspected reactions in children and severe suspected reactions in adults should be reported to the Commission on Human Medicines using the Yellow Card scheme.

Safety of VZIG

VZIG is well tolerated. Very rarely anaphylactoid reactions occur in individuals with hypogammaglobulinaemia who have IgA antibodies, or in those who have had an atypical reaction to blood transfusion.

No cases of blood-borne infection acquired through immunoglobulin preparations designed for intramuscular use have been documented in any country.

Treatment

VZIG has no place in the treatment of severe disease.

Supplies

Vaccines

- Varivax® – manufactured by Sanofi Pasteur MSD (Tel: 0800 085 5511).
- Varilrix® – manufactured by GlaxoSmithKline (Tel: 0808 100 9997).

VZIG

England and Wales: available from the Communicable Disease Surveillance Centre (CDSC) (Tel: 020 8200 6868), HPA laboratories and selected NHS hospitals.

Northern Ireland: available from Specialist Medicines, Pharmacy Department, Royal Group of Hospitals Trust, Grosvenor Road, Belfast BT12 6BA (Tel: 028 9063 5872).

Scotland: available from regional transfusion centres.

Aberdeen and North East of Scotland Blood Transfusion Centre
Foresterhill Road
Foresterhill
Aberdeen AB9 2ZW
(Tel: 01224 685685)

North of Scotland Blood Transfusion Centre
Raigmore Hospital
Inverness IV2 3UJ
(Tel: 01463 704212)

Dundee and East of Scotland Blood Transfusion Centre
Ninewells Hospital
Dundee DD1 9SY
(Tel: 01382 645166)

The West of Scotland Blood Transfusion Centre
Gartnavel General Hospital
25 Shelly Road
Glasgow G12 0XB
(Tel: 0141 357 7700)

Edinburgh and South East of Scotland Blood Transfusion Centre
Royal Infirmary of Edinburgh
51 Little France Crescent
Edinburgh EH16 4SA
(Tel: 0131 242 7520 (Irene McKechnie))

VZIG is issued free of charge to patients who meet the criteria given above. Clinicians who wish to issue VZIG for patients not meeting these criteria should approach the manufacturer directly to purchase a dose.

No other licensed VZIG preparations for intramuscular use apart from the BPL and PFC products are available in the UK.

References

American Academy of Pediatrics (2003) Active immunization. In: Pickering LK (ed.) *Red Book: 2003 Report of the Committee on Infectious Diseases,* 26th edition. Elk Grove Village, IL: American Academy of Pediatrics, p 33.

Annunziato PW and Gershon AA (2000) Primary vaccination against varicella. In: Arvin AM and Gershon AA (eds) *Varicella-zoster virus*. Cambridge: Cambridge University Press.

Balfour HH, Rotbart HA, Feldman S *et al.* (1992) Aciclovir treatment of varicella in otherwise healthy adolescents. The Collaborative Aciclovir Varicella Study Group. *J Pediatr* **120**: 627–33.

Bohlke K, Davis RL, DeStefano F *et al.* (2003) Vaccine Safety Datalink Team. Postpartum varicella vaccination: is the vaccine virus excreted in breast milk? *Obstet Gynecol* **102** (5 Pt 1): 970–7.

Breuer J (2003) Monitoring virus strain variation following infection with VZV: is there a need and what are the implications of introducing the Oka vaccine? *Commun Dis Public Health* **6**(1): 59–62.

British HIV Association (2006) *Immunisation guidelines for HIV-infected adults:* www.bhiva.org/pdf/2006/Immunisation506.pdf.

Dunkle LM, Arvin AM, Whitley RJ *et al.* (1991) A controlled trial of aciclovir for chickenpox in normal children. *N Engl J Med* **325**: 1539–44.

Enders G and Miller E (2000) Varicella and herpes zoster in pregnancy and the newborn. In: Arvin AM and Gershon AA (eds) *Varicella-zoster virus*. Cambridge: Cambridge University Press.

Enders G, Miller E, Cradock-Watson JE *et al.* (1994) The consequences of chickenpox and herpes zoster in pregnancy; a prospective study of 1739 cases. *Lancet* **343**: 1548–51.

Evans EB, Pollock TM, Cradock-Watson JE and Ridehalgh MK (1980) Human anti-chickenpox immunoglobulin in the prevention of chickenpox. *Lancet* **i**: 354–6.

Ferson MJ (2001) Varicella vaccine in post-exposure prophylaxis. *Commun Dis Intell* **25**: 13–15.

Gold WL, Boulton JE, Goldman C *et al.* (1993) Management of varicella exposures in the neonatal intensive care unit. *Pediatr Infect Dis J* **12**: 954–5.

MacMahon E, Brown LJ, Bexley S *et al.* (2004) Identification of potential candidates for varicella vaccination by history: questionnaire and seroprevalence study. *BMJ* **329** (7465): 551–2.

Merck Research Laboratories (2003) *Pregnancy registry for Varivax®: The 7th annual report, 2002.*

Miller E, Cradock-Watson JE and Ridehalgh MK (1990) Outcome in newborn babies given anti-varicella zoster immunoglobulin after perinatal infection with varicella-zoster virus. *Lancet* **ii**: 371–3.

Miller E, Marshall R and Vurdien JE (1993) Epidemiology, outcome and control of varicella-zoster infection. *Rev Med Microbiol* **4**: 222–30.

Mullooly J and Black S (2001) Simultaneous administration of varicella vaccine and other recommended childhood vaccines – United States, 1995–9. *MMWR* **50**(47): 1058–61.

Paryani SG, Arvin AM, Koropchak CM *et al.* (1984) Comparison of varicella-zoster antibody titres in patients given intravenous immune globulin or varicella-zoster immune globulin. *J Pediatr* **105**: 200–5.

Pasturszak AL, Levy M, Schick B *et al.* (1994) Outcome of maternal varicella infection in the first 20 weeks of pregnancy. *N Engl J Med* **330**: 901–5.

Patou G, Midgely P, Meurisse EV and Feldman RG (1990) Immunoglobulin prophylaxis for infants exposed to varicella in a neonatal unit. *J Infection* **29**: 207–13.

Tan MP and Koren G (2006) Chickenpox in pregnancy: Revisited. *Reprod Toxicol* **21**(4): 410–20.

35

Yellow fever

NOTIFIABLE

The disease

Yellow fever is an acute flavivirus infection spread by the bite of an infected mosquito. The disease occurs in tropical Africa and South America (see maps on the website of the National Travel Health Network and Centre (NaTHNaC), www.nathnac.org); it has never been reported in Asia despite the presence of the vector. Two epidemiological patterns of yellow fever are recognised – urban and jungle – although the disease is clinically and aetiologically identical. In urban yellow fever, the viral reservoir is man and the disease is spread between humans by the *Aedes aegypti* mosquitoes that live and breed in close association with humans. Jungle yellow fever is transmitted among non-human hosts (mainly monkeys) by forest mosquitoes. Humans may become infected when they enter into the forest habitat and can become the source of urban outbreaks. Yellow fever can reappear with outbreaks after long intervals of apparent quiescence. Rural populations are at greatest risk of yellow fever but in recent years urban outbreaks have occurred both in West Africa and South America.

Yellow fever ranges in severity from non-specific, self-limited symptoms of fever, malaise, photophobia and headache to an illness of sudden onset with fever, vomiting and prostration which may progress to jaundice and haemorrhage. In local populations in endemic areas, the overall fatality ratio is about 5%, rising to 20 to 30% once jaundice and severe symptoms occur. In non-immune travellers and migrants, and during epidemics in areas that have low levels of yellow fever activity, the case fatality rate can exceed 50% (Monath, 2004). The incubation period is generally three to six days but may be longer. Death usually occurs seven to ten days after the onset of illness.

There is no specific treatment for yellow fever. Preventive measures such as the eradication of *Aedes* mosquitoes, protection from mosquito bites, and immunisation reduce the risk. Jungle yellow fever can only be prevented by immunisation and personal protection against mosquito bites because of the wide range and distribution of mosquito vectors and mammalian hosts.

There is no risk of transmission in the UK from imported cases since the mosquito vector does not occur in the UK.

History and epidemiology of the disease

Sequence analysis of the viral genome suggests that yellow fever virus originated in Africa about 3000 years ago (Zanotto *et al.*, 1996). However, the earliest record of an epidemic was in the Yucatan in Mexico in 1648. The term 'yellow fever' was first used in an outbreak that occurred in Barbados in 1750. The disease became a major problem in the colonial settlements of the Americas and West Africa in the 1700s and was repeatedly introduced into sea ports of the United States and Europe during this time (Monath, 2004).

Transmission of yellow fever by mosquitoes was first postulated by Josiah Clark Nott in 1848 and confirmed by Walter Reed and colleagues in Cuba in 1900. The live, attenuated vaccine that remains in use today was developed in the 1930s. Control of the urban vector, combined with a highly effective vaccine, had reduced human cases, particularly in South America, but there has been a resurgence of the disease in the last decade with at least 200,000 cases estimated to occur annually (Robertson *et al.*, 1996; Monath, 2001).

The yellow fever vaccination

Yellow fever vaccine is a live, attenuated preparation of the 17D strain of yellow fever virus grown in specific pathogen-free embryonated chick eggs. Each 0.5ml dose contains not less than 1000 mouse LD_{50} units.

Storage

Vaccines should be stored in the original packaging at +2˚C to +8˚C and protected from light. All vaccines are sensitive to some extent to heat and cold. Heat speeds up the decline in potency of most vaccines, thus reducing their shelf life. Effectiveness cannot be guaranteed for vaccines unless they have been stored at the correct temperature. Freezing may cause increased reactogenicity and loss of potency for some vaccines. It can also cause hairline cracks in the container, leading to contamination of the contents.

Presentation

The yellow fever vaccine is available as a lyophilised powder for reconstitution with a diluent.

Yellow fever vaccines are thiomersal-free. They contain live organisms which have been attenuated (modified).

Dosage and schedule

First dose is 0.5ml. Further doses should be given at the recommended intervals if required.

Administration

The vaccines should be reconstituted with the diluent supplied by the manufacturer and either used within an hour or discarded.

Doses of 0.5ml of yellow fever vaccine should be given by deep subcutaneous injection irrespective of age.

Yellow fever vaccine can be given at the same time as other inactivated and live vaccines. The vaccines should be given at separate sites, preferably in a different limb. If given in the same limb, they should be given at least 2.5cm apart (American Academy of Pediatrics, 2003). The site at which each vaccine was given should be noted in the patient's records.

If yellow fever vaccine cannot be given at the same time as another live vaccine, it should be given at an interval of four weeks.

Disposal

Equipment used for vaccination, including used vials or ampoules, should be disposed of at the end of a session by sealing in a proper, puncture-resistant 'sharps' box (UN-approved, BS 7320).

Recommendations for the use of the vaccine (including re-immunisation)

The objectives of the immunisation programme are to provide a minimum of one dose of yellow fever vaccine for individuals at risk of yellow fever and to prevent the international spread of yellow fever. The latter aims to prevent infected individuals introducing the virus into areas where the presence of mosquito vectors and an appropriate host could support the establishment of yellow fever.

A single dose correctly administered confers immunity in 95 to 100% of recipients. Immunity persists for at least ten years and possibly for life (Groot and Riberiro, 1962; Rosenzweig *et al.*, 1963; Poland *et al.*, 1981).

The following groups should be immunised:

- laboratory workers handling infected material
- persons aged nine months or older who are travelling to countries that require an International Certificate of Vaccination for entry
- persons aged nine months or older who are travelling to or living in infected areas or countries in the yellow fever endemic zone (see maps on www.nathnac.org), even if these countries do not require evidence of immunisation on entry.

Immunisation should be performed at least ten days prior to travel to an endemic area to allow protective immunity to develop and for the International Certificate of Vaccination (if required) to become valid.

Reinforcing immunisation

Re-immunisation every ten years is recommended for those at risk, although the vaccine is considered to confer longer protection.

Risk assessment for travel

With the recent recognition of rare severe adverse events related to yellow fever vaccine (Centers for Disease Control and Prevention (CDC), 2002; Kitchener, 2004), it is critical to make a careful risk assessment prior to administering vaccine. In general, the risk from yellow fever for travel to a yellow fever endemic region outweighs the risk associated with the vaccine (World Health Organization (WHO), 2004). Itineraries should be scrutinised to ensure that the vaccine is given only to those considered at risk from the disease. In general, the risk of yellow fever from travel to endemic regions of Africa is ten times higher than the risk from travel to South America (Monath, 2004, Monath and Cetron, 2002), but risk depends entirely on itinerary, season of travel and planned activities.

Although the risk is small, infants under nine months are at higher risk of vaccine-associated encephalitis, with the risk being inversely proportional to age. Infants aged six to nine months should only be immunised if the risk of yellow fever during travel is unavoidable; expert opinion should be sought in these situations. Infants aged five months or younger should never be immunised (Monath, 2004). Advice on the avoidance of mosquito bites should be given (see contraindications).

Further details about the recommendations for travellers are contained in *Health information for overseas travel* (Department of Health, 2001) and may be found on the NaTHNaC, www.nathnac.org.

Yellow fever certificate

Under the International Health Regulations (both those of 1969, and those of 2005, which are due to come into force in June 2007), states may require immunisation against yellow fever. A valid International Certificate of Vaccination is required as evidence. Country requirements are published annually by WHO in *International travel and health* (available at www.who.int/ith) (WHO, 2004), and are included in *Health information for overseas travel* (Department of Health, 2001).

The International Certificate of Vaccination is valid for ten years beginning from the tenth day after primary immunisation and immediately after re-immunisation if re-immunisation occurs within the ten-year period.

Contraindications

There are very few individuals who cannot receive yellow fever vaccine when it is recommended. When there is doubt, appropriate advice should be sought from a travel health specialist.

The vaccine should not be given to:

- those aged five months or under
- those who have had a confirmed anaphylactic reaction to a previous dose of yellow fever vaccine
- those who have had a confirmed anaphylactic reaction to any of the components of the vaccine
- those who have had a confirmed anaphylactic reaction to egg
- those who have a thymus disorder

and also to:

- patients considered immunocompromised due to a congenital condition, disease process or treatment (see Chapter 6).

Patients with any of the conditions described above who must travel should be informed of the risk of yellow fever and instructed in mosquito avoidance measures. For those who intend to visit countries where an International Certificate of Vaccination against yellow fever is required for entry, a letter of exemption should be issued by the Yellow Fever Vaccination Centre or by the practitioner treating the patient. This should be taken into consideration by the port health authorities at the destination.

Precautions

Minor illnesses without fever or systemic upset are not valid reasons to postpone immunisation.

If an individual is acutely unwell, immunisation should be postponed until they have fully recovered. This is to avoid confusing the differential diagnosis of any acute illness by wrongly attributing any sign or symptoms to the adverse effects of the vaccine.

People over 60 years of age

The risk for neurologic and viscerotropic adverse events increases with age (see below). The risk assessment needs to take account of this.

Pregnancy

Yellow fever vaccine should not be given to pregnant women because of the theoretical risk of fetal infection from the live virus vaccine. Pregnant women should be advised not to travel to a high-risk area. When travel is unavoidable, the risk from the disease and the theoretical risk from the vaccine have to be assessed on an individual basis. WHO states that the vaccine may be considered after the sixth month of pregnancy and should be administered if the destination risk is high (WHO, 2004). Two studies in which pregnant women have been vaccinated demonstrated no adverse fetal outcomes (Nasidi *et al.*, 1993; Tsai *et al.*, 1993), but transplacental transmission has occurred in early pregnancy (Tsai *et al.*, 1993). A slightly increased risk of spontaneous abortion in women vaccinated in early pregnancy has been suggested (Nishioka *et al.*, 1998). Antibody titres following vaccination are lower in pregnant women (Nasidi *et al.*, 1993). Women who continue to be at risk once the pregnancy is completed should be revaccinated.

Inadvertent vaccination during early pregnancy is not an indication for termination (Monath, 2004).

Breast-feeding

There is no evidence of harm to the baby from vaccination of the breast-feeding mother. While there is a theoretical risk that yellow fever vaccine virus is excreted in breast milk, vaccination should be considered in cases where there is a real risk to the mother from yellow fever disease.

Immunosuppression and HIV infection

Unless the yellow fever risk is unavoidable, asymptomatic HIV-infected persons should not be immunised. There is limited evidence from data, however, that yellow fever vaccine may be given safely to HIV-infected persons with a CD4 count that is greater than 200 and a viral load that is suppressed (Receveur *et al.*, 2000; Tattevin *et al.*, 2004). Specialist advice should be sought in these cases. The antibody response in HIV positive persons may be diminished (Sibailly *et al.*, 1997). (See Chapter 6.)

Further guidance is provided by the Royal College of Paediatrics and Child Health (www.rcpch.ac.uk), the British HIV Association (BHIVA) *Immunisation guidelines for HIV-infected adults* (BHIVA, 2006) and the Children's HIV Association of UK and Ireland (CHIVA) Immunisation guidelines (www.bhiva.org/chiva).

Adverse reactions

Adverse reactions following yellow fever vaccine are typically mild and consist of headache, myalgia, low grade fever and/or soreness at the injection site and will occur in 10 to 30% of recipients (Monath, 2004; Freestone *et al.*, 1977; Lang *et al.*, 1999; Monath *et al.*, 2002). Injection site reactions tend to occur from days one to five after immunisation. Systemic side effects also occur early but may last up to two weeks (Monath *et al.*, 2002). Up to 1% of individuals may need to alter daily activities. Reactions are more likely to occur in persons who have no prior immunity to yellow fever virus (Monath *et al.*, 2002; Moss-Blundell *et al.*, 1981).

Rash, urticaria, bronchospasm and anaphylaxis occur rarely. In a passive surveillance system in the US, the rate of anaphylaxis following yellow fever vaccine was estimated to be one case per 130,000 doses of vaccine (Kelso *et al.*, 1999). Reactions are most likely related to egg protein in the vaccine. It is possible that some persons are sensitive to and react to the gelatin that is used as a stabiliser in this vaccine as well as in other vaccines.

Post-vaccine encephalitis has been recognised as a rare event since the early use of the vaccine. It was particularly seen in infants (see above), and early reports indicated an incidence of 0.5 to 4 cases per 1000 infants under six months of age (Monath, 2004). Since 2001, a new pattern of neurological adverse events was recognised that occurred in older individuals (CDC, 2002; Kitchener, 2004). When this was recognised, a retrospective review revealed other cases that occurred in the 1990s. These events have now been termed yellow fever vaccine-associated neurological disease (YEL-AND). The clinical presentation of this new pattern of neurological events begins four to 23 days following receipt of vaccine with the onset of fever and headache that may progress to include one or more of confusion, focal neurological deficits, coma and Guillain-Barré syndrome. CSF in these cases demonstrates a pleocytosis with increased protein and when, tested, yellow fever virus-specific IgM antibody. The clinical course is usually for complete recovery. All cases have occurred in primary vaccinees who have no underlying yellow fever immunity.

Yellow fever vaccine-associated viscerotropic disease (YEL-AVD) is a newly recognised syndrome of fever and multi-organ failure that resembles severe yellow fever, first described in 2001 (CDC, 2001; Chan *et al.*, 2001; Martin *et al.*, 2001a; Vasconcelos *et al.*, 2001). Two to seven days following vaccination, patients develop fever, malaise, headache and myalgias that progress to hepatitis, hypotension and multi-organ failure; death has occurred in more than 60% of reported cases. Vaccine-derived virus has been isolated from several of the cases and yellow fever viral antigen has been detected in post-mortem samples (Martin *et al.*, 2001a). As with YEL-AND, all cases have occurred in primary vaccinees without underlying yellow fever immunity. In the reports of viscerotropic disease, 17% have had a history of thymus disease with subsequent thymectomy (Barwick Eidex, 2004). Thus, all patients with thymus disorders should not receive vaccine (see Contraindications on p 447).

Based on reported cases and the number of doses of yellow fever vaccine distributed, the US has estimated the risk of neurological disease to be about four cases per million doses and viscerotropic disease to be three cases per million doses (Cetron *et al.*, 2002). These estimates are similar to those made based on cases reported in Europe (Kitchener, 2004). Based on the current evidence, for individuals who are aged 60 years or older, the risk of neurological and viscerotropic adverse events increases several-fold, such that neurological events occur at a rate of about 17 cases per million doses and viscerotropic events at a rate of 20.5 cases per million doses (Martin *et al.*, 2001b; Marfin *et al.*, 2005).

All suspected reactions in children and severe suspected reactions in adults should be reported to the Commission on Human Medicines through the Yellow Card scheme.

Yellow fever vaccination centres

Yellow fever vaccine may be administered only at 'designated' centres as established by the International Health Regulations of WHO.

In England and Wales, the Department of Health and Welsh Assembly Government have devolved responsibility for administering yellow fever vaccination centres (YFVCs) to NaTHNaC, an organisation established in 2003 that is dedicated to providing information to health professionals and setting standards in travel medicine.

A listing of approved YFVCs in England and Wales may be found at: www.nathnac.org/yellowfevercentres.aspx?comingfrom=professional.

Information on becoming a YFVC, including attendance at a yellow fever vaccine training seminar and clinical information about travel medicine, can be obtained on the NaTHNaC website, www.nathnac.org.

Practitioners in Scotland should apply to:

Chris Sinclair
Public Health Policy Unit 1
Scottish Executive
3E South
St Andrews Building
Regent Road
Edinburgh EH1 3DG
(Tel: 0131 2442501
E-mail: chris.sinclair2@scotland.gsi.gov.uk)

Practitioners in Northern Ireland should apply to:

Linda Hutcheson
Health Protection Team
Department of Health
Social Services and Public Safety
Room C4.22
Castle Buildings
Stormont
Belfast BT4 3PP
(Tel: 028 9052 2118
E-mail: Linda.Hutcheson@dhsspsni.gov.uk)

Supplies

All vaccines used to protect against yellow fever must be approved by WHO. One WHO-approved licensed vaccine is currently available in the UK – Stamaril™ (Sanofi Pasteur MSD, Tel: 0800 085 5511).

The vaccine is supplied to designated centres only for injection as freeze-dried powder and solvent.

References

American Academy of Pediatrics (2003) Active immunization. In: Pickering LK (ed.) *Red Book: 2003 Report of the Committee on Infectious Diseases*, 26th edition. Elk Grove Village, IL: American Academy of Pediatrics, p 33.

Barwick Eidex R (2004) History of thymoma and yellow fever vaccination (letter) for the Yellow Fever Vaccine Safety Working Group. *Lancet* **364**: 931.

British HIV Association (2006) *Immunisation guidelines for HIV-infected adults:* www.bhiva.org/pdf/2006/Immunisation506.pdf.

CDC (2001) Fever, jaundice, and multiple organ system failure associated with 17D-derived yellow fever vaccination, 1996–2001. *MMWR* **50**: 643–5

CDC (2002) Adverse events associated with 17D-derived yellow fever vaccination – United States, 2001–2002. *MMWR* **51**: 989–93.

Cetron MS, Marfin AA, Julian KG *et al.* (2002) Yellow fever vaccine. Recommendations of the Advisory Committee on Immunization Practices (ACIP). *MMWR* **51** (No. RR-17): 1–10.

Chan RC, Penney DJ, Little D *et al.* (2001) Hepatitis and death following vaccination with 17D-204 yellow fever vaccine. *Lancet* **358**: 121–2.

Department of Health (2001) *Health information for overseas travel,* 2nd edition. London: TSO.

Freestone DS, Ferris RD, Weinberg AL and Kelly A (1977) Stabilized 17D strain yellow fever vaccine: dose response studies, clinical reactions and effects on hepatic function. *J Biol Stand* **5**: 181–6.

Groot H and Riberiro RB (1962) Neutralizing and haemagglutination-inhibiting antibodies to yellow fever 17 years after vaccination with 17D vaccine. *Bull World Health Organ* **27**: 699–707.

Kelso JM, Mootrey GT and Tsai TF (1999) Anaphylaxis from yellow fever vaccine. *J Allergy Clin Immunol* **103**: 698–701.

Kengsakul K, Sathirapongsasuti K and Punyagupta S (2002) Fatal myeloencephalitis following yellow fever vaccination in a case with HIV infection. *J Med Assoc Thai* **85**: 131–4.

Kitchener S (2004) Viscerotropic and neurotropic disease following vaccination with the 17D yellow fever vaccine, ARILVAX((R)). *Vaccine* **22**: 2103–5.

Lang J, Zuckerman J, Clarke P *et al.* (1999) Comparison of the immunogenicity and safety of two 17D yellow fever vaccines. *Am J Trop Med Hyg* **60**: 1045–50.

Marfin AA, Eidex RS, Kozarsky PE and Cetron MS (2005) Yellow fever and Japanese encephalitis vaccines: indications and complications. *Infect Dis Clin North Am* **19**(1): 151–68.

Martin M, Tsai TF, Cropp B *et al.* (2001a) Fever and multisystem organ failure associated with 17D-204 yellow fever vaccination: a report of four cases. *Lancet* **358**: 98–104.

Martin M, Weld LH, Tsai TF *et al.* (2001b) Advanced age a risk factor for illness temporally associated with yellow fever vaccination. *Emerg Infect Dis* **7**: 945–51.

Monath TP (2001) Yellow fever: an update. *Lancet Infect Dis* **1**: 11–20.

Monath TP (2004) Yellow fever vaccine. In: Plotkin SA and Orenstien WA (eds) *Vaccines*, 4th edition Philadelphia: WA Saunders Company, pp 1095–176.

Monath TP and Cetron MS (2002) Prevention of yellow fever in persons travelling to the tropics. *Clin Infect Dis* **34**:1369–78.

Monath TP, Nichols R, Archambault WT *et al.* (2002) Comparative safety and immunogenicity of two yellow fever 17D vaccines (ARILVAX and YF-VAX) in a phase III multicenter, double-blind clinical trial. *Am J Trop Med Hyg* **66**: 533–41.

Moss-Blundell AJ, Bernstein S, Shepherd WM *et al.* (1981) A clinical study of stabilized 17D strain live attenuated yellow fever vaccine. *J Biol Stand* **9**: 445–52.

Nasidi A, Monath TP, Vandenberg J *et al.* (1993) Yellow fever vaccination and pregnancy: a four-year prospective study. *Trans R Soc Trop Med Hyg* **87**: 337–9.

Nishioka SD, Nunes-Araujo FRF, Pires WP *et al.* (1998) Yellow fever vaccination during pregnancy and spontaneous abortion: a case-control study. *Trop Med Int Health* **3**: 29–33.

Poland JD, Calisher CH, Monath TP *et al.* (1981) Persistence of neutralizing antibody 30–35 years after immunization with 17D yellow fever vaccine. *Bull World Health Organ* **59**: 895–900.

Receveur MC, Thiebaut R, Vedy S *et al.* (2000) Yellow fever vaccination of human immunodeficiency virus-infected patients: report of two cases. *Clin Infect Dis* **31**: E7–8.

Robertson SE, Hull BP, Tomori O *et al.* (1996) Yellow fever. A decade of re-emergence. *JAMA* **276**: 1157–62.

Rosenzweig EC, Babione RW and Wisseman CL, Jr (1963) Immunological studies with group B arthropod-borne viruses. IV. Persistence of yellow fever antibodies following vaccination with 17D strain yellow fever vaccine. *Am J Trop Med Hyg* **12**: 230–5.

Sibailly TS, Wiktor SZ, Tsai TF *et al.* (1997) Poor antibody response to yellow fever vaccination in children infected with Human Immunodeficiency Virus Type 1. *Pediatr Infect Dis J* **16**: 1177–9.

Tattevin P, Depatureaux AG, Chapplain JM *et al.* (2004) Yellow fever vaccine is safe and effective in HIV-infected patients. *AIDS* **18**: 825–7.

Tsai TF, Paul R, Lynberg MC and Letson GW (1993) Congenital yellow fever virus infection after immunization in pregnancy. *J Infect Dis* **168**: 1520–3.

Vasconcelos PF, Luna EJ, Galler R *et al.* (2001) Serious adverse events associated with yellow fever 17DD vaccine in Brazil: a report of two cases. *Lancet* **358**: 91–7.

World Health Organization (2004) *International Travel and Health. Vaccination Requirements and Health Advice*. Geneva: World Health Organization, p 210.

Zanotto PM, Gould EA, Gao GF *et al.* (1996) Population dynamics of flaviviruses revealed by molecular phylogenies. *Proc Natl Acad Sci USA* **93**: 548–53.

Index

Vaccines by proprietary name indexed by chapter

Vaccines by common name indexed by chapter

Notes

Notes

Notes

Notes

Notes

Notes